Transport and
Inherited Disease

Previous Symposia of the Society for the
Study of Inborn Errors of Metabolism*

1. Neurometabolic Disorders in Childhood. Ed. K. S. Holt and J. Milner 1963
2. Biochemical Approaches to Mental Handicap in Children. Ed. J. D. Allan and K. S. Holt 1964
3. Basic Concepts of Inborn Errors and Defects of Steroid Biosynthesis. Ed. K. S. Holt and D. N. Raine 1965
4. Some Recent Advances in Inborn Errors of Metabolism. Ed. K. S. Holt and V. P. Coffey 1966
5. Some Inherited Disorders of Brain and Muscle. Ed. J. D. Allan and D. N. Raine 1969
6. Enzymopenic Anaemias, Lysosomes and other papers. Ed. J. D. Allan, K. S. Holt, J. T. Ireland and R. J. Pollitt 1969
7. Errors of Phenylalanine Thyroxine and Testosterone Metabolism. Ed. W. Hamilton and F. P. Hudson 1970
8. Inherited Disorders of Sulphur Metabolism. Ed. N. A. J. Carson and D. N. Raine 1971
9. Organic Acidurias. Ed. J. Stern and C. Toothill 1972
10. Treatment of Inborn Errors of Metabolism. Ed. J. W. T. Seakins, R. A. Saunders and C. Toothill 1973
11. Inborn Errors of Skin, Hair and Connective Tissue. Ed. J. B. Holton and J. T. Ireland 1975
12. Inborn Errors of Calcium and Bone Metabolism. Ed. H. Bickel and J. Stern 1976
13. Medico-Social Management of Inherited Metabolic Disease. Ed. D. N. Raine 1977
14. The Cultured Cell and Inherited Metabolic Disease. Ed. R. A. Harkness and F. Cockburn 1977
15. Inborn Errors of Immunity and Phagocytosis. Ed. F. Güttler, J. W. T. Seakins and R. A. Harkness 1979
16. Inherited Disorders of Carbohydrate Metabolism. Ed. D. Burman, J. B. Holton and C. A. Pennock 1980

The Society exists to promote exchanges of ideas between workers in different disciplines who are interested in any aspect of inborn metabolic disorders. Particulars of the Society can be obtained from the Editors of this Symposium.

*Symposia 1–10 published by E. & S. Livingstone

Transport and Inherited Disease

Monograph based upon Proceedings
of the Seventeenth Symposium of The Society
for the Study of Inborn Errors of Metabolism

Edited by
N. R. Belton
and
C. Toothill

MTP PRESS LIMITED · LANCASTER · BOSTON · THE HAGUE
International Medical Publishers

Published in the UK and Europe by
MTP Press Limited
Falcon House
Lancaster, England

British Library Cataloguing in Publication Data

Transport and inherited disease. – (Symposia/Society
for the Study of Inborn Errors of Metabolism; 17)
1. Metabolism, Inborn errors of – Congresses
I. Belton, N.R.   II. Toothill, C.
III. Symposium of the Society for the Study of
Inborn Errors of Metabolism (17th: 1979: Leeds)
IV. Series
616.3'9042   RC627.8

Published in the USA by
MTP Press
A division of Kluwer Boston Inc
190 Old Derby Street
Hingham, MA 02043, USA

Library of Congress Cataloging in Publication Data

Main entry under title:

Transport and inherited disease.

Includes index.
1. Metabolism, inborn errors of—congresses.
2. Biological transport, active—congresses.
3. Epithelium—congresses. I. Belton, N. R.
(Neville R.), 1937–   . II. Toothill, C. (Colin),
1928–   . III. Society for the study of inborn
errors of metabolism. [DNLM: 1. Biological transport—congresses. 2. Hereditary diseases—congresses. QZ 50 T772 1979]
RC627.8.T7   1981   616.3'9042   81–15575
                                                AACR2

ISBN-13: 978-94-009-7318-3   e-ISBN-13: 978-94-009-7316-9
DOI: 10.1007/978-94-009-7316-9

Contents

SECTION THREE

Transport in Brain

SECTION FOUR

Renal Transport

SECTION FIVE

Transport in Red Blood Cells

List of Contributors

N. R. BELTON
Department of Child Life and Health, University of Edinburgh, 17, Hatton Place, Edinburgh

J. BRODEHL
Kinderklinik der Medizinischen Hochschule Hannover, Karl-Wiechert-Allee 9, D-3000 Hannover 61, West Germany

C. E. BROWNE
Department of Biology, Wake Forest University, Winston-Salem, NC 27021, USA

D. E. C. COLE
The Human Genetics Center, Department of Biology and Department of Pediatrics, McGill University and The De Belle Laboratory for Biochemical Genetics, Montreal Children's Hospital Research Institute, 2300 Tupper Street, Montreal, Quebec, Canada

R. COLEMAN
Department of Biochemistry, University of Birmingham, P. O. Box 363, Birmingham

B. DEUTICKE
Abteilung Physiologie, RWTH Medizin Theoret Institute, Schneebergweg 211, D-5100 Aachen, West Germany

R. FRASER
MRC Blood Pressure Unit, Western Infirmary, Glasgow, Scotland

J. W. FOREMAN
Children's Hospital of Philadelphia, 34th Civic Center Boulevard, Philadelphia, Pennsylvania 19104, USA

C. GARNER
Department of Chemical Pathology and Child Health, University of Manchester

S. M. JARVIS
ARC Institute of Animal Physiology, Babraham, Cambridge [Present address: University of Alberta Cancer Research Unit, McEachern Laboratory, Edmonton, Alberta T6G 2H7, Canada]

A. J. KENNY
Department of Biochemistry, University of Leeds, Leeds

A. K. KHULLAR
Department of Chemical Pathology and Child Health, University of Manchester

R. KINNE
Department of Physiology, Albert Einstein College of Medicine, 1300 Morris Park Avenue, Bronx, NY 10461, USA

A. LARSSON
Department of Paediatrics, Karolinska Institute, St Göran's Children's Hospital, Box 12500, 11281 Stockholm, Sweden

J. LENARD
Department of Physiology and Biophysics, College of Medicine and Dentistry of New Jersey, Rutgers Medical School, Piscateway, New Jersey 08854, USA

E. R. LOVE
Department of Neuropathology, Institute of Psychiatry, De Crespigny Park, London

P. D. McNAMARA
Children's Hospital of Philadelphia, 34th Civic Center Boulevard, Philadelphia, Pennsylvania 19104, USA

O. E. PRATT
Department of Neuropathology, Institute of Psychiatry, De Crespigny Park, London

L. E. ROSENBERG
Department of Human Genetics, Yale University School of Medicine, 333 Cedar Street, New Haven, Connecticut 06510, USA

V. SCHWARZ
Department of Chemical Pathology and Child Health, University of Manchester, Stopford Building, Oxford Road, Manchester

C. R. SCRIVER
The Human Genetics Center, Department of Biology and Department of Pediatrics, McGill University and The De Belle Laboratory for Biochemical Genetics, Montreal Children's Hospital Research Institute, 2300 Tupper Street, Montreal, Quebec, Canada

S. SEGAL
Children's Hospital of Philadelphia, 34th Civic Centre Boulevard, Philadelphia, Pennsylvania 19104, USA

N. I. M. SIMPSON
Department of Chemical Pathology and Child Health, University of Manchester

A. L. STEINER
Division of Endocrinology, PO Box 20708, University of Texas School of Medicine, Houston, Texas 77025, USA

G. W. STEWART
St Mary's Medical School, Paddington, London

H. S. TENENHOUSE
The Human Genetics Center, Department of Biology and Department of Pediatrics, McGill University and The De Belle Laboratory for Biochemical Genetics, Montreal Children's Hospital Research Institute, 2300 Tupper Street, Montreal, Quebec, Canada

C. TOOTHILL
Department of Chemical Pathology, Old Medical School, Thoresby Place, Leeds

J. D. YOUNG
Agricultural Research Council, Insitute of Animal Physiology, Babraham, Cambridge [Present address: Department of Biochemistry, The Chinese University of Hong Kong, Shatin, N.T., Hong Kong]

Preface

Many clinical problems of transport have been known for decades, particularly those disorders involving the liver and kidney. As a result of the dramatic increase in interest in transport at the membrane level the Society devoted its Seventeenth Symposium, held at Leeds during September 1979, to Transport and Inherited Disease, the result of that meeting forming the basis of this monograph. For the occasion over a hundred members and guests of the Society were joined by many invited speakers from Europe and the USA to discuss this rapidly developing field with special reference to the direct interests of the Society – inherited metabolic disease.

The major theme of the meeting was opened with formal scientific presentations on membrane structure, synthesis and the regulation of epithelial transport. These were followed by discussions of specific problems of transport in brain, kidney and red blood cells. Almost all of these later lectures had clinical applications with cystic fibrosis and nephrogenic diabetes insipidus featuring as examples of the common inherited diseases.

The Hudson Memorial Lecture was delivered by Professor H. Bickel (Heidelberg). This outstanding review lecture on 'Phenylketonuria – past, present and future' is reproduced in the Journal of the Society – the *Journal of Inherited Metabolic Disease* (Volume 3 No. 4, pp.123–132).

The members' papers (both oral and poster) are also being reprinted in various issues of the Journal (published by MTP Press Ltd., Lancaster, UK).

As on previous occasions our thanks for support are due to colleagues in commerce and particularly to Mr Gordon Jones of Scientific Hospital Supplies for financial support and other help, all of which contributed to the success of the meeting and this consequent report. Mr Milner, the 'pillar of strength' of the Society from its origins, was again honoured by the Society in their invitation to Professor L. E. Rosenberg (Yale) to give the Milner Lecture on 'The Inherited Methylmalonic Acidaemias'.

The editors wish to record their appreciation of colleagues in the Society who gave much of their time to the organization of the meeting, and to various staff of the University of Leeds who made the meeting the successful 'get-together'. Not least, we are grateful to Mrs Doreen Jobbins who not only helped with the organization but who bore the burden of the secretarial work before and after the meeting.

N. R. Belton
C. Toothill

SECTION ONE

1

The inherited methylmalonic acidaemias: a model system for the study of vitamin metabolism and apoenzyme–coenzyme interactions

L. E. Rosenberg

INTRODUCTION

It is now 25 years since Flavin et al.[1] and Katz and Chaikoff[2] demonstrated that methylmalonic acid is an intermediate in the glycogenic pathway by which propionate is converted to succinate. In the ensuing decade much was learned about the biochemistry of this pathway (reviewed by Rosenberg[3]). Propionyl coenzyme A (CoA) was shown to be an intermediate in the catabolism of several essential amino acids, odd-chain fatty acids and the side chain of cholesterol, whereas methylmalonyl CoA was said to be formed directly from valine and thymine, as well as being a product of propionyl CoA carboxylation (Figure 1.1); specific enzymes were found to catalyse the carboxylation of propionyl CoA to D-methylmalonyl CoA, the racemization of D- to L-methylmalonyl CoA, and the isomerization of L-methylmalonyl CoA to

succinyl CoA (Figure 1.1). Adenosylcobalamin (AdoCbl), that deriva-
tive of cobalamin (Cbl; vitamin B_{12}) in which a 5'-deoxy-5'-adenosyl
moiety is linked to the central cobalt nucleus by a carbon–cobalt bond
(Figure 1.2), was a cofactor found to be required for the mitochondrial
matrix enzyme, methylmalonyl CoA mutase, which catalyses the inter-
conversion of L-methylmalonyl CoA and succinyl CoA; and methylcobalamin (MeCbl) was demonstrated to be the specific Cbl coenzyme
needed by methyltetrahydrofolate: homocysteine methyltransferase, a
cytosolic enzyme which is responsible for the synthesis of tetrahydrofol-
ate and methionine from methyltetrahydrofolate and homocysteine, respectively (Figure 1.1).

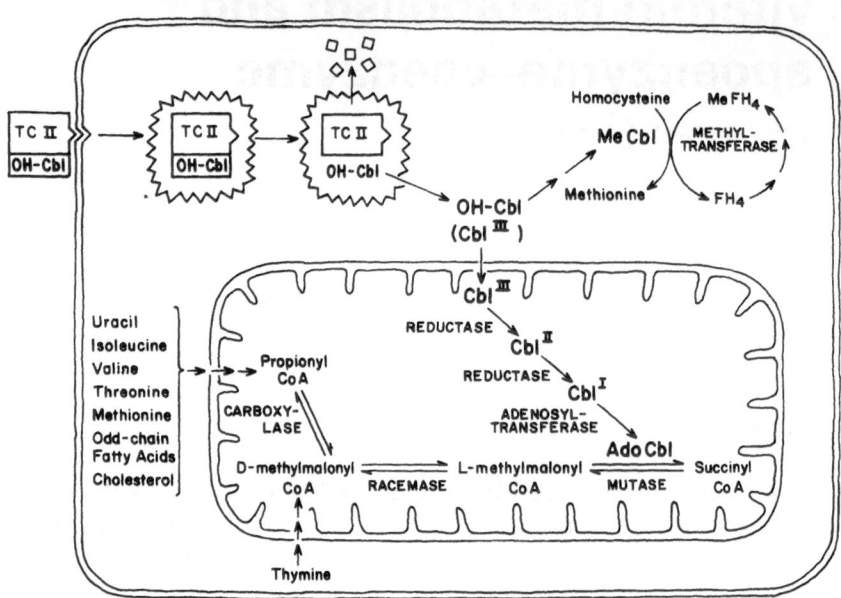

Figure 1.1 Cellular pathways relevant to the inherited methylmalonic acidaemias. Key features include transcobalamin II (TC II)-mediated adsorptive
endocytosis of cobalamin (Cbl), intralysosomal degradation of TC II, multiple
precursors of propionyl CoA, intramitochondrial localization of methylmalonyl
CoA mutase and of the pathway leading from cob(III)alamin (Cbl^{III}) to adenosylcobalamin (AdoCbl) synthesis, and cytosolic localization of methyltetrahydrofolate ($MeFH_4$):homocysteine methyltransferase and of methylcobalamin
(MeCbl) formation. Series of sequential arrows indicate the presence of multiple
steps. See text for detailed discussion

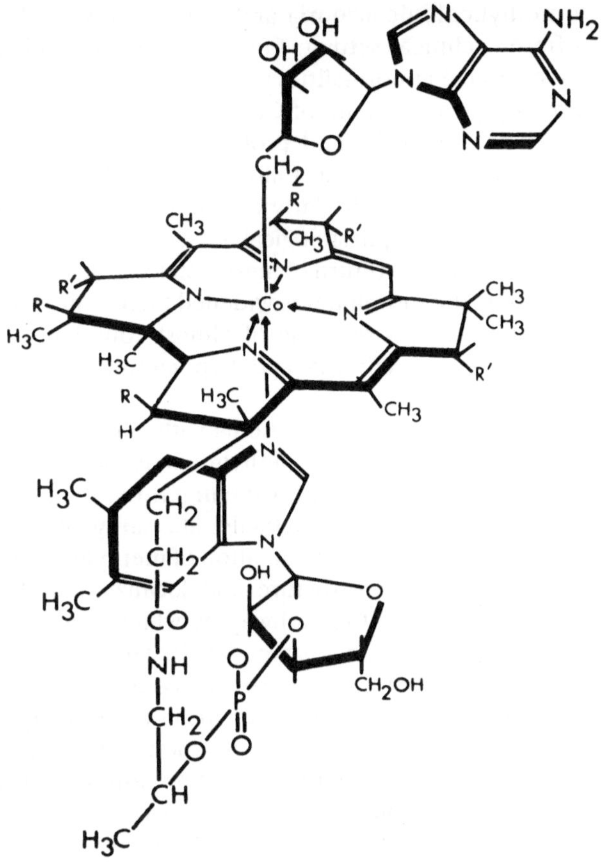

Figure 1.2 Structure of adenosylcobalamin (AdoCbl). R = CH₂CONH₂; R' = CH₂CH₂CONH₂. Note co-ordination of planar corrin rings around central cobalt nucleus and bond between cobalt nucleus and 5'-deoxyadenosyl moiety

Since neither propionate nor methylmalonate are found in human blood, urine, or cerebrospinal fluid in more than trace amounts, their clinical significance was not even hinted at until the early 1960s when Cox and White[4] and Barness et al.[5] showed that patients with typical pernicious anaemia due to Cbl deficiency excreted large amounts of methylmalonate in the urine. This form of methylmalonic aciduria was rapidly and completely reversed by administration of physiological doses of Cbl; it was, therefore, correctly attributed to an acquired block in methylmalonyl CoA mutase activity produced by inadequate amounts of the necessary Cbl coenzyme.

In 1967 methylmalonic aciduria and acidaemia were described in an entirely different clinical setting. Oberholzer et al.[6] and Stokke et al.[7] noted these chemical abnormalities in neonates or infants who had none of the haematological stigmata of Cbl deficiency but who, instead, had metabolic acidosis, ketosis, and protein intolerance of lethal or life-threatening proportions. In the following years Rosenberg et al.[8] and Lindblad et al.[9] described similarly affected infants who responded to pharmacological, but not physiological, doses of Cbl vitamers with a pronounced, yet incomplete, return of methylmalonic acid excretion toward normal. The clinical panorama was widened further in 1969 when Mudd et al.[10] described a newborn dying of almost complete developmental arrest who had homocystinuria and hypomethioninaemia as well as methylmalonic aciduria.

These descriptions of the first patients with what we now know to be different variants of inherited methylmalonic acidaemia were truly seminal in that they proclaimed, for the first time, the physiological significance of the propionate–methylmalonate pathway in man and triggered a burst of inquiry into the regulation of methylmalonate formation and degradation, into the structure and localization of the involved enzyme proteins, and into the pathway by which inactive Cbl vitamers are converted to their active coenzyme forms. This trail of research, conducted in numerous laboratories in several countries, has depended on the use of many modern technologies including gas–liquid chromatography, mass spectrometry, nuclear magnetic resonance, stable and radioactive isotopes, subcellular fractionation, affinity chromatography, gel filtration, and electrophoresis. It has employed an equally wide range of biological substrates: whole humans and animals; physiological fluids; intact leukocytes and cultured fibroblasts; interspecific and intraspecific somatic cell heterokaryons and hybrids; crude cell extracts; subcellular organelles; and purified proteins.

In this presentation I shall attempt to summarize the salient biochemical, genetic and clinical findings which have accrued from our own studies of the inherited methylmalonic acidaemias over the past dozen years. In the name of clarity, and with more than a little regret, I shall take several literary liberties. Rather than detailing methods, I shall stress strategies; rather than describing specific results, I shall emphasize conclusions; rather than citing all primary publications, I shall rely on recently published reviews[11-13] for all contributions except those too current to have been so cited; and rather than identifying publications by first authors, I shall rely on the collective, 'we'. I hope that, in this way, I shall be able to illustrate what we have learned, and, as importantly, what remains to be discovered about both the normal metabolic processes concerned with methylmalonate and Cbl utilization, and the pathobiology observed in the inherited methylmalonic acidaemias.

BIOCHEMICAL OBSERVATIONS

Normal processes

To illustrate the principle that the study of rare inborn errors of metabolism often provides new insights into normal metabolic processes, I shall discuss contributions in three areas: the route of methylmalonate formation from valine; the pathway of cellular Cbl metabolism; and the structure and function of methylmalonyl CoA mutase.

Methylmalonate formation from valine   As stated earlier, methylmalonyl CoA is an intermediate in the catabolic pathway for four essential amino acids (isoleucine, methionine, threonine, and valine). Earlier work had established that isoleucine, methionine, and threonine are first converted to D-methylmalonyl CoA (Figure 1.1). There were, however, two contradicting views on the pathway by which valine breakdown led to methylmalonyl CoA. As noted in Figure 1.3, this controversy involved the steps from methylmalonic acid semialdehyde (MMS) to methylmalonyl CoA. According to one hypothesis (Route I, Figure 1.3), MMS is oxidized directly to methylmalonyl CoA; according to the second (Route II, Figure 1.3) MMS is first decarboxylated to propionate, then carboxylated to methylmalonyl CoA.

To resolve this matter, we used valine labelled with the stable isotope of carbon, ^{13}C. [α-^{13}C]- and [α,β-^{13}C]valine were administered, at different times, to a child with methylmalonic acidaemia, methylmalonate was isolated from multiple urine samples, and these specimens were analysed by Fourier-transform ^{13}C-nuclear magnetic resonance to determine the intramolecular labelling[14] of methylmalonate with ^{13}C. If MMS metabolism proceeded via route I, the carboxyl carbon would have been enriched with ^{13}C after administration of either compound; if route II were followed, only the methine (—CH—) carbon of MMA would be enriched after [α,β-^{13}C]valine administration. The results showed unequivocally that only the methine carbon was enriched with ^{13}C after use of the dual-labelled compound; no ^{13}C enrichment was observed at the carboxyl carbons. These results prove that propionate is an obligate in-

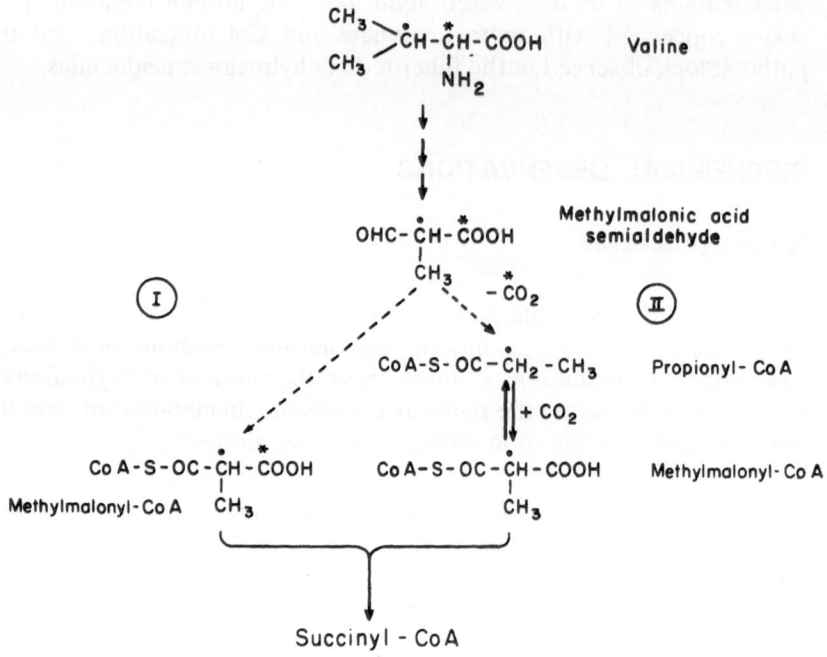

Figure 1.3   Two possible routes (I and II) of valine catabolism after formation of methylmalonic acid semialdehyde. The α and β carbons of valine are marked with ★ and ●, respectively, to illustrate labelling patterns of methylmalonyl CoA expected for each of the routes. See reference 14 for details

termediate in the pathway by which valine is converted to methylmalonate, a conclusion confirmed by subsequent animal studies.

Pathway of cellular uptake and metabolism of cobalamins   As mentioned earlier, mammalian cells contain only two Cbl-dependent apoenzymes (Figure 1.1): methylmalonyl CoA mutase (referred to as mutase), an AdoCbl-requiring enzyme located in the mitochondrial matrix; and methyltetrahydrofolate:homocysteine methyltransferase (referred to as methyltransferase), a MeCbl-requiring enzyme found in the cytosol. The existence of these two Cbl-dependent apoenzymes, each requiring a different coenzyme form of Cbl, poses three interesting cell biological and biochemical problems for the cell. First, the Cbl vitamers must be transported across the plasma membrane from the extracellular space to the intracellular space. Second, the inactive precursor vitamin (in most instances, hydroxocobalamin, abbreviated OH-Cbl) must be converted to AdoCbl and to MeCbl. Thirdly, the coenzymes must bind to their respective apoproteins to form functional holoenzyme complexes.

Previous work had demonstrated that, under physiological circumstances, Cbl vitamers newly absorbed from the gastrointestinal tract circulate bound to a specific β-globulin, transcobalamin II (TC II), which facilitates the uptake of Cbl by cells[3,12]. When TC II is absent, however, or when the concentration of Cbl in plasma exceeds the binding capacity of TC II, then free Cbl both circulates in plasma and is taken up by cells.

To define the processes by which human cells transport either TC II-bound or free Cbl, we have followed the uptake of free or TC II-bound [57Co]Cbl or of [125I-]TC II by intact fibroblast monolayers. Our data demonstrate that the uptake of TC II-bound Cbl is accomplished by receptor-mediated, adsorptive endocytosis[15,16], shown schematically in Figure 1.1. The TC II–Cbl complex binds to a high affinity cell-surface receptor which recognizes a site on TC II and which requires Ca^{2+}. Next, the TC II–Cbl complex is internalized via adsorptive endocytosis which results in the fusion of the endocytotic vacuole with a primary lysosome to form a secondary lysosome. Lysosomal proteases then degrade the TC II and liberate the Cbl which moves, by processes still to be defined, from the lysosome to the cytosol and to the mitochondrion. The TC II receptor has a half-life of approximately 8 h and its activity does not appear to be regulated by exposure to high concentrations of either TC II–Cbl or free Cbl[16].

Free Cbl is transported quite differently. It is taken up by a saturable, Ca^{2+}-independent process whose capacity to accumulate Cbl intracellularly is only a small fraction of that noted for the TC II-mediated process[17]. Neither endocytosis nor the participation of lysosomal proteases appears to be involved. Yet, the end result of this probably vestigial system is similar to that accomplished by the TC II-mediated one, namely, delivery of the Cbl moiety to the cytosol and mitochondrion for the subsequent formation of MeCbl and AdoCbl.

The conversion of precursor vitamin (e.g. OH-Cbl) to MeCbl has not been studied in detail in either bacteria or higher organisms. Presumably this sequence takes place in close association with, or perhaps as a result of the action of, the MeCbl-dependent methyltransferase (Figure 1.1). On the other hand, the conversion of OH-Cbl (also denoted cob(III)alamin) to AdoCbl has been studied in detail – in micro-organisms, rat liver mitochondria, and human fibroblasts[12]. Mitochondria take up OH-Cbl by a process which is concentrative, saturable, and specific but does not depend on either mitochondrial energy metabolism or specific ion transport (Figure 1.1). Since the specificity and saturability of the uptake process result from the binding of the Cbl to one or more intramitochondrial proteins, and since large magnitude mitochondrial swelling is required for such OH-Cbl accumulation, we believe that the uptake is accomplished by passive diffusion. The intramitochondrial AdoCbl-forming reaction sequence appears to contain three enzymatic steps. First, two separate one-electron transfers catalysed by cob(III)alamin reductase and cob(II)alamin reductase reduce the cobalt atom from Co(III) to Co(I); then ATP:cob(I)alamin adenosyltransferase (to be denoted adenosyltransferase) carries out the adenosylation of cob(I)alamin by ATP to form AdoCbl. Preliminary studies suggest that the adenosyltransferase is located in the mitochondrial matrix, but the suborganellar distribution of the reductases is unclear. Although we have shown that AdoCbl is not an intermediate in MeCbl formation or vice versa, there is no information as to the nature or number of specific or non-specific reductase systems in the cytosol or mitochondrion, nor is it known whether cob(II)alamin or cob(I)alamin traverse the mitochondrial membranes in either direction.

Finally the coenzymes bind specifically to their respective apoenzymes, methyltransferase and mutase. In studies with both rat liver and human fibroblasts, virtually all of the intracellular binding of cobalamins could be accounted for by attachment to these two proteins[18, 19]. Since OH-Cbl and MeCbl were recovered from methyltransferase whereas only AdoCbl was found with mutase, it seems likely that methyltransferase initially binds an oxidized Cbl species and reduces it *in situ*, while mutase normally binds only AdoCbl.

Enzyme structure and function   Of the five known enzymes required for normal intracellular Cbl metabolism (two reductases, adenosyltransferase, methyltransferase, and mutase), detailed structural and functional information is available only for mutase. Neither reductase species nor adenosyltransferase has been purified from mammalian sources. Methyltransferase has been partially purified. In our laboratory a four-step protocol led to a 200–300-fold purification of the enzyme from human placenta; the molecular weight of the most purified fraction was estimated to be 180 000 (Gertler and Rosenberg, unpublished observations).

We have learned considerably more about the structure of methylmalonyl CoA mutase. This enzyme has now been purified to homogeneity from human liver and appears to be a dimer of identical subunits, each having a molecular weight of approximately 75 000 and each binding one molecule of AdoCbl (Fenton *et al.*, unpublished observations). The pure enzyme has a K_m for DL-methylmalonyl CoA of 1–4 mM. Its association constant for AdoCbl has yet to be determined because satisfactory resolution of the pure holoenzyme has not yet been accomplished.

The two Cbl-dependent enzymes exist in cells either complexed with coenzyme (holoenzyme) or free of coenzyme (apoenzyme). In fibroblasts grown in basal medium containing approximately 30 pg/ml Cbl, holomethyltransferase accounts for approximately 50% of total activity whereas holomutase accounts for <10%[19, 20]. When the medium is supplemented with 1 μg OH-Cbl, however, nearly all methyltransferase and mutase activity exists in the holoenzyme form. Total activity sometimes rises concomitantly, probably because the holoenzymes turn over more slowly than do their respective apoenzymes.

Kinetic studies of mutase activity in crude fibroblast extracts indicate that its two binding sites for AdoCbl are not equivalent. Under some extraction and assay conditions, AdoCbl binding to one of the two sites markedly impedes binding of coenzyme to the second site[21]. This negative co-operativity is modulated by the presence of methylmalonyl CoA and by the cationic and anionic environment of the enzyme. Thus, as shown in Figure 1.4, it appears that mutase can exist in three forms – one in which AdoCbl is bound to neither active site; a second in which AdoCbl is bound to a single site; and a third in which AdoCbl is bound to both sites. Furthermore, OH-Cbl has been shown to be a potent inhibitor of the human enzyme – probably acting both as a competitive inhibitor at the AdoCbl binding site and as an irreversible inactivator[13, 22].

Localization of defects in the methylmalonic acidaemias

Even the first handful of case reports of children with inherited methylmalonic acidaemia spoke loudly for biochemical and genetic heterogeneity – some children had methylmalonic acidaemia and aciduria only, while others had disordered sulphur amino-acid metabolism as well; some responded to pharmacological doses of Cbl, while others did not[6-10]. Although each of these early reports suggested that methylmalonyl CoA mutase activity was deficient in affected patients, the first *in vitro* demonstration of mutase deficiency was provided by Morrow *et al.*[23]. They assayed mutase activity in liver homogenates of four affected patients. In three, holomutase activity was approximately 1% of control and addition of saturating amounts of AdoCbl yielded no significant increase; in the fourth, holomutase activity was again markedly

Relative activity

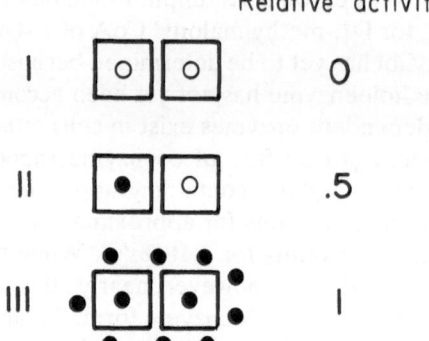

Figure 1.4 Proposed forms of methylmalonyl CoA mutase. Mutase is depicted as a dimer of identical subunits each containing one AdoCbl binding site (□). AdoCbl molecules (●) may bind to neither subunit (I), one subunit (II) or, in the presence of saturating amounts of cofactor, both subunits (III) yielding three possible species of enzyme with relative catalytic activities of 0, 0.5, and 1.0, respectively. See text and reference 21 for details

decreased, but addition of AdoCbl restores total activity to normal. These findings were interpreted as evidence for a defective mutase apoenzyme in the first three patients and for defective AdoCbl synthesis in the fourth. That Cbl coenzyme synthesis was, in fact, impaired in some patients with methylmalonic acidaemia alone and in all reported patients with methylmalonic acidaemia and homocystinuria was demonstrated by our subsequent studies[3, 24, 25] and those of Mudd and colleagues[10, 26]. The use of cultured fibroblasts was instrumental in these studies and we have since used this tissue source to define the nature and extent of the currently recognized biochemical heterogeneity in the inherited methylmalonic acidaemias.

Our strategy in this quest may be summarized as follows[3, 11–13]. First, we collected fibroblast cell lines from 80 affected patients from many parts of the world. Second, we demonstrated that intact cells from each of these lines was deficient in propionate pathway activity, using as a screening test the ability to oxidize [^{14}C]propionate to $^{14}CO_2$ or to convert labelled propionate to trichloracetic acid-precipitable material. Third, we measured holo- and total mutase and methyltransferase activities and adenosyltransferase activity in crude fibroblast extracts. And, fourth, we quantitated in intact cells the conversion of ^{57}Co-labelled CN-Cbl to OH-Cbl, that of OH-Cbl to AdoCbl and MeCbl, and the binding of these labelled cofactors to their respective apoenzymes[12, 13, 19, 27].

This series of experimental protocols enabled us to identify six different mutant classes among the inherited methylmalonic acidaemias. Their distinguishing characteristics, summarized in Table 1.1, are as follows. Those in the largest group, designated *mut* and accounting for half of all mutant lines, have primary abnormalities in the mutase apoenzyme. Whereas Cbl metabolism is normal in all *mut* mutants, this group can be subdivided into mut^0 and mut^- classes as will be discussed below. Four others, designated *cbl A, cbl B, cbl C* and *cbl D*, owe their deficient mutase holoenzyme activity to different abnormalities in the pathway by which precursor Cbl vitamin is converted to active Cbl coenzymes. In each of these mutants, the mutase and methyltransferase apoproteins are normal.

TABLE 1.1   Biochemical features of cultured fibroblasts from patients with the methylmalonic acidaemias

	Mutant class*					
	mut^0	mut^-	cbl A	cbl B	cbl C	cbl D
¹⁴C-Substrate utilization						
Propionate	−	−	−	−	−	−
Methyltetrahydrofolate	+	+	+	+	−	−
Enzyme activities in cell extracts						
Mutase holoenzyme	−	−	−	−	−	−
Mutase total enzyme	−	±	+	+	+	+
Methyltransferase holoenzyme	+	+	+	+	−	−
Methyltransferase total enzyme	+	+	+	+	±	±
Adenosyltransferase	+	+	+	−	+	+
Cobalamin metabolism in intact cells						
AdoCbl synthesis	+	+	−	−	−	−
MeCbl synthesis	+	+	+	+	−	−
Binding to methyltransferase and mutase	+	+	+	+	−	±
Conversion of CN-Cbl to OH-Cbl	+	+	+	+	−	±

*+ = normal; − = markedly deficient or undetectable; ± = partially deficient

Mutase apoenzyme mutants   In those *mut* mutants designated mut^0, mutase activity in cell extracts is undetectable (<0.1% of normal) even when assayed in the presence of AdoCbl concentrations greatly in excess of that required to saturate the enzyme[13,28]. It has not yet been determined whether mutant protein devoid of catalytic activity is present within cells belonging to this class. The *mut⁻* mutants, on the other hand, contain a structurally-altered mutase apoprotein which has a markedly reduced affinity for AdoCbl and is more thermolabile than the normal enzyme[13, 28, 29]. In the six *mut⁻* lines examined in detail, the K_m for AdoCbl has ranged from 200 to 5000 times normal, and the V_{max} from 2 to 75% of control activity. Affinity for methylmalonyl CoA, however, is normal.

cbl C *and* cbl D *mutants*   As noted in Table 1.1, the biochemical phenotypes of these two mutant classes generally differ quantitatively rather than qualitatively, the *cbl C*s being the more severely affected. In both classes, synthesis of AdoCbl and of MeCbl is defective; accordingly, binding of coenzymes to apoenzymes is deficient and holomutase and holomethyltransferase activities are impaired[3, 13, 19]. Although the precise site of the primary biochemical defect in both classes remains unclear, much progress has been made. Thus, we have shown that neither TC II-mediated binding to the cell surface, nor internalization of the TC II–Cbl complex, nor intralysosomal degradation of TC II are impaired in either class[12, 13, 15]. These negative results make it seem likely that the molecular block in *cbl C* and *cbl D* cells occurs at some proximate enzymatic step(s) in the intracellular Cbl pathway which converts newly absorbed Cbl to a form capable both of being utilized for coenzyme synthesis and of being bound by methyltransferase and mutase. Evidence for such an enzymatic defect in *cbl C* cells has recently been obtained[27]. Whereas normal cells and *cbl D* cells were able to effect the removal of the cyanide ion from CN-Cbl, *cbl C* cells were not. This 'cyanide-removing' or 'processing' activity exhibits characteristics expected for a cob(III)alamin reductase, and it seems likely that deficiency of such a reductase could block subsequent reduction and alkylation of the cobalt nucleus, and, thereby, interfere with coenzyme formation. It remains to be determined whether *cbl D* cells have a less severe defect at the same site, or alternatively, are defective at some step beyond this early reduction but one still common to the synthesis of AdoCbl and MeCbl.

cbl A *and* cbl B *mutants*   In these classes only AdoCbl synthesis is defective; therefore, only holomutase activity is impaired. Since MeCbl synthesis is normal, and since the reduction of Cbl and its adenosylation to AdoCbl occurs intramitochondrially (Figure 1.1), it seems certain that the biochemical defect in both *cbl A* and *cbl B* cells involves a mitochondrial function. We have demonstrated a specific deficiency of adenosyl-transferase activity in extracts of *cbl B* cells[12,30]. This activity is normal in *cbl A* cells, however, implying either that they are deficient in one of the intra-mitochondrial reductases which convert cob(III)alamin to cob(I)alamin or that they are defective in the process by which Cbl is transported from cytosol to the mitochondrion. Since mitochondria from *cbl A* cells accumulate Cbls as well as normal mitochondria do, however, a transport defect seems much less likely than a reductase deficiency.

The presumptive or proven location of the defects in the various *mut* and *cbl* mutant classes is shown schematically in Figure 1.5. It should be mentioned that although only one site is shown for each mutant class, there is surely biochemical heterogeneity within each mutant class as well as between them. For example, some *mut⁻* mutants have a K_m for AdoCbl which is approximately 200 times the normal value, whereas others have a K_m approximately 5000 times that of the control. Similarly, some *cbl B* mutants have no detectable adenosyltransferase activity, whereas others have up to 5% of normal activity.

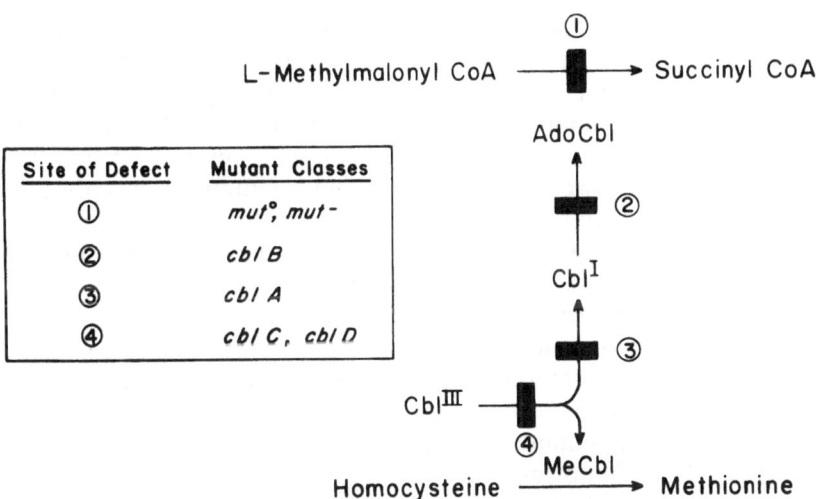

Figure 1.5 Localization of defects leading to different forms of the inherited methylmalonic acidaemias. The metabolic blocks numbered 1–4 correspond to the mutant classes shown in the inset. See text and references 3 and 12 for details

Effects of cobalamin supplementation in culture

As mentioned above, some of the earliest reported children with inherited methymalonic acidaemia responded to pharmacological doses of Cbl *in vivo*, whereas others did not. Since such supplementation has important therapeutic implications, it is not surprising that several groups of workers, including our own, have attempted to define its mechanism, frequency, and extent [3,11,12]. To those matters, let me add a fourth – its potential danger. Our experimental strategy has involved contrasting measurements of mutase and methyltransferase activities in control and mutant fibroblasts grown in basal medium (containing <50 pg/ml of Cbl) to those in medium supplemented with as much as 1 μg of OH-Cbl for as long as 30 days. Fixation of [^{14}C] from labelled propionate or methyltetrahydrofolate by intact cells has been taken as an index of mutase and methyltransferase activity, respectively; enzyme activity in cell extracts was measured directly.

Correlation between mutant class and response to supplementation
There was, in general, a close correlation between the nature of the biochemical defect in the mutant lines and their qualitative response to Cbl supplementation in culture, particularly when enzyme activity was estimated in intact cells (Figure 1.6). Thus, propionate fixation increased in none of the 16 *mut*^{0} mutants grown in supplemented medium, whereas fixation increased in all seven *mut*$^-$ cell lines [28]. In like fashion each of eight *cbl A*, four *cbl C*, and two *cbl D* lines responded with distinct increases in propionate, and where appropriate, in methyltetrahydrofolate fixation [13,20]. Those *cbl B* mutants devoid of residual adenosyltransferase activity showed no response to supplementation, while those with some residual activity demonstrated increased propionate fixation. In essence, then, it appears that 'leaky' mutants do respond to Cbl supplementation in culture, whereas 'tight' ones do not.

The term 'responsive' must not be equated with 'correction', however. Propionate fixation increased in *mut*$^-$, *cbl A*, and some *cbl B* mutants following supplementation, but never to normal values. Furthermore, holomutase activity in cell extracts never rose to >3% of control. Only in *cbl C* and *cbl D* mutants did supplementation truly correct propionate fixation. It is important, however, that mutase activity in extracts increased only to 5–10% of paired controls, implying that stimulation of mutase activity to this degree is sufficient to overcome the block in propionate pathway activity observed in patients with the inherited methylmalonic acidaemias.

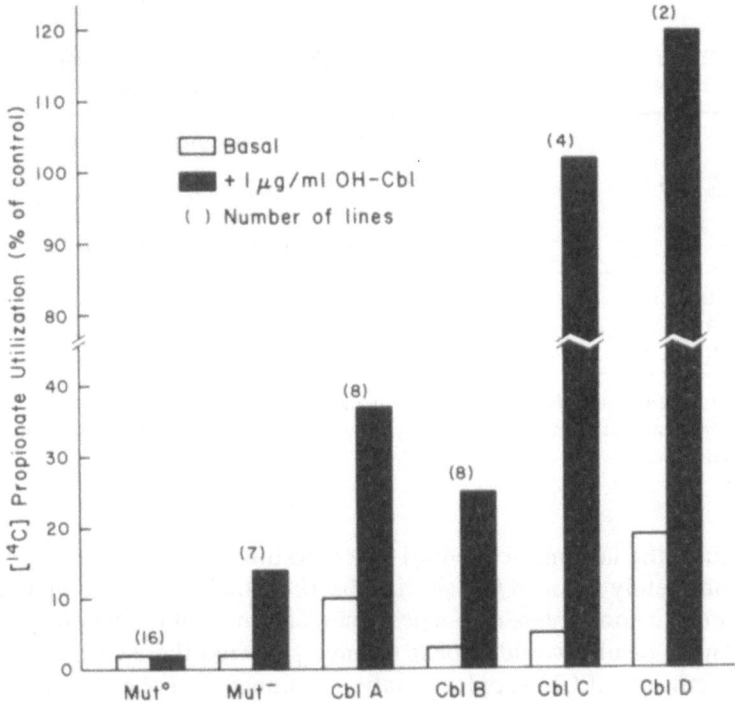

Figure 1.6 Effect of supplementation in culture with 1 μg/ml hydroxocobala-min (OH-Cbl) on incorporation of [1-¹⁴C]propionate into trichloroacetic acid-precipitable material by intact fibroblasts belonging to various *mut* and *cbl* complementation groups. Basal medium contained <50 pg/ml Cbl. Values are shown as percentage of those in control cells. See text and references 20 and 28 for details

Contrasting effects of supplementation with OH-Cbl and AdoCbl in cbl A *and* cbl B *mutants*   When normal cells are cultured in medium supplemented with 1 μg/ml OH-Cbl, holomutase activities measured in cell extracts increase approximately 20-fold; total activity is unchanged or may rise as much as two-fold (see Table 1.2). Similar results are obtained when AdoCbl is used instead of OH-Cbl[13]. Very different findings were noted in *cbl A* and *cbl B* cells, however (Table 1.2). Following supplementation with OH-Cbl, total mutase activity fell by 80–90% in *cbl A* extracts and 30–50% in *cbl B* extracts. Since we have shown that OH-Cbl is a potent competitive and irreversible inhibitor of mutase activity, and since *cbl A* and *cbl B* mutants are defective in steps required to convert OH-Cbl to AdoCbl, it seems likely that, following supplementation in

TABLE 1.2   Effect of Cbl supplementation in culture on methylmalonyl CoA mutase activity in extracts of representative normal, *cbl A* and *cbl B* cell lines

| Cells | *Mutase activity after growth in** | | | | | |
| | *Basal medium* | | *1 μg/ml OH-Cbl* | | *1 μg/ml AdoCbl* | |
	Holo-	*Total*	*Holo-*	*Total*	*Holo-*	*Total*
Control	37	1459	780	1512	625	1335
cbl A	7	2281	16	299	315	1753
cbl B	7	2927	42	1222	186	1849

*Cells were grown for 4 days in basal medium containing <50 pg/ml Cbl or in the supplemented medium indicated. Enzyme activity is expressed as pmol succinate formed/min/mg protein

culture, the intramitochondrial concentration of OH-Cbl (or some other incompletely reduced Cbl species) becomes high enough so that binding to mutase apoenzyme molecules occurs, thereby inhibiting their activity.

These results would appear to have potential therapeutic relevance. The efficacy of Cbl supplementation treatment in patients with methylmalonic acidaemia due to a defect in AdoCbl synthesis may not simply be a matter of how much AdoCbl can be produced in the tissues. Rather it may reflect a delicate balance struck between activation of mutase apoenzyme by newly synthesized AdoCbl and inhibition by the high concentrations of OH-Cbl or its metabolites which are administered in an attempt to stimulate the inherently limited synthesis of AdoCbl. Prolonged administration of very high doses of OH-Cbl, could, in such a setting, prove harmful by reducing mutase activity through pharmacological means to an even greater extent than it is impaired by nature's experiment. Administration of lower doses of OH-Cbl, or, more attractively, of AdoCbl itself could prove to be more effective. To explore the latter possibility, *cbl A* and *cbl B* cells were grown in medium supplemented with 1 μg/ml AdoCbl (Table 1.2). Significantly, holomutase activity increased far more than it did following OH-Cbl supplementation, and total mutase activity declined little. From this study we conclude that at least some AdoCbl can be transported into cells and into mitochondria intact, thereby raising the possibility that administration of AdoCbl to patients with certain forms of methylmalonic acidaemia may be of greater therapeutic value than held currently.

GENETIC OBSERVATIONS

At several critical points in our analysis of the inherited methylmalonic acidaemias, genetic techniques have been illuminating. At times these tools have corroborated independently-obtained biochemical findings. On other occasions they have provided insights unappreciated or unavailable from biochemical studies. This mutually beneficial cross fertilization between biochemical and genetic methodologies has told us much about the number and nature of the loci at which mutations lead to disease and about the Mendelian expression of the inherited methylmalonic acidaemias. It is beginning to tell us, as well, about the chromosomal location of the loci involved.

Complementation analyses

Demonstration of five complementation groups   When two mutant cells which are phenotypically identical but genetically distinct are fused, there is often correction of the mutant phenotype in the resulting heterokaryon or hybrid. No such correction is observed if the two parent cells are genotypically as well as phenotypically identical. We have made extensive use of such complementation tests in our studies of the methylmalonic acidaemias. The strategy of these experiments is straightforward. We formed pairwise crosses, with Sendai virus or polyethylene glycol, between any two fibroblast lines from patients with methylmalonic acidaemia, each having the common phenotype of impaired [14C] propionate fixation. Then we used qualitative radioautographic[31] or quantitative liquid scintillation counting[32] methods to determine whether this phenotypic abnormality had been corrected in the heterokaryotic cell progeny. Our early results demonstrated the existence of four distinct complementation groups, corresponding perfectly with the biochemical evidence above-discussed for discrete *mut, cbl A, cbl B,* and *cbl C* mutant classes. Interclass complementation was always observed, while intraclass and self-complementation were never seen[31]. We then began to use such complementation testing on all new mutant lines received[32]. Crossing each new line with a panel of representative members of the four established groups (Table 1.3) enabled us to classify new lines without more laborious biochemical investigation. Soon, however, we found that lines (line 414 in Table 1.3 as an example) from sibs with methylmalonic acidaemia and homocystinuria reported by Goodman and co-workers[33] complemented members of *all* known mutant classes. This established the existence of a fifth complementation group (cbl D), subsequently shown to be biochemically distinct from the other *cbl* mutants (*vide supra*). Since there are major qualitative biochemical differences between the *mut, cbl A, cbl B,* and *cbl C* groups, the observed complementation among them is almost certainly intergenic. It is not yet clear, however, whether the complementation between *cbl C* and *cbl D* mutants is intergenic or interallelic. Hence, mutations at a minimum of four (and probably five) discrete genetic loci can lead to one of the currently recognized forms of methylmalonic acidaemia.

TABLE 1.3 Use of complementation panels in analysis of cultured human fibroblasts from patients with inherited methylmalonic acidaemia

| Cell line* | Change in [^{14}C] propionate fixation when fused to | | | | | Complementation group assignment |
	Self	cbl A	cbl B	cbl C	mut	
257	−0.02	1.62	1.34	0.96	−0.03	*mut*
287	0.06	2.00	0.76	−0.04	0.73	*cbl C*
311	−0.09	0.45	−0.05	0.76	0.66	*cbl B*
410	0.07	*0.06*	0.77	1.31	0.81	*cbl A*
414	−0.03	1.97	0.97	0.92	0.86	*cbl D*

*Cell lines were mixed 1:1 with a representative of each complementation group, treated with polyethylene glycol (PEG), and assayed for [1-^{14}C] propionate fixation 18–32 h later. Data represent differences in incorporation of ^{14}C into TCA-precipitable material in 10 h between PEG-treated and untreated samples and are expressed as nanoatoms ^{14}C fixed/mg protein.

Interspecific complementation with cbl C *mutants* We have also used cell fusion experiments to focus our biochemical studies aimed at defining the underlying defect in the still elusive *cbl C* mutants. When extracts prepared from normal human fibroblasts or from mouse cells grown in medium containing [^{57}Co]cobalamin were analysed by gel electrophoresis, most of the label co-migrated with the Cbl-dependent methyltransferase[34]. As discussed above, no such binding was observed in extracts of *cbl C* cells (Figure 1.7). Since the mouse and human forms of methyltransferase differed electrophoretically, we were able to test the notion that the lack of binding in *cbl C* cells reflected an abnormality in cellular processing of Cbl rather than an intrinsic abnormality in the methyltransferase protein by forming an interspecific hybrid between mouse cells and *cbl C* cells, and analysing the ^{57}Co-binding pattern of the hybrid. As noted in Figure 1.7, a labelled peak corresponding to human methyltransferase was as prominent in the mouse × *cbl C* hybrid as in the mouse × normal human-cell cross[34]. Thus, the binding defect in the *cbl C* cell had been complemented in the mouse × human hybrid, thereby demonstrating that the *cbl C* mutation does not involve the methyltransferase apoprotein, but rather some metabolic step which must convert Cbl to a chemical form capable of binding to the enzyme.

Mendelian expression

Recessive inheritance   In addition to establishing the existence of five distinct complementation groups, analysis of heterokaryons derived from mutant lines provided direct evidence that the inherited methylmalonic acidaemias are recessively inherited[13,31]. This conclusion derives from the finding that each mutation can be complemented by fusion with cells of a mutant class other than its own, and by the demonstration that fusion of mutant cells with normal human or mouse cells leads to normal activity in the resulting heterokaryons or hybrids[13,34]. Moreover, approximately equal numbers of affected males and females have been described in the *mut⁰*, *mut⁻*, *cbl A*, *cbl B*, and *cbl C* classes, indicating an autosomal mode of inheritance[13] (Matsui *et al.*, unpublished observations). The formal possibility of X-linkage exists only for the *cbl D* group, the only two members of which are male[33].

Additional evidence for autosomal recessive inheritance has come from enzyme assays on cultured cell-extracts from parents of children in the *mut* and *cbl B* classes. We found about half of normal mutase activity in two parents of *mut⁰* mutants and five parents of *mut⁻* mutants, demonstrating that obligate heterozygotes for these disorders can be identified *in vitro*[13,28] though not *in vivo*[3]. Likewise, cells from both parents of a *cbl B* mutant had approximately 30% of normal adenosyltransferase activity[12,30]. Definition of the biochemical phenotype in individuals heterozygous for the *cbl A*, *cbl C*, and *cbl D* mutations must await more precise identification of the specific enzymatic defects in these variants.

Co-dominant expression of mutase apoenzyme alleles   Our studies of mutase activity in obligate heterozygotes for apomutase deficiency also provide considerable evidence that normal and mutant alleles at the *mut* locus are co-dominantly expressed. First, such heterozygotes exhibit about 50% of normal mutase activity. Second, detailed kinetic analyses with extracts of heterozygotes for the *mut* lesion revealed complex patterns consistent with expression of both the normal and the mutant

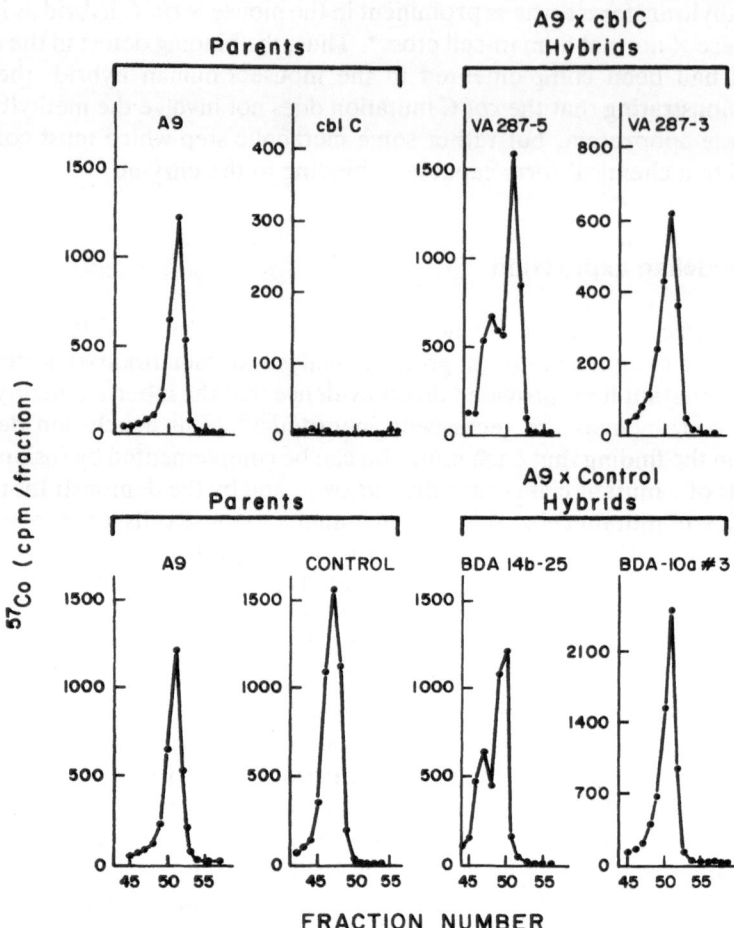

Figure 1.7 Restoration of human intracellular cobalamin binding activity in mouse × *cbl C* hybrids. Hybrids formed between mouse L-cells (line A9) and a human fibroblast line of the *cbl C* class were tested for intracellular [^{57}Co] cobalamin binding by polyacrylamide gel electrophoresis. The binding profiles of both parental lines are shown in the upper left-hand panels; the upper right-hand panels are the binding profiles of two of the hybrid clones. Hybrid VA 287–5 expresses both the human and the mouse intracellular cobalamin binding activities, as well as both methyltransferase isozymes (not shown). For comparison, the bottom panels show the binding profiles of A9, a normal human fibroblast line, and two hybrid clones derived from their fusion. See text and reference 34 for details

alleles (Figure 1.8)[28]. Some enzyme molecules in such cells appear to have a normal K_m for AdoCbl, others a distinctly increased K_m. Third, mutase activity in cells from some mut^- heterozygotes is more thermolabile than control, but less labile than that in cells from the affected homozygote. Presumably these findings reflect the dimeric structure of the mutase apoenzyme and the likelihood that cells from heterozygotes for mut mutants contain three types of enzyme molecules, $\alpha\alpha$, $\alpha\alpha'$, and $\alpha'\alpha'$ (where α is the normal subunit and α' the mutant one).

Evidence for genetic compounds among mut *mutants*　It is generally assumed that individuals affected with autosomal recessively inherited enzyme deficiencies receive the same mutant gene from each heterozygous parent, and are, therefore, true homozygotes for the defect. Genetic compounds (individuals who get one mutant allele from one parent and a different mutant allele at the same locus from the other) are being described with increasing frequency, however. Our studies of mutase apoenzyme deficiency have uncovered at least one such example[28]. The proband's cells contained no detectable activity and were, therefore, called mut^0. Whereas his father's cells had approximately 50% of normal activity with a normal K_m for AdoCbl (mut^0/mut^+), his mother's cells demonstrated a mutant allele with a reduced affinity for cofactor (mut^-/mut^+). Thus the affected child presumably has a mut^0/mut^- genotype rather than the expected mut^0/mut^0. Apparently, neither of the homodimeric species nor the heterodimeric one in his cells retain demonstrable activity.

Chromosome localization of the human methyltransferase locus　As mentioned earlier, human methyltransferase and mouse methyltransferase have different electrophoretic mobilities on polyacrylamide gels. This difference enabled us to detect the human isozyme in interspecific mouse × human hybrids and correlate its presence with the human chromosome complement of such hybrids. From an examination of 12 mouse × human hybrid clones, we assigned, with a high degree of certainty, the gene coding for the human methyltransferase apoenzyme to the human chromosome one[34]. Moreover, since those hybrids expressing both human and mouse forms of the enzyme contained no heteropolymeric band, it seems likely that the methyltransferase is a monomer.

CLINICAL OBSERVATIONS

I have been fascinated by the study of inborn errors of metabolism in

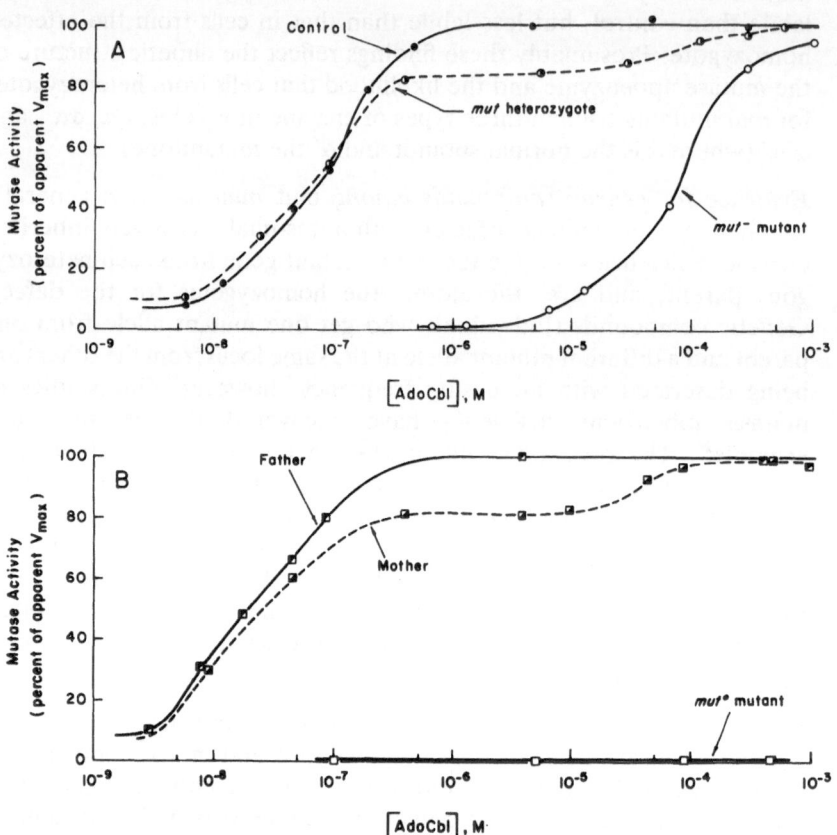

Figure 1.8 Michaelis–Menten plots of effect of AdoCbl concentration on methylmalonyl CoA mutase activity, expressed as percentage of apparent V_{max}, in extracts of cell lines from controls, *mut* mutants, and *mut* heterozygotes. (A) Extracts of control line 87 (●), *mut⁻* mutant 550 (○) and *mut* heterozygote 613 (from the father of *mut⁻* mutant 550 (◐) were incubated at 37°C with the indicated concentrations of AdoCbl for 10 min prior to assay. The respective V_{max}s of these three cell lines were 1770, 510, and 1271 pmol/min/mg protein. (B) Extracts of *mut⁰* mutant 507 (□) and of cell lines from that patient's mother and father, lines 508 (◪) and 509 (◩), respectively, were incubated with varying concentrations of AdoCbl, as above. The respective V_{max}s of these three cell lines were <2, 492, and 836 pmol/min/mg protein. Concentration of DL-methylmalonyl CoA in each experiment was 0.37 mM. See text and reference 28 for details

general and of the inherited methylmalonic acidaemias in particular for two reasons. The first is scientific and selfish. I have been thrilled by the challenge of attempting to solve these elegant, and intrinsically logical mysteries of nature. The second is medical and, hopefully, not so selfish. I have hoped that what we decipher in the laboratory can be translated into improved means of diagnosis, treatment, and prevention. This presentation has, thus far, considered almost exclusively the scientific aspects of our efforts not, I hope, because I am so much more comfortable and adept in the laboratory than I am in the clinic, but rather because much more has been learned from 80 fibroblast cell lines than from the single affected patient whom we have had the opportunity to follow. Nonetheless, I wish to conclude this discussion by returning it to its origin – the clinical manifestations in children affected with the inherited methylmalonic acidaemias.

Natural history

In the dozen years since children with inherited methylmalonic acidaemia were first described, numerous other case reports have appeared (reviewed by Rosenberg[3] and Morrow[35]). Yet, we know little about the natural history of these disorders and less still about the physician's ability to modify that natural history. We are currently attempting to gain this information by collecting from questionnaires detailed information on the clinical course of those patients whose fibroblasts have been sent to us and whose biochemical phenotype we have determined (Matsui et al., unpublished observations). Since only about half of these questionnaires (33 of 58) have been completed to date, and since some of the forms of the methylmalonic acidaemias are represented in the completed survey by no more than four patients (cbl B, cbl C, cbl D), we cannot be very precise. However, certain conclusions can be drawn provisionally. First, patients with isolated mutase deficiency (mut, cbl A and cbl B classes) regularly present with severe metabolic acidosis, ketosis and protein intolerance, whereas those children with defective synthesis of AdoCbl and MeCbl (cbl C and cbl D groups) do not. Second, more than half of the children with isolated mutase deficiency manifested hyperglycinuria and/or hyperammonaemia. Third, about 90% of children in the mut class become clinically ill within the first month of life, whereas a majority of those in the cbl A and cbl B groups do not manifest symptoms until after this interval. Fourth, whereas about 60% of children in the mut class died of their disease some time during the first two years of life and another 30% are alive but with significant neurological or intellectual impairment, >70% of the children in the *cbl A* class are alive and well – their ages ranging from 3 to 12 years. And fifth, although most of the affected children have received a therapeutic trial of Cbl supplementation, benefit has been observed only in children with defects in Cbl metabolism. Clinical responsiveness among the latter group appears to be more impressive in members of the *cbl A, cbl C* and *cbl D* classes than in those from the *cbl B* category.

Pathophysiology

Accumulation of methylmalonate, propionate, and lactate appears to account satisfactorily for the acidosis so often observed in patients with isolated mutase deficiency. Likewise, the long-chain ketones which pile up because the catabolism of branched-chain amino acids is impaired explains the ketosis encountered in this group. Far more complex, however, are the mechanisms responsible for the often noted triad of secondary biochemical disturbances – hypoglycaemia, hyperglycinaemia, and hyperammonaemia. As shown in Figure 1.9, each of these findings can be accounted for by proposing that the increased amounts of propionyl CoA and methylmalonyl CoA (or their respective free acids) which accumulate within the mitochondrion inhibit one or more critical mitochondrial processes relevant to gluconeogenesis, glycine disposal, and ammonia detoxification. Since methylmalonyl CoA is a known inhibitor of pyruvate carboxylase and since methylmalonate inhibits the transmitochondrial shuttle system for malate, interference with either or both of these systems could impair gluconeogenesis and produce hypoglycaemia[3,6,35]. Likewise, reduced activity of the glycine cleavage enzyme (as has been reported in the liver of some patients with methylmalonic acidaemia) could produce hyperglycinaemia[3,35]. Finally, recent findings make it seem likely that the hyperammonaemia results from impaired activity of the first enzyme of the urea cycle, carbamyl phosphate synthetase I (CPS I). Nyhan and colleagues[36] have shown that propionyl CoA is a potent inhibitor of *N*-acetylglutamate synthetase, the mitochondrial enzyme required for the formation of a necessary activator of CPS I activity, *N*-acetylglutamate. We have found that propionyl CoA and methylmalonyl CoA are effective inhibitors of CPS I activity *in vitro* even when saturating amounts of *N*-acetylglutamate are available[37]. Hence, at least two different mechanisms of secondary CPS I deficiency are now at hand.

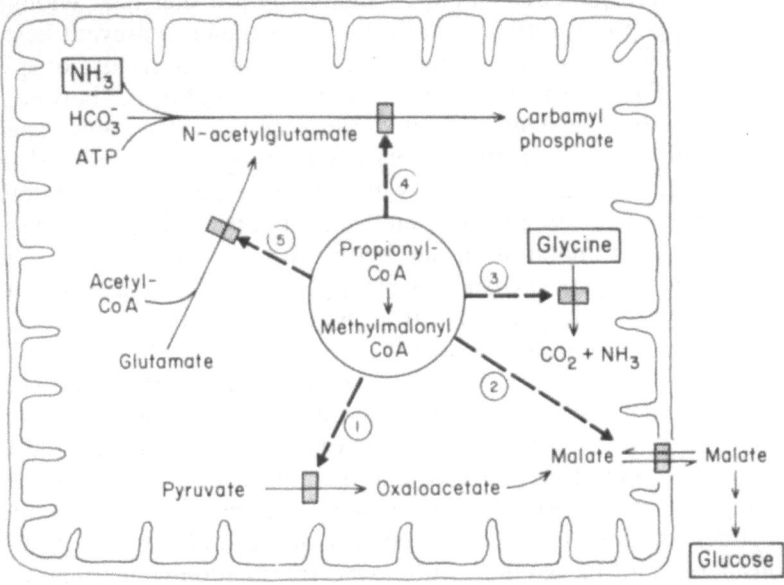

Figure 1.9 Proposed mechanisms of hypoglycaemia, hyperglycinaemia, and hyperammonaemia in patients with the inherited methylmalonic acidaemias. Inhibitory effects of the enlarged intramitochondrial pools of propionyl CoA and methylmalonyl CoA (as well as their respective free acids) on mitochondrial functions are shown by the numbered, dashed lines corresponding to the following enzymatic or carrier-mediated reactions: 1 pyruvate carboxylase; 2 the transmitochondrial malate shuttle; 3 glycine cleavage enzyme; 4 carbamyl phosphate synthetase I; 5 N-acetylglutamate synthetase. See text for discussion

Diagnosis and treatment

Since colorimetric and gas chromatographic assays for urinary and serum methylmalonate are widely available, it should no longer be difficult to make a diagnosis of one of the inherited methylmalonic acidaemias or to distinguish them from acquired Cbl deficiency states. Confirmation and classification can be provided from fibroblast studies by the kinds of complementation tests and biochemical assays discussed earlier. Such assays have also proved beneficial in diagnosing these conditions prenatally. Studies with cultured amniotic fluid cells have identified foetuses at risk with mutations of the mutase apoenzyme (*mut⁰*) and of AdoCbl synthesis (*cbl A* and *cbl B*).

All affected patients should be treated with a diet high enough in protein to support normal growth, but low enough to prevent ketoacidosis. This is, in no way, an easy task and often requires use of special formulae. Even then, it is difficult to 'walk the tightrope' between inanition on the one hand and intoxication on the other. Since specific classification of patients by fibroblast genotyping is laborious and time-consuming, since most children with defects in Cbl metabolism derive benefit from Cbl supplements, and since it appears that children with defects in Cbl metabolism do better than do those with mutase apoenzyme deficiency, a trial of Cbl supplementation seems appropriate in all newly detected patients. It is less easy to define what an appropriate therapeutic trial is. I hold that a patient cannot be deemed 'Cbl-responsive' unless a clearcut fall in serum or urine methylmalonate has been documented, and believe that such an assessment can almost always be achieved after 7–14 days of Cbl supplements (1–2 mg of OH-Cbl/day parenterally), provided that dietary stabilization is maintained during this interval. If responsive patients are noted to relapse while on treatment with OH-Cbl, the possibility of OH-Cbl toxicity should be considered and the vitamin withdrawn. Information concerning the *in vivo* efficacy of AdoCbl is badly needed, as is data concerning the age at which supplements can be discontinued. The parents of our boy with Cbl-responsive methylmalonic acidaemia (of the *cbl A* class) discontinued all dietary restriction and Cbl supplementation against our advice when he was 8 years old. In the ensuing 4 years he has not demonstrated acidosis, ketosis or protein intolerance, has grown well, and is of above normal intelligence. Long-term follow-up of other patients is needed before this impressive result is extrapolated to other affected children. Finally, the feasibility of prenatal therapy with Cbl supplements has been established[38]. When a woman carrying a foetus affected with the *cbl A* mutation was given oral and parenteral OH-Cbl supplements, her urinary excretion of methylmalonate fell significantly. The necessity for such prenatal therapy has not yet, however, been established.

CONCLUDING REMARKS

When one is as close to a subject as I am to the inherited methylmalonic acidaemias, perspective is difficult to achieve. In the 12 years since we made a diagnosis of methylmalonic acidaemia in a little boy named Robby, my emotional response to the subject has ranged from great exhilaration to massive frustration. Far more enduring than these polar positions has been a continuing sense of privilege at having had the great good fortune to stumble into the most rewarding work of my career.

Acknowledgements

The author is deeply indebted to the following colleagues who worked in his laboratory and contributed to some aspect of the study of the inherited methylmalonic acidaemias: L. Ambani, N. Berliner, R. Blunden, J. Durant, M. Feldman, W. Fenton, J. Goldberg, R. Gravel, J. Gruskay, A. Hack, A. Hart, Y. Hsia, A. Lilljeqvist, M. Mahoney, G. Marchant, S. Matsui, I. Mellman, L. Patel, F. Rosenbloom, K. Scully, C. Sennett, M. Seashore, V. Steen, H. Willard, and P. Youngdahl-Turner. Their work has resulted in nearly 40 original publications and reviews, for which the author is acting as spokesman.

The author is also indebted to the many collaborators from other laboratories, including R. Allen, I. Armitage, A. Gertler, P. Lin, B. Lindblad, S. Lipsky, S. Mudd, E. Nakamura, H. Ramsdell, F. Ruddle, K. Tanaka, B. Uhlendorf, J. Waldenstrom, and R. Zetterstrom. Their studies have complemented, and in some important instances, defined the direction of our own.

References

1. Flavin, M., Ortiz, P. J. and Ochoa, S. (1955). Metabolism of propionic acid in animal tissues. *Nature (London)*, **176**, 823
2. Katz, J. and Chaikoff, I. L. (1955). The metabolism of propionate by rat liver slices and the formation of isosuccinic acid. *J. Am. Chem. Soc.*, **77**, 2659
3. Rosenberg, L. E. (1978). Disorders of propionate, methylmalonate and cobalamin metabolism. In J. B. Stanbury, J. B. Wyngaarden and D. S. Fredrickson, (eds.). *The Metabolic Basis of Inherited Disease*, p. 411 (New York: McGraw-Hill)
4. Cox, E. V. and White, A. M. (1962). Methylmalonic acid excretion: Index of vitamin-B_{12} deficiency. *Lancet*, **2**, 853
5. Barness, L. A., Young, D., Mellman, W. J., Kahn, S. B. and Williams, W. J. (1963). Methylmalonate excretion in patient with pernicious anemia. *N. Engl. J. Med.*, **268**, 144
6. Oberholzer, V. G., Levin, B., Burgess, E. A. and Young, W. F. (1967). Methylmalonic aciduria: An inborn error of metabolism leading to chronic metabolic acidosis. *Arch. Dis. Child.*, **42**, 492
7. Stokke, O., Eldjarn, L., Norum, K. R., Steen-Johnsen, J. and Halvorsen, S. (1967). Methylmalonic aciduria: A new inborn error of metabolism

which may cause fatal acidosis in the neonatal period. *Scand. J. Clin. Lab. Invest.*, **20**, 313

8. Rosenberg, L. E., Lilljeqvist, A. C. and Hsia, Y. E. (1968). Methylmalonic aciduria: An inborn error leading to metabolic acidosis, long-chain ketonuria and intermittent hyperglycinemia. *N. Engl. J. Med.*, **278**, 1319

9. Lindblad, B., Lindstrand, K., Svanberg, B. and Zetterstrom, R. (1969). The effect of cobamide coenzyme in methylmalonic acidemia. *Acta Paediatr. Scand.*, **58**, 178

10. Mudd, S. H., Levy, H. L. and Abeles, R. H. (1969). A derangement in B_{12} metabolism leading to homocystinemia, cystathioninemia and methylmalonicaciduria. *Biochem. Biophys. Res. Commun.*, **35**, 121

11. Rosenberg, L. E. and Tanaka, K. (1976). Metabolism of amino acids and organic acids. In N. Freinkel, (ed.). *The Year in Metabolism 1975–1976*, p. 181. (New York: Plenum)

12. Fenton, W. A. and Rosenberg, L. E. (1978). Genetic and biochemical analysis of human cobalamin mutants in cell culture. *Annu. Rev. Genet.*, **12**, 233

13. Willard, H. F. and Rosenberg, L. E. (1979). Inherited deficiencies of methylmalonyl CoA mutase activity: Biochemical and genetic studies in cultured skin fibroblasts. In F. Hommes (ed.). *Models for the Study of Inborn Errors of Metabolism*, p. 297. (Amsterdam: Elsevier/North Holland Biomedical Press)

14. Tanaka, K., Armitage, I. M., Ramsdell, H. S., Hsia, Y. E., Lipsky, S. R. and Rosenberg, L. E. (1975). [^{13}C]Valine metabolism in methylmalonic acidemia using nuclear magnetic resonance: Propionate as an obligate intermediate. *Proc. Natl. Acad. Sci. USA.*, **72**, 3692

15. Youngdahl-Turner, P., Rosenberg, L. E. and Allen, R. H. (1978). Binding and uptake of transcobalamin II by human fibroblasts. *J. Clin. Invest.* **61**, 133

16. Youngdahl-Turner, P., Mellman, I. S., Allen, R. H. and Rosenberg, L. E. (1979). Protein mediated vitamin uptake: Adsorptive endocytosis of the transcobalamin II–cobalamin complex by cultured human fibroblasts. *Exp. Cell. Res.*, **118**, 127

17. Berliner, N. and Rosenberg, L. E. (1981). Uptake and metabolism of free cyanocobalamin by cultured human fibroblasts from controls and a patient with transcobalamin II deficiency. *Metabolism*, **30**, 230

18. Mellman, I. S., Youngdahl-Turner, P., Willard, H. F. and Rosenberg, L. E. (1977). Intracellular binding of radioactive hydroxocobalamin to cobalamin-dependent apoenzymes in rat liver. *Proc. Natl. Acad. Sci. USA*, **74**, 916

19. Mellman, I. S., Willard, H. F. and Rosenberg, L. E. (1978). Cobalamin binding and cobalamin-dependent enzyme activity in normal and mutant human fibroblasts. *J. Clin. Invest.*, **62**, 952

20. Willard, H. F. and Rosenberg, L. E. (1979). Inborn errors of cobalamin metabolism: Effect of cobalamin supplementation in culture on methylmalonyl CoA mutase activity in normal and mutant human fibroblasts. *Biochem. Genet.*, **17**, 57

21. Willard, H. F. and Rosenberg, L. E. (1980). Interactions of methylmalonyl CoA mutase from normal human fibroblasts with adenosylcobalamin and

methylmalonyl CoA: Evidence for non-equivalent active sites. *Arch. Biochem. Biophys.*, **200**, 130

22. Willard, H. F. and Rosenberg, L. E. (1979) Irreversible enzyme inhibition by hydroxocobalamin: possible mechanism of water-soluble vitamin toxicity. *Clin. Res.*, **27**, 508A (abstract)

23. Morrow, G., Barness, L. A., Cardinale, G. J., Abeles, R. H. and Flaks, J. G. (1969). Congenital methylmalonic acidemia: Enzymatic evidence for two forms of the disease. *Proc. Natl. Acad. Sci. USA*, **63**, 191

24. Rosenberg, L. E., Lilljeqvist, A. C., Hsia, Y. E. and Rosenbloom, F. M. (1969). Vitamin B_{12} dependent methylmalonicaciduria: Defective B_{12} metabolism in cultured fibroblasts. *Biochem. Biophys. Res. Commun.*, **37**, 607

25. Mahoney, M. J., Rosenberg, L. E., Mudd, S. H. and Uhlendorf, B. W. (1971). Defective metabolism of vitamin B_{12} in fibroblasts from patients with methylmalonicaciduria. *Biochem. Biophys. Res. Commun.*, **44**, 375

26. Mudd, S. H., Uhlendorf, B. W., Hinds, K. R. and Levy, H. L. (1970). Deranged B_{12} metabolism: Studies of fibroblasts grown in tissue culture. *Biochem. Med.*, **4**, 215

27. Mellman, I., Willard, H. F., Youngdahl-Turner, P. and Rosenberg, L. E. (1979). Cobalamin coenzyme synthesis in normal and mutant human fibroblasts: Evidence for a processing enzyme activity deficient in *cbl C* cells. *J. Biol. Chem.*, **254**, 11847

28. Willard, H. F. and Rosenberg, L. E. (1980). Inherited methylmalonyl CoA mutase apoenzyme deficiency in human fibroblasts: Evidence for allelic heterogeneity, codominant expression, and the existence of genetic compounds. *J. Clin. Invest.*, **65**, 690

29. Willard, H. F. and Rosenberg, L. E. (1977). Inherited deficiencies of human methylmalonyl CoA mutase activity: Reduced affinity of mutant apoenzyme for adenosylcobalamin. *Biochem. Biophys. Res. Commun.*, **78**, 927

30. Fenton, W. A. and Rosenberg, L. E. (1981). The defect in the *cbl B* class of human methylmalonic acidemia: deficiency of cob(I)alamin adenosyltransferase activity in extracts of cultured fibroblasts. *Biochem. Biophys. Res. Commun.*, **98**, 283

31. Gravel, R. A., Mahoney, M. J., Ruddle, F. H. and Rosenberg, L. E. (1975). Genetic complementation in heterokaryons of human fibroblasts defective in cobalamin metabolism. *Proc. Natl. Acad. Sci. USA*, **72**, 3181

32. Willard, H. F., Mellman, I. S. and Rosenberg, L. E. (1978). Genetic complementation among inherited deficiencies of methylmalonyl-CoA mutase activity: Evidence for a new class of human cobalamin mutant. *Am. J. Hum. Genet.*, **30**, 1

33. Goodman, S. I., Moe, P. G., Hammond, K. B., Mudd, S. H. and Uhlendorf, B. W. (1970). Homocystinuria with methylmalonic aciduria: Two cases in a sibship. *Biochem. Med.*, **4**, 500

34. Mellman, I. S., Lin, P.-F., Ruddle, F. H. and Rosenberg, L. E. (1979). Genetic control of cobalamin binding in normal and mutant cells: Assignment of the gene for 5-methyltetrahydrofolate:L-homocysteine S-methyltransferase to human chromosome 1. *Proc. Natl. Acad. Sci. USA*, **76**, 405

35. Morrow, G. III (1974). Methylmalonic acidemia. In W. L. Nyhan (ed.).
     Heritable Disorders of Amino Acid Metabolism, p. 61. (New York: John
     Wiley)
36. Coude, F. X., Sweetman, L. and Nyhan, W. L. (1979). The inhibition by
     propionyl CoA of *N*-acetylglutamate synthetase in rat liver mitochondria:
     A possible explanation for hyperammonemia in propionic and methyl-
     malonic acidemia. *J. Clin. Invest.*, **64**, 1544
37. Gruskay, J. and Rosenberg, L. E. (1979). Inhibition of hepatic mitochon-
     drial carbamyl phosphate synthetase (CPS I) by acyl CoA esters: Possible
     mechanism of hyperammonemia in the organic acidemias. *Pediat. Res.*, **13**,
     475 (abstract)
38. Ampola, M. G., Mahoney, M. J., Nakamura, E. and Tanaka, K. (1975).
     Prenatal therapy of a patient with vitamin B_{12} responsive methylmalonic
     acidemia. *New Engl. J. Med.*, **293**, 313

SECTION TWO

Biochemistry of Membranes

2

Membrane structure

R. Coleman

Insight into the structure of membranes came initially from physiologists interested in the transport of molecules into cells, and from lipid biochemists. Their studies emphasized the lipid bilayer as an important feature of membrane structure. The application of new techniques in the mid 1960s caused initial conflict with these views by stressing a variety of protein-dominated structures. A consensus was reached which viewed membranes as being built on a common plan, composed of a fluid bilayer in which were embedded biologically active proteins capable of independent movement in the plane of the bilayer. More recent work has stressed the constraints on movement of particular membrane components and the local order which may exist within this basic plan, and thus is slowly indicating the basis for the differences between individual membranes. In this account I shall attempt to outline some aspects of our understanding of membrane structure, in the hope that it might form a rational basis on which to build the more detailed discussions of what membranes can do, how they do it, and what may go wrong with their contribution to cellular function.

MEMBRANES AS LIPOPROTEIN BARRIERS OF SELECTIVE PERMEABILITY

Membranes were recognized initially as general permeability barriers to both large and small molecules. As such, intracellular membranes separate regions of the cytoplasm and the plasma membrane separates the cytoplasm from the environment. The main purpose of these barriers is to retain specific protein and metabolite complements in the various sub-cellular compartments. Leakage of cytoplasmic enzymes from cells is therefore taken as a diagnostically specific indicator of cell (and membrane) damage; in a reciprocal way the entry of normally-excluded dye molecules is an indicator of membrane damage in isolated cells[1].

These general permeability studies and the high capacitances shown by membranes indicated that they possessed a layer of lipid. The presence of lipid, i.e. phospholipids and in some cases cholesterol and glycolipids, was confirmed directly by analyses of isolated membranes. In addition, isolated membrane preparations contained substantial amounts of protein; protein had been previously implicated in the structure of membranes in order to explain both their low surface tensions and their high permeabilities to specific small molecules and ions. These specific permeabilities are the properties of individual proteins, several of which have now been characterized in some detail and, in some cases, isolated. The presence of such proteins in membranes allows for the selective uptake of nutrients and key substrates, for the selective elimination of wastes, and for the generation of ion gradients.

Metabolism and protein biosynthesis also require regulatory signals from the environment, and thus specific proteins are present in the otherwise exclusive lipid layer to receive the message (e.g. from hormones, transmitters, antigens or drugs) and to transduce it into the cell.

The membrane also provides a platform for many enzyme activities: not only does this give a local concentration of the particular metabolism (and increase efficiency), but the general impermeability of the membrane ensures that location on one side or the other of the lipid layer restricts the activity to a single compartment and gives to the cell an overall metabolic topology. In some cases, there may even be a regional specialization of functions in the plane of the membrane, e.g. in epithelial cells the plasma membrane has a distinct composition and function according to whether it borders the lumenal or basal aspect of the cell. (For a more detailed account of the functions of membranes see Finean et al.[2].)

MEMBRANE LIPID, A FLUID BILAYER

A wide variety of evidence now supports the view that membrane lipid exists as a bilayer, i.e. two apposed monolayers, back to back, creating a central hydrophobic core of hydrocarbon chains, with their outer surfaces bearing the polar head groups of the various lipid molecules. Initial indications for the nature and molecular dimensions of this bilayer came from capacitance studies, from the area occupied by lipids extracted from erythrocyte membranes, from the appearance of membranes by transmission electron microscopy and, more particularly, from X-ray diffraction studies; these latter gave the approximate molecular dimensions and also the electron density profile showed a central region of low electron density, sandwiched between two higher density regions. Later studies compared the properties of the lipid in a wide variety of isolated membranes with those in artificially-prepared lipid bilayers and showed close correlations by X-ray diffraction, freeze-fracture electron microscopy, differential thermal calorimetry, electron spin and nuclear magnetic resonance spectroscopy[3-6].

Several of these techniques (ESR, NMR, calorimetry, X-ray diffraction) and fluorescence polarization can be used to measure the motions of molecules or parts of molecules in the membrane, or the viscosity (fluidity) of the lipid environment. They have shown that the lipid is in a relatively fluid state and that individual lipid molecules can diffuse in the plane of the membrane at about the same speed as in lipid bilayers, exchanging with their lateral neighbours about a million times a second. In addition, there exists a flexibility gradient down the lipid molecules with the centre of the bilayer having the highest flexibility (i.e. the most fluid).

In model bilayers containing a restricted range of lipids, the fluidity decreases with decreasing temperature (often with the separation of a discrete gel phase); at a given temperature, fluidity is greater with unsaturated lipids than with saturated ones and with short fatty-acid chains than longer ones. The situation in membranes is more complex, however, due to the large number of lipid species, to the presence of cholesterol (which smooths out the phase transitions and ensures membrane fluidity over a greater temperature range) and to the influence of membrane proteins[5,7-9].

Interruption of the bilayer was envisaged initially to explain the specific high permeabilities to a variety of molecules. The advent of freeze fracture techniques, which are thought to cleave bilayers through the middle of the hydrophobic core showed, by electron microscopy, that membranes bore particles on one or both of the fracture faces; in contrast, the freeze fracture replicas of pure lipid bilayers were uninterrupted by such particles. These particles have been equated with proteins penetrating into the hydrophobic core of the membrane and in some membranes the extent of bilayer penetration is quite high[4]. More direct evidence of the penetration of the bilayer by protein comes, however, from the use of reagents specific for protein composition and function.

ASYMMETRIC DISTRIBUTION OF PROTEINS

In the cell the membrane separates two distinct environments, each with its own characteristic metabolism; functional proteins of the membrane make their own contributions to such metabolism. It is therefore of relevance to ask whether membrane proteins are exposed only on the side of the membrane relevant to their function, or are to be found on both sides of it.

The answers to these questions have been investigated using a variety of reagents: substrates, inhibitors, hormones, transmitters, drugs, antibodies, modifying enzymes and chemical labels for particular groups on the protein molecule. One prerequisite for the usefulness of such reagents is that the membrane is essentially impermeable to them in the time scale of the experiment, and thus they will act only on the side of the membrane to which they are presented; some of the most definitive information has therefore been obtained using macromolecules. The sensitivity of detection is often increased by using radiolabelled reagents and in a few instances, direct morphological detection of the bound reagent has been possible by the use of ferritin-labelled antibodies.

In some cases it has been possible to present the reagent to either side of the membrane separately. One way is by the use of membrane preparations of normal (outside out) or reversed (inside out) orientation, which are often made as vesicles; it is important that all membranes in the preparation have the same orientation and are impermeable, or ambiguous results will be obtained. Another method is by introducing the reagent inside an appropriate permeable membrane preparation, resealing the membrane, washing away the excess reagent from the outside and then initiating the reaction, e.g. by photoactivation or introduction of an initiator compound. Appropriate controls using permeable or solubilized preparations are needed in all of these studies to indicate the total capacity of the system.

These techniques have demonstrated very clearly that all molecules of a particular protein have the same orientation in the membrane, e.g. that the active centre of a given enzyme is only presented to one metabolic compartment. They also show that proteins do not readily invert from

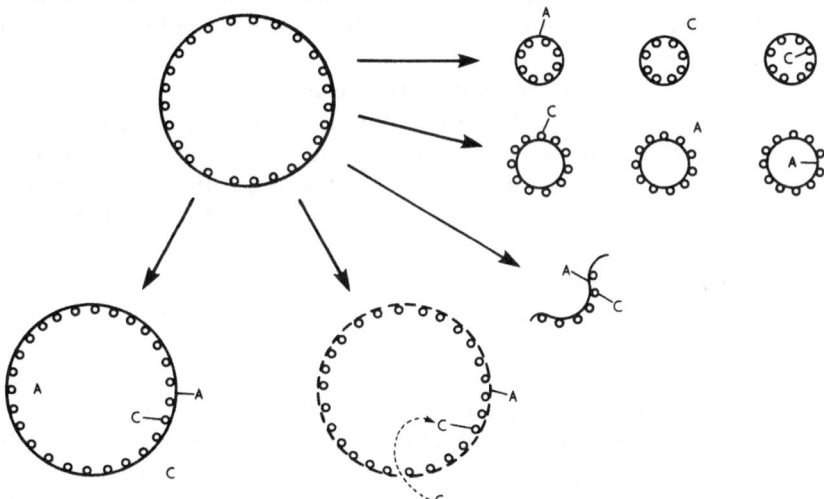

Figure 2.1 Determination of membrane protein topography by the use of impermeant reagents and membrane preparations of different orientations. A and C represent reagents for different biological activities

one face of the bilayer to the other, since this would result in a more symmetrical distribution of functions across the membrane than is observed in practice.

Whilst yielding information on the disposition of the functional region of a membrane protein, these techniques yield little information about the location of the remainder of the molecule. Such information has been obtained, in a few cases, by using them in conjunction with polypeptide separations (sodium dodecyl sulphate–polyacrylamide gel electrophoresis) and peptide mapping ('fingerprinting' of labelled peptide fragments). Some polypeptides have been found to be labelled by appropriate reagents in different specific regions of the polypeptide chain, according to the side of the membrane exposed to the labelling reagent. These polypeptides therefore span the membrane, exposing different regions of the chain to the two metabolic compartments, and can maintain this asymmetrical distribution. The regions exposed on the different faces of the membrane must, therefore, be connected by a peptide sequence spanning the hydrophobic interior of the lipid layer.

It is much more difficult, however, to conclude that other polypeptides may only penetrate the membrane, but not span it, since non-labelling from the alternate face of the membrane could also be due to a chemically unreactive or shielded sequences; many controls with different labelling reagents, and comparison with the solubilized protein, would be needed to improve the prediction[7,8,10-13].

Labelling and selective-modification techniques have given a clear indication of the asymmetric distribution of carbohydrate sequences associated with membranes; most of these are found on the external (i.e. non-cytoplasmic) face of the plasma membrane and the non-cytoplasmic) face of other related membranes, e.g. endoplasmic reticulum, Golgi. Since many carbohydrate sequences are attached to specific regions of individual proteins their asymmetry confirms that of the protein. Lipids appear to be asymmetrically distributed in the two leaflets of the lipid bilayer, but here the situation is more complex and less well understood. Glycolipids appear to be located in the external leaflet of the plasma membrane, but the distribution of the phospholipid classes, whilst characteristic for a given membrane, is much less absolute, e.g. phosphatidylcholine may appear in both leaflets, but in different proportions in each; these proportions may differ from those in the two leaflets of other membranes[12].

ISOLATION AND CHARACTERIZATION OF MEMBRANE PROTEINS

Early attempts to understand the molecular characteristics of membrane proteins were complicated by the large number of polypeptide species in many membranes. This, together with their various extents of penetration of the bilayer, tended to average out both amino acid compositions and protein conformational studies, such that there appeared to be little difference between the characteristics of membrane and of cytosol proteins. Significant advances were made once individual proteins had been purified and could be studied separately.

One group of proteins can be removed from membranes by using (relatively) mild treatments, e.g. extremes of ionic strength or pH, chelating agents, chaotropic agents; these perturb polar interactions (i.e. ionic and hydrogen bonds) of components at the membrane surface. The removal of these extrinsic (also called peripheral) proteins leaves the lipid bilayer intact together with another group of proteins, the intrinsic (integral) proteins. In order to disperse the intrinsic proteins from the membrane, reagents such as detergents or organic solvents are required; these reagents perturb hydrophobic interactions within the lipid bilayer

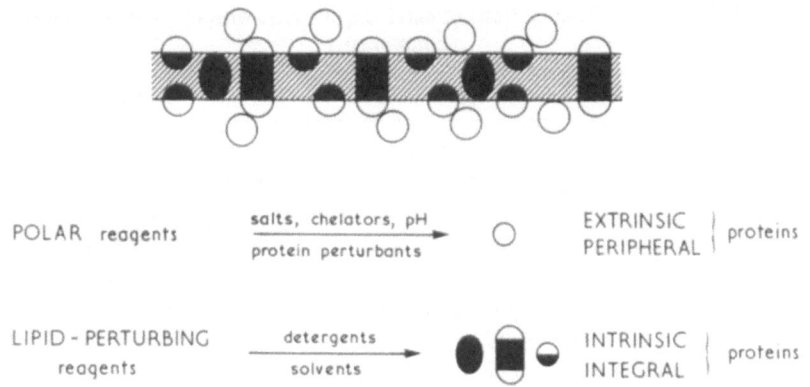

POLAR reagents · salts, chelators, pH / protein perturbants → ○ EXTRINSIC PERIPHERAL ⎱ proteins

LIPID - PERTURBING reagents · detergents / solvents → ● ▢ ● INTRINSIC INTEGRAL ⎱ proteins

Figure 2.2 Solubilization of membrane proteins

and their use suggests that intrinsic proteins penetrate the hydrophobic interior of the membrane[7,8,14-18].

Once removed from the membrane, the extrinsic proteins form stable solutions in water. They can be purified by the techniques applicable to soluble proteins, they are lipid free, and their amino-acid composition and general properties are similar to those of other soluble proteins. Within this group there exists a wide spectrum of intensity of attachment to the membrane; partial purification may therefore be achieved, in some cases, by releasing different proteins with progressively more vigorous reagents. Bonding of the protein to the membrane may be due either to interaction with the polar head groups of membrane lipids, or to general or specific interaction with other membrane proteins, extrinsic or intrinsic. The number of examples of specific interactions with other membrane proteins is increasing; these are detected by functional co-operation of the two proteins by cross-linking studies, or by inhibiting the binding by antibody directed at the more firmly bound membrane component[14,16-18] (see also Table 2.1).

Removal of intrinsic proteins from membranes by organic solvents often gives rise to denatured, inert material due to the unfavourable dielectric constant of the solvent. Since they liberate proteins into an aqueous medium and thereby preserve biological activity, detergents such as deoxycholate and Triton X100 have largely been the reagents of choice for the solubilization of intrinsic proteins. In most cases the protein has been 'solubilized' rather than rendered truly soluble, since removal of the detergent by dilution, dialysis, or during column chromatography gives rise to high molecular weight, often insoluble aggregates.

TABLE 2.1   Associations of extrinsic proteins with other membrane components

Extrinsic	Associate	Evidence
Spectrin	{ Band 3 (intrinsic) { Actin (extrinsic)	{ antibodies, cross linking { co-isolation
Cytochrome c	{ Succ–cyt c reductase (intrinsic) { Cyt oxidase (intrinsic)	{ enzymology, { antibody blocking
F_1 ATPase	{ OSCP (extrinsic) { Hydrophobic peptides { (intrinsic)	{ selective solubilization { reconstitution, antibodies
α Lactalbumin	Galactosyltransferase (intrinsic)	lactose synthesis
Ca^{2+} binding protein	ATPase (intrinsic)	high affinity Ca^{2+} ATPase (rbc)
Fibronectin	Membrane glycoproteins (intrinsic)	binding studies

All purification and handling procedures of the 'solubilized' proteins are therefore carried out in detergent-containing media to avoid this aggregation[15,19].

In many cases, the initial stages of detergent solubilization involve disaggregation of membrane structure and the formation of protein–lipid–detergent complexes, which can no longer be sedimented at centrifugal forces appropriate to membranes. At higher detergent levels the detergent can often completely substitute for the lipid to yield a 'solubilized', 'lipid-free' protein. The role of the detergent in this solubilization process appears to be the provision of a protective shell for that part of the protein originally inserted into the hydrophobic region of the lipid layer. The polar regions of the detergent molecules are thus exposed to the aqueous medium, whereas their hydrophobic regions cover the hydrophobic region of the protein, replacing its layer of protecting lipids.

Evidence for this shell of detergent molecules comes from the binding of radioactive detergents during protein isolation procedures. The various intrinsic proteins bind different, but characteristic amounts of detergents such as deoxycholate or Triton X100; in contrast, soluble and extrinsic proteins bind little or none of these detergents (but all proteins bind denaturing detergents such as dodecylsulphate due to the unfolding of the protein molecule). The amount of detergent bound to each intrinsic protein probably depends upon factors such as the amount of hydrophobic surface in relation to the total molecular weight. It is obvious that if this shell of detergent is removed, then the hydrophobic surfaces so exposed will aggregate with those of other proteins to form oligomeric protein complexes; if lipid is available, they may even re-form membrane-like structures[19,20].

The detergent molecules are associated with sequences of apolar amino acids exposed as an α helix. The α-helix content of some intrinsic proteins is high; these proteins may have much of their mass inserted in the bilayer. Other proteins, however, have a relatively small content of α helix; this may mean that most of the protein is exposed at the membrane surface. Only a relatively short sequence of 35–40 Å is required to traverse the hydrophobic region of the lipid bilayer; this is equivalent to 3500–4000 daltons and may represent only a relatively small contribution to the total mass of the protein. Such hydrophobic sequences have been identified more directly by peptide analysis following proteolytic digestion, and by their specific labelling with a recently developed labelling reagent, iodonaphthylazide[21].

The following are some examples of intrinsic proteins which illustrate various features of their structure.

Cytochrome b_5

Cytochrome b_5 can be obtained from the membrane by detergent extraction and, in detergent solution, has a molecular weight of approximately 15 000. The protein aggregates on detergent removal to an octomer of molecular weight approximately 120 000. Treatment of the membrane or detergent-solubilized form with trypsin, releases a biologically-active polypeptide of molecular weight approximately 10 000, which is water soluble and non-aggregating. This fragment contains the N-terminal sequence of the original protein. Remaining in the membrane, after trypsin treatment, is a detergent-soluble peptide fragment of molecular weight approximately 4500 containing the C-terminal sequence. This peptide is extremely hydrophobic, containing approximately 60% of apolar amino-acid residues and aggregates on removal of the detergent. Thus, it appears that the protease-released fragment was originally exposed at the membrane surface and carried out the biological activity and that the hydrophobic fragment was a 'foot' which anchored the protein into the membrane. Cytochrome b_5 is only labelled from one side of the membrane, indicating but not proving that it is merely anchored in the membrane rather than spanning it[22].

Glycophorin

Glycophorin (PAS-I, MN glycoprotein) of human erythrocytes (Figure 2.3) is accessible to labelling reagents from both sides of the membrane, but in different regions of the polypeptide chain: it is therefore a spanning polypeptide. The N-terminal sequence is exposed on the outer surface of the erythrocyte and bears 16 oligosaccharide chains of total molecular weight about 15 000. The C-terminal sequence is exposed on the cytoplasmic surface and is rich in acidic amino acids and proline. Trypsin cleaves the polypeptide, giving water-soluble peptides and a hydrophobic peptide which is only soluble in detergents; this has a molecular weight of approximately 3700, contains 35 amino acids, and bears no sugar residues. Compared to the 19% in the original protein, this peptide has approximately 83% α-helical character. It is labelled by iodonaphthylazide and contains the sequence of 23 hydrophobic amino acids which crosses the non-polar domain of the membrane. Glycophorin has a total polypeptide molecular weight of approximately 30 000 and thus the transmembrane sequence represents only approximately 10% of the total amino acid complement[16,21,23].

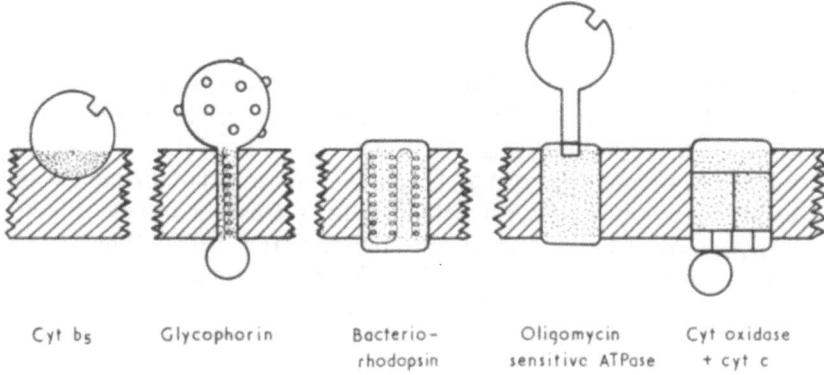

| Cyt b$_5$ | Glycophorin | Bacterio-rhodopsin | Oligomycin sensitive ATPase | Cyt oxidase + cyt c |

Figure 2.3 Diagrammatic representation of some intrinsic proteins

Bacteriorhodopsin

This protein (see Figure 2.3) is found in the patches of purple membrane of *Halobacterium*. The polypeptide molecular weight is approximately 26 000 and the protein has a high content of hydrophobic amino acids.

X-ray diffraction analysis shows a high content of α-helix in the protein, in regions oriented across the membrane and having dimensions of 40 Å. There appear to be seven such regions per molecule of protein and the N-terminal and C-terminal sequences are located on opposite sides of the membrane. This polypeptide chain therefore appears to span the membrane with seven sequences, which must be connected together with short, less hydrophobic segments located at the surface of the membrane. The X-ray diffraction pattern shows that three polypeptide chains form a unit cell in the membrane[24].

A second protein spanning the membrane with several sequences, is the anion transport protein (Band 3) of human erythrocyte membranes. Carbohydrate sequences, labelling reactions and binding sites are asymmetrically distributed across the membrane on different regions of the 90 000 dalton polypeptide chain. Proteolysis of the exposed sequences cleaves the molecule, but leaves the peptide fragments embedded in the membrane. This has been taken as evidence for multiple insertion points and, though there is still controversy, the polypeptide chain probably spans the membrane with at least two sequences[25–29].

Mitochondrial oligomycin-sensitive ATPase

This is made up of a complex of polypeptide subunits. Some of these (the extrinsic polypeptides) form the F_1 ATPase and stalk (which can be seen by negative staining) and make specific interaction with a series of very hydrophobic (intrinsic) polypeptides embedded in the lipid bilayer, which together span the membrane forming the proton-conducting channel. These have a high proportion of apolar amino acids and a high content of α-helix; they present a relatively large amount of hydrophobic surface since they can be taken up not only in detergent, but also in chloroform–methanol[30].

Cytochrome oxidase

Cytochrome oxidase (see Figure 2.3) is also formed from a complex of intrinsic polypeptides which spans the membrane overall; the asymmetric distribution of the complex is due to that of individual polypeptides. The distribution of these has been established from labelling patterns with impermeable reagents[31].

Oligomeric associations

Some intrinsic proteins are isolated from membranes as small oligomers or in association with specific other proteins[17]. Such associations may have pre-existed in the membrane or may have been created as a result of the isolation or identification procedures. Cross-linking studies on the intact membrane can sometimes give evidence of a pre-existing association, but they, too, can create apparent associations, thus band 3 polypeptide probably exists in the membrane as a dimer, whereas studies on the sarcoplasmic reticulum Ca^{2+} ATPase have yet to give a clear result[32]. The smallest active Na^+–K^+ ATPase complex which can be isolated from the shark rectal gland contains two molecules of the catalytic polypeptide unit and four molecules of an accompanying glycoprotein. Further dissociation of the complex results in loss of activity[33]; such studies suggest an association in the membrane but do not prove it. X-ray diffraction has given clear evidence of a unit cell of three bacteriorhodopsin molecules in the *Halobacterium* membrane[24].

PROTEIN MOVEMENT IN A FLUID LIPID BILAYER

A variety of studies have indicated that lateral movement occurs, or can occur, in the plane of the fluid lipid bilayer[7,34-36]. Thus, two populations of tissue culture cells were labelled at their surfaces with antibodies bearing different fluorescent colours. Fusion of the cells with Sendai virus resulted in randomization of the two labels over the surface of the heterokaryon; this occurred at 37°C but not at 4°C. There was, however, no dependence upon metabolic energy and thus the temperature effect is probably related to other factors, probably membrane fluidity. Other illustrations of this random movement include the randomization of bleached and non-bleached rhodopsin molecules in retinal rod membranes following local illumination; the movement and aggregation of intra-membranous particles by multivalent ligands in erythrocyte membranes previously treated with protease or low ionic strength; the spreading of labelled bound univalent antibodies after spot application to the surfaces of muscle fibres and the aggregation into patches of labelled divalent antibodies applied to lymphocytes. In this last example, the divalent antibody is thought to bring together the membrane antigens on the surface by cross-linking reactions, since monovalent (Fab) antibodies do not bring about aggregation.

Perhaps the most striking example of protein movement is found where diffusion of hormone receptors from one cell type confers hormone sensitivity to the adenylate cyclase of a second cell type. In these experiments (i) turkey erythrocyte adenylate cyclase was inactivated by n-ethylmaleimide leaving functional catecholamine (β-adrenergic) receptors unaffected; (ii) the treated turkey erythrocytes were fused by Sendai virus to one of several cell types which possessed a functional adenylate cyclase but which had no catecholamine receptor; (iii) the adenylate cyclase of the heterokaryon was then responsive to catecholamines, suggesting movement of the receptor and adenylate cyclase in the plane of the membrane[37]. Incorporation of cis-vaccenic acid into the membrane of native turkey erythrocytes brought about both an increase in membrane fluidity and the rate of activation of adenylate cyclase by occupied p-adrenergic receptor molecules. This result gives support for the activation being by an increased rate of 'collision-coupling' between receptor and cyclase, since there was a much smaller effect upon the activity of fluoride-sensitive cyclase[38,39].

On cooling some membranes, especially those lacking cholesterol, the lipids reach a transition point and form a gel phase; by freeze fracture techniques many intramembranous particles are seen to be excluded from the smooth-lipid gel regions and to form clusters. The relative fluidity of the lipid bilayer appears to affect markedly some biological activities; thus on cooling membranes, several enzymes and transport systems show a change in activation energy at temperatures close to the phase transition point of the membrane lipid. Manipulation of the lipid composition of several membranes, e.g. by fatty acid substitution, brings about parallel changes in both the lipid phase transitions and the activation energies of particular membrane functions, and is probably due to the influence of the fluidity of the lipid layer upon the conformation of the protein.

Studies on the lipid depletion of membranes, and the reconstitution of lipid-free proteins with lipid, indicate that a minimum amount of lipid is required to support the activity of particular proteins. This is thought to represent the shell of lipid molecules covering the hydrophobic surface region of the protein, and has been termed the boundary lipid. In many cases there is little difference in composition between the boundary lipid and the remainder of the bilayer, and individual lipid molecules appear to equilibrate readily; in a few cases the boundary layer may differ, due probably to specific lipid head-group interactions. Discrepancies between the temperature, showing a change in activation energy, and the overall transition temperature of the bulk of the membrane lipid have been interpreted as due to the existence of regions of lipid of different fluidities, but this is too complex and controversial to be discussed briefly[5,8,40,41].

CONTROL OF PROTEIN MOBILITY

Whilst the previous studies indicate that some proteins move randomly in the plane of the bilayer, or will move so after perturbation by external agents, there are also many indications of non-random distributions of proteins in various membranes; this would suggest that factors may be operating to suppress or control the random lateral movement[7,35,36]. Examples of these phenomena include (i) the presence of large patches of protein, e.g. in *Halobacterium* plasma membrane and in junctional complexes of solid tissues; (ii) the existence of two functional domains, brush border and basolateral, in the plasma membranes of epithelial cells; (iii) the directed flow of proteins in some membranes; (iv) the apparent immobility of discrete proteins in the membranes of some cells, e.g. human erythrocytes; (v) the specialization of protein content during vesicle formation.

PROTEIN PLAQUES

The plaques of bacteriorhodopsin in *Halobacterium* membranes, of the acetylcholine receptor in neuromuscular junctions, of the specific proteins of gap junctions, tight junctions and desmosomes, and of the coat proteins of enveloped viruses, all appear to be maintained by specific protein–protein interactions which exclude the penetration of other proteins into the plaque. Diffusion of these huge islands in the plane of the membrane may be reduced on the grounds of size, though in the case of the various junctions there may also be some anchoring due to attachment, either to extracellular or to cytoplasmic proteins. A more transient form of protein aggregates may also be formed by exclusion of proteins from the gel phase when some membranes are cooled, though these aggregates disaggregate again when the temperature is raised.

EPITHELIAL CELL POLARITY

Epithelial cells show a marked polarity in terms of composition and function due to distinct domains of the plasma membrane[42]. Thus the lumenal (brush border) region of intestinal epithelial cells possesses terminal digestive hydrolases, Na^+/solute symport systems and heavily glycosylated high-weight polypeptides. In contrast, the basolateral domain possesses high Na^+–K^+ ATPase activity, hormone receptor/effector mechanisms, and its polypeptide profile shows lightly glycosylated species of a wide molecular-weight range[43]. The mechanism responsible for maintaining this regional specialization is not known, but a strong possibility is that the continuous plaque of protein molecules, which forms a collar round the cell at the junctional complex, may exclude other proteins (as discussed above), thereby preventing random mixing of the protein populations of the two domains. This collar of proteins may also be a lateral diffusion barrier to lipids, since the two domains of the membrane have distinct lipid compositions[43]. Other contributors to the regional protein distributions may be specific protein–protein interactions in the plane of the membrane and the anchoring of intrinsic proteins by specific interactions with skeletal elements of the cytoplasm. In this context, the brush border region possesses an appreciable amount of actin and α-actinin[13], but it is not known whether these interact with the digestive hydrolases.

INVOLVEMENT OF MICROFILAMENTS AND MICROTUBULES

The 'capping' and pinocytosis phenomena observed initially in lymphocytes, but now in many other tissue culture cells, showed that the movements of membrane proteins could be controlled, and also that this control was exercised by elements of the cytoskeleton[7,35,36]. Capping was observed as a rapid energy-dependent process following the initial patching of immunoglobulin receptors by divalent antibodies; the patches moved to one end of the cell forming a cap and were subsequently pinocytosed. Application of independent ligands to patched and capped cells demonstrated that, in most cases, the various membrane proteins were capped independently; capping was therefore a demonstration of controlled movement of one protein relative to others. Cytochalasin B, which disassembles microfilaments, inhibits cap formation. Networks of microfilaments have been observed on the cytoplasmic side of the plasma membrane in many cells and this region can be shown to respond to labelled anti-actin antibody and to be decorated with arrowheads of heavy meromyosin. The involvement of actin and myosin-like molecules probably explains the energy expenditure of the lateral movement of

membrane proteins. Actin-like molecules have been identified in isolated plasma membrane preparations, but it is not known how the interaction for the specific intrinsic protein undergoing directed movement is
determined.

   In addition to the control of movement exercised by the microfilament
system, the location of some membrane proteins may be determined by
the cytoplasmic microtubular system. Many membrane glycoproteins
can be indiscriminately cross-linked by the lectin, Concanavalin A (Con
A), but this does not result in cap formation. When colchicine or vinblastine, which disassemble microtubules, are added cap formation is initiated. This has been interpreted as an indication that some membrane
proteins may be anchored to the microtubular system (though the molecular details of this are not known) and that cross-linking of other proteins to these will not allow movement; disassembly of the microtubular
system by colchicine may then release the anchoring and allow microfilament movement to produce cap formation. It is interesting in this
context that studies using the technique of fluorescence photobleaching
recovery have shown two classes of Con A receptors in a variety of cells;
some are mobile, but the remainder appear to be immobile[44].

   Since the cytoskeletal system also appears to interact with intracellular
membranes, it may form a functional link between plasma membrane
and cytoplasm and has long been suspected to be involved in such
phenomena as migration of cytoplasmic vesicles to the cell surface.
Moreover, the assembly and disassembly of the cytoskeleton can be controlled by the levels of cytoplasmic Ca^{2+} and certain drugs and therefore
suggest further ways of cytoplasmic control over cell surface properties.

SPECTRIN IN ERYTHROCYTES

In contrast to the plasma-membrane proteins of many other types of
cells, the intrinsic proteins of intact human erythrocytes show little
movement. Thus multivalent ligands do not produce patching and
capping phenomena or the aggregation of intramembranous particles[7,35,36] and the proteins appear to be immobile when the technique of
fluorescence photobleaching recovery is used[44]. Mobility has been
observed, however, in membrane preparations in which the extrinsic
protein complex, spectrin, had been depleted or damaged by preparation of the membrane at low ionic strength, at extremes of pH, and
where the cytoplasmic surface had been exposed to proteases[7,35,36,45].
The movement could then be observed by application of labelled multi-

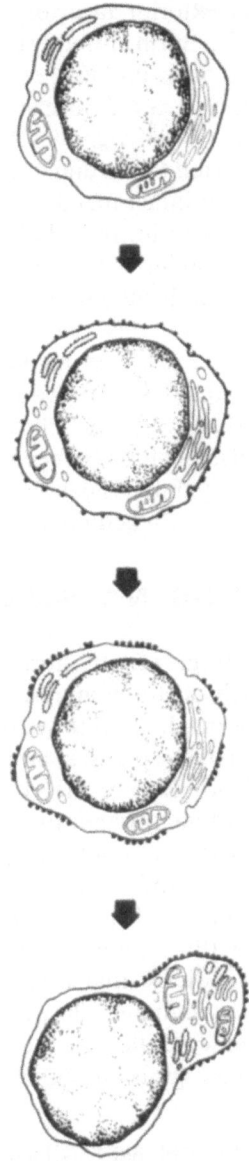

Figure 2.4 Patching and capping of lymphocytes using ferritin-labelled anti-body. Reproduced by permission of Blackwell Scientific Publications, Oxford from *Membranes and Their Cellular Functions*, 2nd Edn. 1978, p. 39

valent ligands to the exterior face, or by antispectrin antibody to the cytoplasmic face; antispectrin antibody does not have this effect on membranes in which spectrin is undamaged, and will even protect spectrin from proteolytic attack[46]. Spectrin can be isolated as a tetramer, but more usually as dimer (of polypeptides 240 000 and 220 000 daltons); the tetramer can be converted to the dimer at low ionic strength and involves some refolding[46]. In the intact membrane, spectrin may exist as a tetramer in association with actin, the whole complex forming a meshwork below the surface interacting with band 3[47].

Several studies have indicated that band 3 can be readily cross-linked to spectrin; the extent of this cross-linking is reduced at low ionic strength and in spectrin-depleted membranes two thiol groups in the cytoplasmic region of band 3 polypeptides are exposed and become susceptible to oxidation[28]. Since band 3 bears most of the binding capacity for multivalent ligands, and has also been equated with the intramembranous particles, it is likely that it is band 3 mobility which may be observed upon damage to the spectrin/actin network.

PROTEIN MOVEMENTS IN VESICULATION

Several procedures (e.g. raised intracellular Ca^{2+} [48], ageing[49,50], bile salts[51]) cause the erythrocyte membrane to form a series of membrane projections which are pinched off to yield a population of microvesicles; the residual cell is smaller, spherical and less flexible due to this loss of membrane material. Analysis of the vesicle membrane shows them to differ from the original membrane; they are greatly depleted in protein relative to lipid and possess a simple polypeptide profile greatly depleted in (particularly) spectrin and band 3, but relatively enriched in a few other components, e.g. acetylcholinesterase and a polypeptide, concentrated particularly in the region possibly originating from the fusion neck[50]. Such studies indicate that a few proteins may move independently of the spectrin/actin/band 3 network, but it is not known what may determine their movement, allowing them to become relatively enriched in the protein depleted regions of the membrane.

DIFFERENCES BETWEEN MEMBRANES

Analyses of isolated membrane preparations show wide differences in the relative amounts of lipids and proteins between different membranes, e.g. myelin is lipid-rich, protein-poor, whereas the mitochondrial membrane is protein-rich, lipid-poor. At one time this was interpreted as different protein-dominated structures incorporating different amounts of lipid. With our present state of knowledge, it is probably more correct to view differences in gross composition as related to a relatively constant amount of lipid bilayer. Since the actual amount of polypeptide mass of the intrinsic proteins inserted into the bilayer may be relatively small (see discussion on glycophorin), it is probable that the differences in protein : lipid ratio between most membranes are due to the relative sizes of the hydrophilic regions of the intrinsic proteins and to the number and size of the extrinsic proteins associated with them.

Simple insertion of intrinsic proteins into lipid bilayers yields morphologically simple 'membrane' preparations. Likewise, after exposure to low ionic strengths, or the stresses of sonication or excessive homogenization, membrane preparations tend to form simple vesicular structures. In the cell, however, membranes are found in a whole variety of forms, large sheets, brush borders, stacked plates, etc. due probably to the association of the simple interrupted bilayer with a range of extrinsic proteins which then determine its shape and distensibility.

The varied functions of membranes in the cell are reflected by their complement of different intrinsic proteins. Thus some membranes are highly specialized in their function and contain one, or only a small number, of polypeptide species. Examples of this are the (i) sarcoplasmic reticulum where the Ca^{2+}–Mg ATPase is almost the only polypeptide species in the membrane, (ii) the plasma membrane of the electroplax of electrogenic fishes which contains mainly the acetylcholine receptor and the Na^+–K^+ ATPase. These must be compared to other membranes performing a wider range of functions, e.g. in mitochondria, erythrocytes etc., these have a much wider polypeptide profile with each polypeptide present in relatively smaller amounts.

How these different patterns arise and are maintained is a difficult problem. Is it merely some form of biosynthetic programming or is it due also to specific protein–protein interactions which maintain one structure and exclude the entry of other protein species? Membrane structure is not, however, static since, for example, the membrane of the erythrocyte precursor cell does not always possess glycophorin, spectrin etc.; these appear later in the life of the cell and must displace other proteins from the precursor membrane.

The lipid layer is equally complex but there are considerable similarities from cell to cell; thus mitochondria have a lipid profile containing cardiolipin, whereas plasma membranes are usually rich in cholesterol, glycolipids and sphingomyelin. Even within membranes of the same type there are individual differences, since within the mammalian erythrocyte series there is a substantial variation in the relative amounts of sphingomyelin and phosphatidyl choline. These differences are evident from different permeabilities to a variety of small molecules[52] and by their susceptibility to bile salt-induced lysis[53].

MEMBRANE PATHOLOGY

It is now appropriate to consider very briefly some of the circumstances in which membrane function may be impaired.

Defective coding of membrane components

It is clear that if a membrane polypeptide is coded defectively, some individual function of the membrane may be reduced or altered; the metabolic effects of this will depend upon the importance of the defective system. Such defects may encompass enzyme activities and their regulatory subunits, transport systems, and information receptors. These defects have been studied in the intestine, kidney, erythrocyte and a variety of other tissues; they will be discussed later in this volume and some are also summarized elsewhere[53-55].

Inefficient metabolic support
to maintain normal membrane structure

Inefficient general metabolism from a variety of causes will lead to inadequate production of ATP and consequent decline in biosynthetic and transport activities. Amongst the effects of this are the accumulation of cell $[Ca^{2+}]$, which possibly has far reaching effects on membranes in relation to activation of degradative processes and effects on transport systems[1]. Defective metabolism may also be unable to ensure a continuous supply of thiol groups to protect against oxidation of protein thiol groups, necessary for protein conformation, or to counteract the production of free radicals[54-56].

Damage to membranes caused by other molecules

Antibodies produced against membrane proteins will cause the decline in membrane function and several auto-immune diseases of membrane components have now been recognized, e.g. myasthenia gravis, insulin resistance, etc. Enveloped viruses produce proteins which substitute for membrane proteins and, in a late stage of the infection, membrane lipid is used in providing the virus envelope. A wide variety of toxins range in their effects from degradative enzymes to receptor-blocking agents. The effects of drugs range from receptor blockers, enzyme inhibitors, fluidizing agents for the lipid bilayer, ionophores (ion transporting molecules)[2,54-57].

Amongst endogenous compounds affecting membrane structure are the bile salts. These are secreted at very high concentrations into the bile; it is one of our current interests as to what factors are involved in determining the resistance of membranes to damage by these natural detergents[51,53,58,59].

References

1. Michell, R. H. and Coleman, R. (1979). Structure and permeability of normal and damaged membranes. In D. J. Hearse and J. de Lieris (eds.). *Enzymes in Cardiology: Diagnosis and Research*, pp. 59–79. (Chichester: John Wiley)
2. Finean, J. B., Coleman, R. and Michell, R. H. (1978). *Membranes and their Cellular Functions*. 2nd Edn. (Oxford: Blackwell Scientific)
3. Stockenius, W. and Engleman, D. M. (1969). Current models for the structure of biological membranes. *J. Cell Biol.*, **42**, 613
4. Finean, J. B. (1972). The development of ideas on membrane structure. *Sub-Cell. Biochem.*, **1**, 363
5. Jain, M. K. and White, H. B. (1977). Long range order in biomembranes. *Adv. Lipid Res.*, **15**, 1
6. Robertson, J. D. (1978). The anatomy of biological interfaces. In T. E. Andreoli, J. F. Hoffman and D. D. Fanestil (eds.). *Physiology of Membrane Disorders*, pp. 1–26. (New York: Plenum Medical)
7. Bretscher, M. S. and Raff, M. C. (1975). Mammalian plasma membranes. *Nature (London)*, **258**, 43
8. Lenard, J. and Landsberger, F. R. (1976). A perspective on models of membrane structure. In G. A. Jamieson and D. M. Robinson (eds.). *Mammalian Cell Membranes*, Vol. I, pp. 244–264. (London: Butterworths)
9. Thompson, T. E. and Huang, C. (1978). Dynamics of lipids in biomembranes. In T. E. Andreoli, J. F. Hoffman and D. D. Fanestil (eds.). *Physiology of Membrane Disorders*, pp. 27–48. (New York: Plenum Medical)
10. Steck, T. L. (1974). The organization of proteins in the human red blood cell membrane. *J. Cell Biol.*, **62**, 1
11. Hubbard, A. L. and Cohn, Z. A. (1976). Specific labels for cell surfaces. In A. H. Maddy (ed.). *Biochemical Analysis of Membranes*, pp. 427–501. (London: Chapman and Hall)

12. Rothman, J. E. and Lenard, J. L. (1977). Membrane asymmetry. *Science*, **195**, 743

13. Kenny, A. J. and Booth, A. G. (1979). Microvilli: their ultrastructure, enzymology and molecular organization. *Essays Biochem.*, **14**, 1

14. Singer, S. J. (1974). The molecular organization of membranes. *Annu. Rev. Biochem.*, **43**, 805

15. Coleman, R. (1974). Solubilization of membrane components. *Biochem. Soc. Trans.*, **2**, 813

16. Furthmayr, H. (1977). Erythrocyte proteins. In P. Cuatrecasas and M. F. Greaves (eds.). *Receptors and Recognition*, Vol. 3A, pp. 101–132. (London: Chapman and Hall)

17. Capaldi, R. A. (1977). The structural properties of membrane proteins. In R. A. Capaldi (ed.). *Membrane Proteins and their Interactions with Lipids*, pp. 1–19. (New York: Marcel Dekker)

18. Guidotti, G. (1978). Membrane proteins: structure and arrangement in the membrane. In T. E. Andreoli, J. F. Hoffman and D. D. Fanestil (eds.). *Physiology of Membrane Disorders*, pp. 49–60. (New York: Plenum Medical)

19. Helenius, A. and Simons, K. (1975). Solubilization of membranes by detergents. *Biochem. Biophys. Acta*, **415**, 29

20. Tanford, C. and Reynolds, J. A. (1976). Characterization of membrane proteins in detergent solutions. *Biochim. Biophys. Acta*, **457**, 133

21. Kahane, I. and Gitler, C. (1978). Red cell membrane glycophorin labelling from within the lipid layer. *Science*, **201**, 351

22. Scott-Matthews, F. and Czerwinski, E. W. (1976). Cytochrome b_5 and cytochrome b_5 reductase from a chemical and X-ray diffraction point of view. In A. Martonosi, (ed.). *The Enzymes of Biological Membranes*, Vol. 4, pp. 143–197. (London: John Wiley)

23. Furthmayr, H. (1977). Structural analysis of a membrane glycoprotein: Glycophorin A. *J. Supramolec. Structure*, 7, 121

24. Stockenius, W., Lozier, R. H. and Bogomolni (1979). Bacteriorhodopsin and the purple membrane of halobacteria. *Biochim. Biophys. Acta*, **505**, 215

25. Rothstein, A. (1978). The function roles of band 3 protein of the red blood cell. In A. K. Solomon and M. Karnovsky (eds.). *Molecular Specialization and Symmetry in Membrane Function*, pp. 128–155. (Cambridge, MA: Harvard University Press)

26. Rothstein, A., Grinstein, S., Ship, S. and Knauf, P. A. (1978). Asymmetry of functional sites of the erythrocyte anion transport protein. *Trends Biochem. Sci.*, **3**, 126

27. Tanner, M. J. A. (1978). Erythrocyte glycoproteins. *Curr. Topics Membr. Transp.*, **11**, 279

28. Rao, A. (1979). Disposition of the band 3 polypeptide in the human erythrocyte membrane. *J. Biol. Chem.*, **254**, 3503

29. Drickamer, A. (1978). Orientation of band 3 protein. *J. Biol. Chem.*, **253**, 7242

30. Kozlov, I. A. and Skulachev, V. P. (1977). H^+ adenosine triphosphatase and membrane energy coupling. *Biochim. Biophys. Acta*, **463**, 28

31. Cabral, F., Birchmeier, W., Kohler, C. E. and Schatz, G. (1978). Molecu-

lar architecture of oligomeric membrane proteins. In A. K. Solomon and M. Karnovsky (eds.). *Molecular Specialization and Symmetry in Membrane Function*, pp. 61–77. (Cambridge, MA: Harvard University Press)

32. Ji, T. H. (1979). The application of chemical crosslinking for studies on cell membranes and the identification of surface reporters. *Biochim. Biophys. Acta*, **559**, 39

33. Hastings, D. F. and Reynolds, J. A. (1979). Molecular weight of (Na$^+$K$^+$) ATPase from shark rectal gland. *Biochemistry*, **18**, 817

34. Singer, S. J. and Nicholson, G. L. (1972). The fluid mosaic model of the structure of membranes. *Science*, **175**, 720

35. Nicolson, G. L. (1976). Transmembrane control of the receptors on normal and tumour cells 1. *Biochim. Biophys. Acta*, **457**, 57

36. Nicolson, G. L., Poste, G. and Ji, T. H. (1977). The dynamics of cell membrane organization. In G. Poste and G. L. Nicolson (eds.). *Dynamic Aspects of Cell Surface Organization*, pp. 1–126. (Amsterdam: North-Holland)

37. Schramm, M., Orly, J., Eimerl, S. and Korner, M. (1977). Coupling of hormone receptors to adenylate cyclase of different cells by cell fusion. *Nature (London)*, **268**, 310

38. Hanski, E., Rimon, G. and Levitzki, A. (1979). Adenylate cyclase activation by the β-adrenergic receptors as a diffusion controlled process. *Biochemistry*, **18**, 846

39. Levitzki, A. and Helmreich, E. J. M. (1979). Hormone–receptor-adenylate cyclase interactions. *FEBS Lett.*, **101**, 213

40. Sandermann, H. (1978). Regulation of membrane enzymes by lipids. *Biochim. Biophys. Acta*, **515**, 209

41. Chapman, D., Gomez-Fernandex, J. C. and Goni, F. M. (1979). Intrinsic protein-lipid interactions. *FEBS Lett.*, **98**, 211

42. Kinne, R. and Kinne-Saffran, E. (1978). Differentiation of cell faces in epithelia. In A. K. Solomon and M. Karnovsky (eds.). *Molecular Specialization and Symmetry in Membrane Function*, pp. 272–293. (Cambridge, MA: Harvard University Press)

43. Michell, R. H., Coleman, R. and Lewis, B. A. (1976). Biochemical differentiation of the plasma membrane of intestinal epithelial cells. *Biochem. Soc. Trans.*, **4**, 1019

44. Lee, A. G. (1978). Fluorescence and N.M.R. studies of membranes. In P. Cuatrecas and M. F. Greaves (eds.). *Receptors and Recognition*, Vol. 5A, pp. 89 131. (London: Chapman and Hall)

45. Elgsaeter, A., Shotton, D. and Branton, D. (1976). Intramembrane particle aggregation in erythrocyte ghosts. *Biochim. Biophys. Acta*, **426**, 101

46. Lalazar, A. and Loyter, A. (1979). Involvement of spectrin in membrane fusion: induction of fusion in human erythrocyte ghosts by proteolytic enzymes and its inhibition by antispectrin antibody. *Proc. Natl. Acad. Sci. USA*, **76**, 318

46. Ralston, G. B. and Dunbar, J. C. (1979). Salt and temperature-dependent conformational changes in spectrin from human erythrocyte membranes. *Biochim. Biophys. Acta*, **579**, 20

47. Ralston, G. B. (1978). The structure of spectrin and the shape of the red blood cell. *Trends Biochem. Sci.*, **3**, 195

48. Allen, D., Billah, M. M., Finean, J. B. and Michell, R. H. (1976). Release of diacylglycerol-enriched vesicles from erythrocytes with increased intracellular Ca^{2+}. *Nature (London)*, **261**, 58

49. Rumsby

50. Shukla, S. D., Berriman, J., Coleman, R., Finean, J. B. and Michell, R. H. (1978). Membrane protein segregation during release of microvesicles from human erythrocytes. *FEBS Lett.*, **90**, 289

51. Billington, D. and Coleman R. (1978). Effects of bile salts on human erythrocytes. *Biochim. Biophys. Acta*, **509**, 33

52. Van Deenen, L. L. M., De Gier, J., Houtsmuller, U. M. T., Montfoort, A. and Mulder, E. (1963). Dietary effects on the lipid composition of biomembranes. In A. C. Frazer (ed.). *Biochemical Problems of Lipids*, pp. 401–414. (Amsterdam: Elsevier)

53. Rosenberg, L. E. (1969). Hereditary diseases with membrane defects. In R. M. Dowben (ed.). *Biological Membranes*, pp. 255–295. (London: Churchill)

54. Bolis, L., Hoffman, J. F. and Leaf, A. (1976). *Membranes and Disease*. (New York: Raven Press)

55. Andreoli, T. E., Hoffman, J. F. and Fanestil, D. D. (1978). *Physiology of Membrane Disorders*. (New York: Plenum Medical Book Company)

53. Coleman, R. and Billington, D. (1979). Membrane composition affects characteristics of glycocholate-induced lysis of erythrocytes. *Biochem. Soc. Trans.*, **7** (In press)

56. Miller, M. W. and Shamoo, A. E. (1977). *Membrane Toxicity*. (New York: Plenum Press)

57. Jaljaszewicz, J. and Wadstrom, T. (1978). *Bacterial Toxins and Cell Membranes*. (London: Academic Press)

58. Coleman, R., Holdsworth, G. and Vyvoda, O. S. (1977). Hepatocyte surface enzymes and their appearance in bile. In H. Popper, L. Bianci and W. Reutter (eds.). *Membrane Alterations as Basis of Liver Injury*, pp. 143–156. (Lancaster: MTP Press)

59. Billington, D., Evans, C. E., Godfrey, P. P. and Coleman, R. (1979). Effects of bile salts on the plasma membrane of isolated hepatocytes. *Biochem. Soc. Trans.*, **7** (In press)

3

Synthesis of membranes
J. Lenard

WHAT IS SYNTHESIZED?

A wealth of experimental information now permits several generalizations to be made, which seem to apply to all biological membranes[1]. Membranes are non-covalent complexes consisting chiefly of lipids and proteins. Membrane lipids exist mainly as bilayers, structures that can be extended indefinitely in two dimensions, and that contribute the passive permeability properties to biological membranes.

Each of the membrane proteins, like the soluble proteins, has a well-defined three-dimensional structure that characterizes the native, functional form. As part of this structure, each membrane protein has its own characteristic interaction with the lipid bilayer. Some membrane proteins span the bilayer from side to side; of these, some cross only once, others cross several times. Other membrane proteins simply dip into the fluid hydrocarbon centre of the bilayer from one side. Some of these integral proteins extend several hundred angstroms from the bilayer surface on one side, so that the membrane-associated portion is only a small fraction of the polypeptide chain. Still another class of membrane proteins is only peripherally associated with one surface of the bilayer, and does not penetrate into the interior at all[2]. But regardless of the nature of the interaction of the membrane protein with the bilayer interior, all membrane proteins extend into the aqueous environment on one or both sides; proteins that lie exclusively in the hydrocarbon interior of the bilayer are not known.

Every membrane component is unequally distributed between the two sides of the membrane in a characteristic way[3]. Protein asymmetry is absolute. That is, every protein molecule of a particular kind is identically oriented in the membrane. No known membrane proteins are symmetrically oriented or distributed between the two sides of a membrane. Phospholipid asymmetry, on the other hand, is only relative. Molecules of each lipid type may be found on either surface, but the proportion present on each surface may be different.

Membranes are dynamic rather than static structures. The individual molecules, both proteins and lipids, undergo constant lateral diffusion at quite a rapid rate. Thus, in the absence of specific structures that anchor membrane components in one place, rapid randomization of membrane components occurs over the entire membrane surface. In contrast to this rapid lateral diffusion, however, transverse diffusion from one side of the bilayer to the other does not occur at a measurable rate, especially for membrane proteins. The absolute asymmetry of membrane proteins is thus maintained by their inability to undergo transverse diffusion.

These generalizations have emerged in answer to a general question that stimulated research for many years, "What is the structure of biological membranes?" However, further insights require either that we narrow our focus to consider the particular properties of one specific membrane, or that we broaden it to consider the role of membranes in the whole cell. The latter approach quickly leads to a consideration of how membranes form.

The problem was graphically, if implicitly, posed by the earliest electron micrographs, which showed a multitude of intracellular organelles, each surrounded by a membrane[4]. Endoplasmic reticulum, Golgi apparatus, mitochondria and lysosomes are examples of ubiquitous membrane-bound organelles, although possessing different morphology in different cell types. These organelles are not disrupted during cell division, so that the compartmentalization imposed by their membranes is passed on undisrupted from generation to generation, a significant extra-genetic reservoir of organizational information.

Membrane lipids and proteins are synthesized in the cytoplasm, where the necessary metabolites and precursors are found, utilizing conventional pathways. Membranes are never formed *de novo*, but rather grow by insertion of membrane components, molecule by molecule, into pre-existing membrane structures. The permeability barrier of the parent membrane is not breached by this insertion process. Thus membrane biogenesis, like cell division, proceeds in a manner that permits maintenance of intracellular compartmentalization.

The pertinent features of membrane synthesis can now be recognized to be problems of insertion, topology, and membrane specificity. The location of newly inserted membrane components in one particular area of a membrane is not a problem, since lateral diffusion will result in rapid transfer from the insertion site to any other site. But we do want to know how new components are inserted into a membrane with the correct asymmetric orientation. For example, how do many membrane proteins end up with most of their mass present in the aqueous environment on the extracytoplasmic side of the bilayer permeability barrier?

The other important problem in membrane synthesis relates to the diversity of cellular membranes. Since the structural generalizations discussed above apply to all biological membranes, we need to know how the appropriate components end up in each of the different cellular membranes, so as to maintain their structural and functional distinctiveness.

GENERAL CONSIDERATIONS
OF BIOLOGICAL ASSEMBLY

The study of soluble proteins has led to a fundamental concept of biological assembly. This is that proteins carry in their genetically determined primary amino acid sequence the information required to fold correctly into their native (biologically functional) conformation under the appropriate conditions[5-7]. Experiments that prove this assertion consist of completely disrupting non-covalent interactions within a protein while leaving the covalent bonds intact. This is usually accomplished by dissolving the protein in an aqueous denaturing medium such as a concentrated guanidine hydrochloride solution, and then gradually re-establishing physiological conditions, e.g. by removing the denaturing agent by dialysis. Complete recovery of biological activity after this treatment shows that the protein has spontaneously re-formed the unique three-dimensional structure that defines its native conformation. In thermodynamic terms, the equation

$$(NATIVE)_{PC} \rightleftharpoons (DENATURED)_{PC}$$

proceeds spontaneously to the left under physiological conditions (PC), indicating that this conformation represents a minimum free energy for the molecule. In other words, the native conformation is the most stable, and can form spontaneously given the information contained in the primary sequence. This statement is generally true of soluble proteins, and has also been demonstrated for more complex biological structures, such as ribosomes and muscle fibres. This property of biological macromolecules (nucleic acids also undergo spontaneous self-assembly into helices) makes it unnecessary to postulate any special catalytic mechanisms for the formation of functional proteins from newly synthesized polypeptides. Indeed, soluble proteins do appear to adopt their native conformation spontaneously upon completion of synthesis of their polypeptide chain(s).

Membrane lipids and proteins can also undergo successful self-assembly. Bilayers form spontaneously from phospholipid molecules in the presence of water. Functional re-assembly of biological membranes has been achieved from many different kinds of membranes after complete disruption of membrane structure with detergents. Several of these reconstituted membrane systems have been shown, by both functional and structural criteria, to have their membrane proteins asymmetrically inserted in the membrane bilayer. Such findings show that for membrane proteins, as for soluble proteins, the native conformation represents the most stable state, which will form spontaneously under appropriate conditions.

The big difference between membrane and soluble proteins, however, is that membrane proteins need to interact with a lipid phase as well as with an aqueous phase in their native state. New membrane proteins must be inserted from the cytoplasmic side into pre-formed lipid bilayers during membrane synthesis, rather than into bilayers in the process of assembling, as in the membrane reconstitution experiments just described. This imposes a formidable energy barrier to the adoption of the native state, often expressed as the energy that would be required to transfer polar amino-acid residues from one side of the bilayer through the hydrophobic centre into the aqueous compartment on the other side[8]. The polar head group of a lipid synthesized on the cytoplasmic side of a membrane faces a similar problem in getting to the extracytoplasmic surface of the bilayer.

Recent evidence has provided strong indications that, both for lipids and at least for some membrane proteins, special catalytic mechanisms exist to solve this problem by transferring newly synthesized material to the appropriate side of the bilayer.

MEMBRANE LIPIDS

Membrane phospholipids are synthesized on the cytoplasmic side of the endoplasmic reticulum membrane. Translocation of newly synthesized phospholipids to the luminal side occurs rapidly in this membrane, as it does also in the membranes of rapidly dividing bacteria. Translocation of phospholipids from one side to the other is not an intrinsic property of bilayers, since it does not proceed at a measurable rate in protein-free synthetic bilayers, regardless of lipid composition. It occurs only very slowly in red blood-cell membranes, where net lipid synthesis is not taking place. It is therefore inferred that lipid translocation is catalysed specifically in those membranes that support active synthesis. Experiments with bacterial membranes have shown that translocation still occurs under conditions where lipid synthesis is completely inhibited, suggesting that the catalytic machinery is separate from the biosynthetic machinery[3,9]. The translocation machinery has not yet been isolated, probably owing to the difficulty in devising a convenient assay for the translocation function. A study of its properties should show how lipid assymmetry in membranes is established and maintained in the face of rapid translocation.

MEMBRANE PROTEINS

Synthesis of membrane proteins may be of more general interest than synthesis of lipids, since all membrane properties except the passive permeability properties are conferred by the proteins. Structural asymmetry of membrane proteins leads directly to asymmetry of function, e.g. vectorial transport. Thus, asymmetric insertion of newly synthesized membrane proteins is essential for appropriate function, while the asymmetry of lipid (as far as is known) has little if any functional significance. In this regard, exciting information has recently been obtained regarding the mechanism of insertion of at least one class of membrane proteins.

The signal hypothesis[10-12]

The extent to which the mechanisms discussed below mediate insertion of different classes of membrane proteins is currently a matter of controversy. Evidence has been obtained for a group of plasma membrane glycoproteins that span the bilayer but have most of their mass, including their sugars, extending into the aqueous environment on the external, i.e. extracytoplasmic, side of the membrane. They also possess a much smaller, non-glycosylated segment that protrudes into the aqueous environment on the cytoplasmic side of the membrane. A single segment of the polypeptide chain crosses the bilayer, connecting the two hydrophilic segments. This class of membrane proteins includes the digestive hydrolases of intestinal brush border, the histocompatibility antigens and a variety of viral glycoproteins. This last group has proved to be most important experimentally since viral infection often shuts off host-cell protein synthesis, leaving only the one or two viral membrane proteins to be synthesized and processed by the normal host-cell mechanisms[13, 14].

It has been established that the synthesis and processing of this class of plasma membrane glycoproteins proceeds by mechanisms that are essentially the same as those used for secreted proteins. They are synthesized exclusively on membrane-bound ribosomes, on the cytoplasmic side of the endoplasmic reticulum. Translocation of the entire molecule of secreted protein, or of the external segment of membrane protein, occurs concomitantly with synthesis. If microsomal membranes are added to a cell-free protein synthesizing system containing messenger RNA for one of these membrane proteins, appropriate insertion into the added membrane can be demonstrated. If synthesis of the protein by the cell-free system is allowed to proceed to more than about 15% completion before addition of microsomal membranes, normal insertion of the newly synthesized protein does not occur[15]. Thus the translocation event must occur in strict temporal association with synthesis, i.e. before substantial folding of the polypeptide chain can occur. When the same cell-free system synthesizes proteins that are normally present in the cell cytoplasm, translocation across the microsomal membrane does not occur.

The membrane-bound ribosomes that synthesize these proteins are identical with those synthesizing soluble proteins. Association of the ribosome with the membrane does not arise from a structural difference in the ribosome, or in the RNA message, but is mediated by the first 16–20 amino-acid residues synthesized, the 'signal sequence'. This sequence is thought to direct attachment of the growing polypeptide chain, with associated ribosomes, to a specific site on the endoplasmic reticulum that facilitates the translocation process. Proteolytic cleavage usually removes the signal sequence shortly after it appears at the lumenal surface of the membrane, before polypeptide synthesis is completed, although this need not occur in all cases.

Secreted proteins differ from membrane proteins in that the entire secreted protein is extruded in this fashion across the membrane. The membrane protein, on the other hand, must get 'stuck' after about 80% of the protein has crossed the membrane. This might be accomplished by a specific amino-acid sequence (the same segment that spans the bilayer in the completed protein) that dissociates the translocating machinery, leaving the growing chain embedded in the bilayer[3].

As yet, the translocation structure has not been isolated. Its characterization will be extremely interesting, both because it will serve to prove the hypothesis outlined above, and because of the unusual reaction that it catalyses. It must be capable of extruding a polypeptide chain, consisting of all the different amino acids in various sequences, at a constant rate across the interior of a lipid bilayer, but must be specifically disrupted by the appropriate sequence in a membrane protein. There are no precedents in protein chemistry for the protein–protein interactions implicit in such a structure.

The sequence of events as outlined leads to two predictions about this class of membrane proteins. Firstly, since protein synthesis always proceeds from the N- to the C-terminus, it would be expected that the N-terminus should be in the external (extracytoplasmic) portion of the protein, while the C-terminus should be in the cytoplasmic segment. This prediction has been confirmed for the few most-thoroughly studied proteins of this type. Secondly, the three major conformational domains, the hydrophilic domain on the extracytoplasmic side of the membrane, the hydrophilic domain in the membrane, and the hydrophilic domain on the cytoplasmic side, should be colinear with sequence domains located progressively from the N- to the C-terminus. This is in contrast to soluble proteins, in which conformational domains are generated upon correct folding of the chain, and are not colinear with sequence. This also has been confirmed in a few specific cases.

Other possibilities for insertion

It is not yet clear whether the signal hypothesis applies to a broad range of membrane proteins, or is limited to the fairly restricted class for which it has been demonstrated. The hypothesis provides a mechanism by which a membrane protein can span the membrane once, but many proteins actually span the membrane several times in their native state. This might be accomplished by spontaneous insertion of the folded protein into the bilayer, either with or without prior translocation of all or part of the polypeptide chain by the signal mechanism. As one example, the coat protein of a bacterial virus has been found to insert spontaneously into a bacterial membrane with the same functionally appropriate asymmetric orientation, regardless of whether it is introduced from without or from within. Here the interaction occurs between the completed, folded protein and the membrane bilayer; no catalytic mechanism is required for the development of the appropriate conformation. On the basis of these observations, it has been suggested that many membrane proteins may be capable of spontaneous insertion into membranes, after completion of synthesis, in the appropriate functional and asymmetric orientation[16].

If some proteins do insert into membranes by spontaneous self-assembly, they need not be synthesized on membrane-bound ribosomes, nor need the translocation process start before synthesis is completed. However, in order not to aggregate in the cytoplasm, such membrane proteins would have to be capable of assuming a water-soluble conformation as well as a membrane-associated conformation. It has been suggested that the signal sequence (also referred to as the 'leader' or 'trigger' depending upon the viewpoint of the author) could mediate between a water-soluble and a membrane-soluble form of a given protein. Once a protein was appropriately inserted into the proper membrane this sequence would be proteolytically removed, stabilizing the correct configuration.

Thus the old question of whether the native conformation of a protein molecule is determined by thermodynamic properties of the completed molecule, or by kinetically controlled events during synthesis, has moved on from soluble to membrane proteins. While the precedent of the soluble proteins, and the successful self-assembly of many membrane proteins, argues for a thermodynamic basis, a kinetic mechanism is strongly supported by the recent evidence, in at least some cases.

Glycosylation

Glycosylation of secreted and membrane proteins occurs simultaneously with synthesis and translocation by the signal mechanism. Glycosylation occurs on the luminal side of the endoplasmic reticulum membrane, on specific amino-acid side chains of the growing polypeptide chain. Initial glycosylation occurs by the transfer of a large oligosaccharide of defined structure from a membrane-bound lipid intermediate to a glycosylation site on the protein[17, 18]. From the time of synthesis to the time the protein arrives at its final destination (at the plasma membrane, or out of the cell for secreted proteins) it is subjected to a highly specific and complex remodelling of its oligosaccharide chains. It has been argued that the attachment of the water-soluble oligosaccharide may serve to anchor the protein in the correct asymmetric orientation in the membrane, but the purpose of the remodelling is currently one of the great mysteries of biochemistry. Although some glycoproteins have been shown to be protected from intracellular proteolysis by their oligosaccharides, this is not true of all of them, and in any event would not account for the extraordinary specificity of the remodelling. It would appear from the considerable metabolic energy expended in these alterations that an important property is being conferred by the carbohydrate structure, but firm evidence is almost totally lacking as to what this property might be.

POST-SYNTHETIC PROCESSING[19]

How do the membrane proteins that are synthesized in the endoplasmic reticulum get to the plasma membrane, or to the appropriate intracellular membranous organelles where they function? Once again, the outlines of the process resemble those used by the secretory proteins very closely[12,20]. Plasma membrane proteins take about 45 min to reach the plasma membrane after completion of their synthesis in the endoplasmic reticulum. The protein follows a closely programmed series of steps, involving pinching off from one membrane followed by fusion with a different membrane. These processes appear to be mediated by the protein clathrin, which interacts with the membrane to form highly characteristic 'coated vesicles' of uniform size. Transfer proceeds from the endoplasmic reticulum to the Golgi apparatus, which functions as a central sorting organelle for membrane and secreted proteins. Remodelling of the oligosaccharide occurs in the Golgi, leading to the suggestion that this may be related to protein sorting. Sorting is specific and complex; some proteins remain in the Golgi, others are transported to the lysosomes, or to the plasma membrane of one surface or the other of a polarized cell.

A recent discovery promises to make this sorting process experimentally accessible. It was found that one kind of enveloped virus, vesicular stomatitis virus (VSV), buds exclusively from the basolateral surface of epithelial cells, while another, influenza, buds exclusively from the apical surface[20]. The most plausible mechanism for achieving this is if the viral glycoproteins are each directed exclusively to the plasma membrane on the appropriate side of the cell. Preliminary evidence suggests that the signal directing the viral protein to one side or the other does not depend upon the presence of oligosaccharide groups.

The last event in biosynthesis of either membrane or secreted proteins, membrane insertion or exocytosis of secretion products, would tend to increase the area of the plasma membrane. However, the area of plasma membrane tends to remain constant, even in secretory cells that are stimulated to maximal exocytosis. Evidence is now accumulating for the existence of a membrane recycling system that operates actively in all cells. Once again, coated vesicles appear to mediate the endocytosis of membrane material. Subsequent intracellular events are still obscure, although the lysosomes may also play a role.

The picture that emerges, although still in very vague general outline, is of a highly integrated membrane economy that encompasses all the membrane structures of the cell and provides communication between them by means of coated vesicles. This membrane economy recycles old membranes, incorporates newly synthesized material, and sorts and packages the flow so as to maintain the many functional and topological distinctions between membranes that are essential to the normal functioning cell.

SUMMARY

The problem of how membranes are synthesized is currently under intensive study, and answers are emerging that promise great advances in our understanding of the role of different membranes in the overall economy of the cell. The following general summary statements can be made.

(1) Some membrane proteins are synthesized in the endoplasmic reticulum by mechanisms analogous to those used for secretory proteins. Their appropriate asymmetric orientation is determined by translocation of the growing polypeptide-chain during synthesis. This process is initiated by interaction between a signal sequence at the N-terminus of the polypeptide chain and a specialized apparatus in the endoplasmic reticulum membrane.

(2) This scheme is probably not applicable to all membrane proteins. Some may be synthesized in the cytoplasm, where they must exist in a soluble form, and integrate into the appropriate cellular membrane by self-assembly.

(3) Synthesis of membrane proteins in the endoplasmic reticulum is followed by elaborate processing that results in the integration of each protein into the functionally appropriate membrane. Recycling of plasma membrane components seems also to be part of this overall scheme. The Golgi apparatus plays a central role in mem-

brane sorting. The membrane transfer between organelles that is essential to this process is accomplished largely or exclusively through coated vesicles.

NOTE ADDED IN PROOF

Engelman and Steitz (*Cell,* **23,** 411–22 (1981)) have recently proposed a 'helical hairpin hypothesis' to explain the correct insertion of proteins into bilayer membranes. According to this hypothesis, insertion proceeds spontaneously from the free energy arising from burying hydrophobic helical surfaces. The signal peptide sequence is considered to fold into a hydrophobic helical segment with which successive, more polar helical segments can interact to form a 'helical hairpin'. This hypothesis requires no special translocating machinery in the membrane, and can account for the full range of asymmetric orientations actually observed for membrane proteins.

References

1. Stryer, L. (1975), Introduction to biological membranes. *Biochemistry*, Chap. 10, pp. 227–253. (San Francisco: Freeman)
2. Singer, S. J. and Nicolson, G. L. (1972). The fluid mosaic model of the structure of cell membranes. *Science*, **175**, 720
3. Rothman, J. E. and Lenard, J. (1977). Membrane asymmetry. *Science*, **195**, 743
4. Palade, G. (1975). Intracellular aspects of the process of protein synthesis. *Science*, **189**, 347.
5. Anfinsen, C. B. (1973). Principles that govern the folding of protein chains. *Science*, **181**, 223
6. Anfinsen, C. B. and Scheraga, H. A. (1975). Experimental and theoretical aspects of protein folding. *Adv. Protein Chem.*, **29**, 205
7. Welaufer, D. B. and Ristow, S. (1973). Acquisition of three-dimensional structure of proteins. *Annu. Rev. Biochem.*, **42**, 135
8. Singer, S. J. (1971), The molecular organization of biological membranes, In L. Rothfield (ed.). *Structure and Function of Biological Membranes*. pp. 146–223. (New York: Academic Press)
9. Lodish, H. F. and Rothman, J. E. (1979). The assembly of cell membranes. *Scient. Am.*, **240**, 48
10. Blobel, G. and Dobberstein, B. (1975). Transfer of proteins across membranes. *J. Cell Biol.*, **67**, 835; *ibid.*, **67**, 852
11. Blobel, G. and Sabatini, D. D. (1971). Ribosome–membrane interaction in eukaryotic cells. In L. Manson (ed.). *Biomembranes*. Vol. 2, p. 193. (New York: Plenum)

12. Milstein, C., Brownlee, G. G., Harrison, R. M. and Mathews, M. J. B. (1972). A possible precursor of immunoglobin light chains. *Nature New Biol.*, **239**, 117

13. Lenard, J. (1978). Virus envelopes and plasma membranes. *Annu. Rev. Biophys. Bioeng.*, **7**, 139

14. Lenard, J. and Compans, R. W. (1974). The membrane structure of lipid-containing virus. *Biochim. Biophys. Acta*, **344**, 51

15. Rothman, J. E. and Lodish, H. F. (1977). Synchronized transmembrane insertion and glycosylation of a nascent membrane protein. *Nature (London)*, **269**, 775

16. Wickner, W. (1979). The assembly of proteins into biological membranes: The membrane trigger hypothesis. *Annu. Rev. Biochem.*, **48**, 23

17. Lennarz, W. J. (1975). Lipid linked sugars in glycoprotein synthesis. *Science*, **188**, 986

18. Waechter, C. J. and Lennarz, W. J. (1976). The role of polyprenol-linked sugars in glycoprotein synthesis. *Annu. Rev. Biochem.*, **45**, 95

19. Alberts, B., Porter, K., Raff, M., Roberts, K. and Watson, J. (1981). Organization and function of the cytoplasm in the synthesis and breakdown of macromolecules, *Molecular Biology of the Cell*, Chap. 9. (New York: Garland Press) (In press)

20. Rodriguez-Boulan, E. and Sabatini, D. D. (1978). Asymmetric budding of viruses in epithelial monolayers: A model system for the study of epithelial polarity. *Proc. Natl. Acad. Sci. USA*, **75**, 5071

4

Some regulatory principles in epithelial transport*

R. Kinne

INTRODUCTION

This symposium takes place as I am about to leave the Max-Planck-Institute for Biophysics after 13 years of stimulating and rewarding research. Looking through the work done during this period by myself and in collaboration with my colleagues, it becomes evident that almost all of the studies have been linked, more or less closely, to the question of regulatory principles in epithelial transport. In rereading these papers, it is interesting to note how they reflect the change in emphasis that was placed for a long time on the metabolic events occurring in the intracellular compartment to the emphasis that is placed nowadays on the events occurring at the barrier between the extra- and intracellular compartment, the cell membrane. Therefore in this chapter I would like to develop, taking my own work as guideline, some general aspects of regulation of transport. This is not intended to be a complete review; its main intent is to provide a framework of concepts concerning the basic principles of epithelial transport and the sites and selectivity of its regulation that might be useful for studies of transport phenomena in health and disease.

---

* Dedicated to Prof. Dr K. J. Ullrich in deep appreciation of his generous support and scientific and personal advice.

SOME GENERAL COMMENTS

Epithelial transport is, in the simplest approximation, a phenomenon composed of two entities, the paracellular and the trans-cellular transport. It can be described by equation (1) where the passive and active driving forces for the movement of a solute are summarized:

$$J_i = \bar{c}_i \, (1 - \sigma_i) \, J_v - P \, \left(\Delta c_i + \frac{Z \cdot F}{RT} \, \bar{c} \Delta \psi \right) + J_{iact} \tag{1}$$

where σ_i is the reflection coefficient, $\bar{c}_i$ is the mean concentration across the epithelium, Δc_i is the concentration difference, Z is the charge of the molecule, R, T, F the meaning.

This chapter deals exclusively with events related to the trans-cellular transport of solutes. It excludes considerations about regulatory processes affecting the paracellular pathway. In some tissues, like the proximal tubule, the latter pathway is used for the majority of sodium and chloride transport[1] and of calcium transport[2]; this transport route is markedly influenced by changes in volume flow (J_v), permeability (P) and in the electrical potential difference ($\Delta \psi$) across the epithelium. With respect of the trans-cellular transport we shall concentrate on the active processes (J_{act}), where transport of a solute is observed in the absence of any physical driving forces across the epithelium and transport is at some point linked to a chemical reaction. As a consequence of this coupling the active transport is sensitive to inhibition of intracellular energy metabolism. For many years this fact focussed the attention of investigators on questions concerning the energy source for active transport and the possibility that transport through epithelia may be regulated by alterations in intracellular metabolism.

THE ENERGY SOURCE FOR TRANSPORT AND REGULATION OF TRANSPORT BY REGULATION OF ENERGY METABOLISM

The energy source for sodium transport in the proximal tubule

It was, for a long time, difficult to define the metabolic pathways supporting active sodium-transport in the kidney and especially in the renal proximal tubule, because of several technical difficulties. First of all, it is very difficult to determine intracellular levels of ATP or of other metabolites which might provide information on the energy source for transport in the renal cortex. Due to its high metabolic activity, metabolic patterns change considerably during short periods of anoxia, which sometimes occur during experimental manipulation of the kidney[3]. Secondly, when metabolic inhibitors are infused into the kidney, the actual concentration of the inhibitor in the proximal tubule is not known and it is, therefore, very difficult to make conclusions about the action of inhibitors. The latter problem was solved when the technique of the simultaneous perfusion of the tubule and of the capillary network surrounding it was applied. Thereby the concentration of the metabolic inhibitor and its site of application could be well controlled. Two interesting observations were made by György and Kinne.[4] Cyanide and the uncoupler CCCP (carbonylcyanide-m-chlorophenylhydrazone) – metabolic inhibitors which permeate cell layers very easily – show an unequivocal action only when applied peritubularly. Sodium reabsorption in the proximal tubule (measured as isotonic volume reabsorption) is completely inhibited by these inhibitors of oxidative metabolism[4]. It was found, also, that some inhibitors of oxidative phosphorylation such as antimycin A and oligomycin, that are very potent in isolated mitochondrial preparations, enter the tubular cells only very slowly. The inhibitors can, however, be shuttled into the cells in association with the aid of albumin.* The albumin–antimycin A complex[5] is taken up at the luminal membrane by pinocytosis and after a typical lag period of 5 min an almost complete inhibition of the isotonic volume flow is observed. These experiments clearly indicate that the sodium transport in the proximal tubule is dependent on oxidative metabolism taking place in the mitochondria. A direct coupling of transport to the rate of electron flow in the mitochondria seems to be excluded since CCCP, an uncoupler, although stimulating the electron flow in the mitochondria, inhibits the sodium transport.

It could also be demonstrated that, under certain conditions, the inhibition of transport by metabolic inhibitors can be almost completely reversed if phosphoenolpyruvate is applied intratubularly[6]. Inside the tubular cell, phosphoenolpyruvate provides energy via the pyruvate

* In disease states where the permeability of the glomerulus for macromolecules is increased, the tubular cell is exposed to a high concentration of albumin. Due to its pinocytic activity the cell takes up protein avidly. Toxins (either endogenous or exogenous) when bound to these proteins, can enter the tubular cell in these instances and cause specific damage in this region of the nephron. This phenomenon could be of pathophysiological relevance.

kinase reaction in which ADP is phosphorylated to ATP. This indicated that, under conditions of markedly reduced oxidative metabolism, sodium transport can be driven by ATP generated intracellularly by the pyruvate kinase reaction. From these studies, therefore, it can be concluded[6] that ATP generated by oxidative metabolism is the energy source for sodium transport in the renal proximal tubule. The transport system involved in active sodium transport is the Na–K-ATPase, which in the erythrocyte ghost and reconstituted proteoliposomes has been shown to perform active sodium transport at the expense of ATP hydrolysis. According to membrane fractionation studies[7] this enzyme is localized exclusively in the basal lateral plasma membranes of the proximal tubule cell.

Regulation of transport by regulation of metabolism

Since oxidative metabolism is necessary for sodium transport in the proximal tubule, the next step was obviously to look for changes in enzymatic reactions involved in this pathway under conditions where the sodium transport is affected by hormones. It is known from micropuncture studies that adrenalectomy inhibits sodium transport in the proximal tubule of rat kidney by approximately 50% under stopped flow conditions. Biochemical studies of the activities of glycolytic enzymes and the enzymes of the tricarboxylic acid cycle[8] revealed that, in parallel to the transport changes, the activity of the condensing enzyme or citrate synthetase in mitochondria isolated from kidneys of adrenalectomized rats was decreased and could be restored to normal values by the application of aldosterone. Similar findings with more defined techniques were then reported for toad bladder and for rat kidney cortex with physiological doses of aldosterone[9].

An anlysis of the cofactors and metabolites in rat kidney cortex provided additional evidence for a higher activity of the citric acid cycle in the presence of aldosterone[10].

As a general principle, regulation of transport by primary regulation of metabolism seems only a very crude method to adapt the transport of a specific solute to the needs of the animal. One can assume that all transport processes linked directly or indirectly to ATP production are affected and therefore only a very low selectivity of regulation can be achieved. Indeed in toad bladder it is very probable that an additional measure is taken to make the regulation more selective, namely that the sodium permeability of the luminal plasma membrane is increased by aldosterone[9]. By this combined action (and perhaps by other factors as yet unknown) this higher potency of the cell to generate ATP is channelled into the energy-requiring active sodium transport.

ATP-DEPENDENT TRANSPORT SYSTEMS AND THEIR REGULATION

ATP-dependent transport systems in the proximal tubule

The nature and membrane location of ATP-dependent transport systems in the proximal convoluted tubule of rat kidney is summarized in Figure 4.1. There is fair amount of evidence from studies on rat and especially on the ouabain-sensitive Syrian hamster, that the sodium reabsorption by the proximal tubule involves the action of the Na–K-ATPase[11,12]. This enzyme is located at the basal pole of the tubular cell where the energy barrier for trans-cellular sodium transport – the chemical concentration difference and the cell interior negative electrical potential – has to be overcome.*

At the same site of the cell an ATP-dependent transport system for calcium has been recently described[13]. In isolated basal–lateral plasma membrane vesicles addition of Mg-ATP stimulates calcium uptake and provokes an intravesicular accumulation of calcium. In the intact cell this system can extrude calcium from the cell against the concentration gradient and electrical gradient present across the cell membrane; it is probably involved in the fine regulation of the intracellular calcium concentration. In trans-cellular transport of calcium the major pathway is sodium-dependent and proceeds via a sodium–calcium exchange system at the contraluminal membrane[2,13].

An ATP-dependent process is also involved in proton secretion by the proximal tubule. In addition to the Na/H exchange system[14] a Mg-ATPase exists in brush-border membranes which similar to the mitochondrial ATPase, is stimulated by anions[15]. Recently it was demonstrated that the rate of intravesicular ATP-hydrolysis in brush-border membrane vesicles is stimulated by the protonophor CCCP. This finding suggests that the ATP-hydrolysis is accompanied by an extrusion of protons from the vesicles. *In vivo* this process would result in proton secretion by the tubule.

* The choroid plexus of the brain seems to be an exception in this respect. The Na–K-ATPase is located on the pole of the cell facing the intraventricular fluid. An explanation for this phenomenon is not available at the moment.

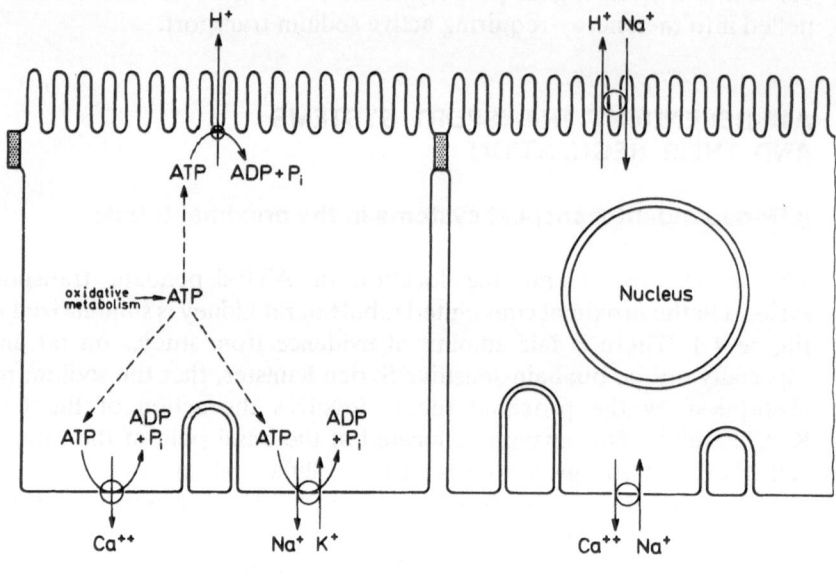

Figure 4.1 Cellular distribution of ATP-dependent transport systems and sodium antiport systems in rat renal proximal convoluted tubule

Regulation of ATP-dependent transport systems

We have studied, as an example of the regulation of an ATP-dependent transport system without an apparent concomitant regulation of metabolic activity, the rat caecum. The rat caecum enlarges when rats are kept on a germ-free diet or when the non-absorbable polymer, polyethylene glycol 4000, is added to the drinking water of adult rats. This hypertrophy is accompanied by an increase of sodium and volume transport rate per unit surface area, the major functional change being an increase in active sodium transport[16].

If the tissue is analysed biochemically, an increase in the Na–K-APTase activity of the cell is observed. Other enzymes, including mitochrondrial ones, remain unchanged. The change in transport and Na–K-ATPase have an identical time course[17]. Since in parallel experiments the solvent drag component and the sodium permeability of the hypertrophied caecum did not change appreciably, it is very likely that the increased Na–K-ATPase activity is the basis for the increased sodium transport.

In the caecum and in other specialized cells such as nasal gland of birds, for example, a regulation of Na–K-ATPase predominantly affects the sodium transport and the volume flow associated with it, therefore the degree selectivity of regulation is already quite high. In the cells described in the next chapter, where sodium-cotransport systems are operating, such a regulation of the Na–K-ATPase would be non-selective because it would affect a great variety of solutes.

THE SODIUM GRADIENT AS DRIVING FORCE FOR EPITHELIAL TRANSPORT AND THE REGULATION OF SODIUM-COTRANSPORT SYSTEMS

The sodium gradient as driving force for epithelial transport

During the last decade it became evident that a number of active transport processes in renal proximal tubule require the presence of sodium in the extra-cellular fluid and are strongly inhibited by ouabain[18]. In transport studies with membrane vesicles isolated from the luminal or contra-luminal pole of the epithelial cells, evidence could be provided that the sodium dependence of the trans-cellular transport is due to the presence of sodium-cotransport systems in the plasma membranes[19].

The sodium-cotransport systems are distributed unevenly (Figure 4.2) between the luminal and the contra-luminal surface of the cell. The properties of the sodium-cotransport systems are as follows:

(a) In the presence of sodium the apparent K_m of the transport system is decreased or the V_{max} is increased.

(b) In the presence of an electrochemical potential difference for sodium across the membrane an electrochemical potential difference for the cotransported solute is established.

(c) The cotransported solute stimulates sodium transport across the membrane.

(d) Depending on the charge of the solute and the stoichiometry of the system, the electrical potential difference across a membrane can influence the rate of sodium-dependent transport. The properties of such systems for sugars, amino acids and phosphate have been reviewed extensively[19].

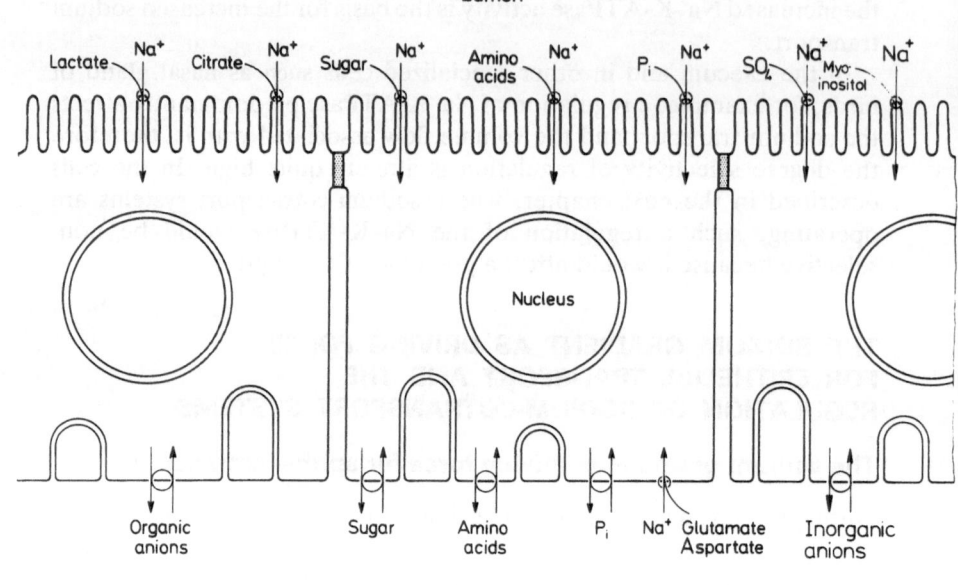

Figure 4.2   Cellular distribution of sodium-dependent and sodium-independent transport systems in rat renal proximal convoluted tubule. The scheme compiles data obtained on isolated luminal or contra-luminal plasma membrane vesicles

Since the vesicles are devoid of intracellular metabolic pathways, they are also well suited for studies of the transport of metabolites of the cell across the two cell borders. Thus, for example, the uptake of L-lactate was found to be sodium-dependent in brush-border membrane vesicles isolated from rat kidney[20]. The basal–lateral plasma membranes of the proximal tubule contain a sodium-independent L-lactate transport system which differs in its sensitivity to inhibitors and stereospecificity from the luminal transport system. Thus L-lactate is taken up primarily from the luminal side of the proximal tubule cell and, if not metabolized, leaves the cell at the contraluminal side. The driving forces involved in such a trans-cellular transport of L-lactate are depicted in Figure 4.3, luminal entry of L-lactate is governed by the electrochemical potential differences for lactate and sodium, whereby an intracellular accumulation of lactate against its electrochemical potential difference is achieved. This electrochemical potential difference drives lactate out of the cell at the contra-luminal cell pole. It should be noted that the stoi-chiometry between sodium and L-lactate in the sodium/lactate cotrans-port system is greater than one, therefore the transport of L-lactate (an anion at physiological pH) is *favoured* by the inside negative electrical potential difference across the brush border.

Sodium gradient coupled transport occurs in a variety of epithelial tissues. Depending on the kind of sodium cotransport system and its location in the cell envelope, absorption or secretion can be achieved. Typical examples for elements involved in absorption are, as depicted in Figure 4.4, sugar and amino symport systems (sodium and the cotrans-ported solute move in the same direction) located in the luminal mem-brane of renal and intestinal cells and the sodium–Ca antiport system (sodium and the cotransported solute move in the opposite direction) located in the contraluminal membrane of the renal epithelial cells.

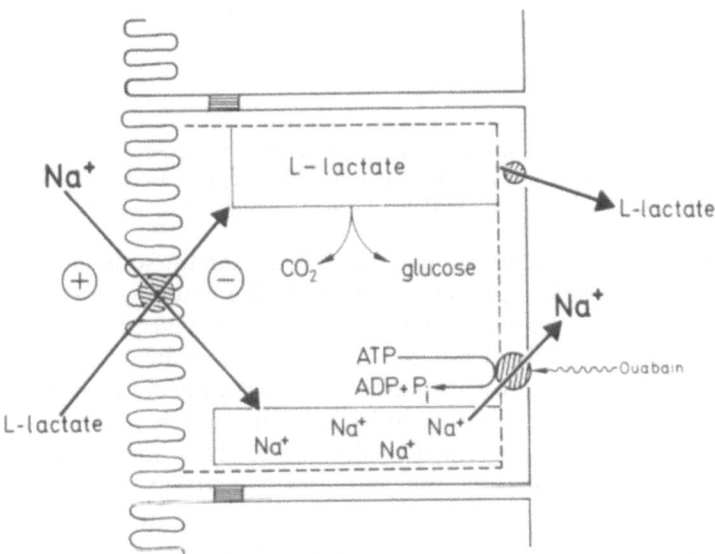

Figure 4.3 Schematic representation of L-lactate reabsorption in the rat renal proximal convoluted tubule

Sodium-dependent secretion, on the other hand, can be elicited by a symport system such as the sodium chloride cotransport system located in the contra-luminal membrane of the shark rectal gland[21] or by the sodium–proton antiport system found in the luminal membrane of the proximal tubule and intestine. In all instances the Na–K-ATPase located at the cell side facing the blood stream is responsible for the maintenance of the sodium-ion gradient and the membrane potential. Both act as driving forces for the sodium cotransport systems.

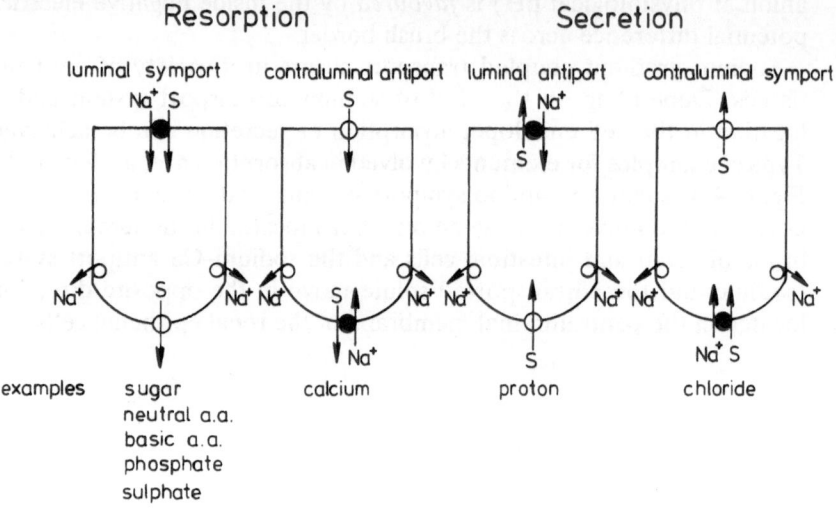

Figure 4.4   Role of sodium-cotransport systems in secretory and absorptive processes in epithelial cells. The Na–K-ATPase represented as Q, Na$^+$ is localized in the basal lateral membrane of the epithelial cells

The most selective regulation is achieved when the sodium cotransport system for the solute proper is regulated. The epithelial system studied most extensively in this respect is the sodium–phosphate cotransport system in the proximal tubule[22,23]. Renal phosphate transport is very well suited for such investigations because a variety of factors are known to influence phosphate transport in the proximal tubule.

Studies with isolated brush-border vesicles have shown that changes observed in the tubular phosphate transport *in vivo* are reflected in – and thus probably caused by – changes in the activity of the sodium–phosphate cotransport system in the brush border membrane. Application of PTH or cAMP to rats, for example, decreased phosphate reabsorption in the proximal tubule and accordingly the rate of phosphate uptake in brush-border membrane vesicles prepared from these animals is decreased[22]. Parathyroidectomy, on the other hand, increases phosphate transport both in the tubule *in vivo* and in the vesicles isolated from these animals. Adaptation of rats to dietary phosphate also affects tubular transport and phosphate transport in the vesicles in parallel[23].

Since other sodium-cotransport systems such as the D-glucose sodium cotransport system are not affected, it can be concluded that the phosphate system in the brush-border membrane* is modified specifically in order to achieve a regulation of the tubular transport of phosphate.

Unfortunately, nothing is known to date about the biochemical basis of this regulation. Several mechanisms are possible, including induction of new transport protein, regulation of the activity of the transport system by phosphorylation or dephosphorylation changes in the lipid boundary surrounding the molecule or changes in the arrangement of the transport system in the membrane by perturbation of the cytoskeleton inside the microvilli (see Kenny, Chapter 7). None of these possibilities has been subjected to a rigorous experimental analysis. There is also no information available about the role of the contraluminal membrane in the regulation of transcellular phosphate transport.

SUMMARY AND OUTLOOK

The experiments discussed above were compiled in order to develop some general principles concerning the analysis of epithelial transport processes and their regulation or disturbance. In the first place, it has to be determined whether the paracellular transport or the trans-cellular transport is affected. For the paracellular pathway, passive driving forces are most important, such as transport by solvent drag, diffusion and electrophoresis. In trans-cellular transport the active transport components become effective. At the cellular level it then becomes important to distinguish between a change in the driving forces for the transport or a modification of the activity of the transport system itself. This problem can be approached by separating the luminal and contraluminal plasma membranes from the intracellular compartments. It should be emphasized, however, that in the isolated membrane system the interplay between membranes and intracellular components has been disturbed and that therefore regulatory phenomena occurring *in vivo* might no longer be observable *in vitro*. Thus the analysis of the intracellular compartment with its ionic composition, metabolite and cofactor concentrations and structural organization is crucial for a complete description of regulatory events in transport.

Another point considered concerns the selectivity of the transport

---

* It should be noted in this context that regulation of sodium phosphate cotransport by parathyroid hormone and dietary phosphate intake are independent. It is therefore possible that multiple transport systems exist for phosphate or several modulators of the transport system.

regulation. Regulation of transport processes by regulation of ATP-generating metabolic reactions exhibits only a limited degree of specificity, except for those instances where the cells in question are highly specialized in their transport function. In multifunctional cells with several ATP-dependent transport processes the regulation is quite non-specific. The same holds for alterations in the driving forces involved in sodium-cotransport systems. Alterations of the electrochemical potential difference for sodium across the membrane affect all sodium-cotransport systems, although some differences in the degree of response might exist because of different properties of the cotransport systems. The highest degree of selectivity is achieved when the transport system itself is regulated, and recent studies on isolated plasma membrane vesicles have demonstrated that this is the case, for example, for renal phosphate transport. The regulation of Na–K-ATPase in avian salt gland, gills and in rat caecum falls in the same category.

In conclusion, it should be emphasized that it is rewarding to see how techniques for studying membrane transport and concepts for analysing epithelial transport processes which have evolved from the work done at the Max-Planck-Institute for Biophysics, are now already widely applied to the analysis of inborn errors of transport. The growing mutual interaction of basic scientists, clinicians and geneticists will hopefully facilitate the understanding of the individual biochemical and biophysical reactions which underlie epithelial transport in health and disease.

References

1. Frömter, E., Rumrich, G. and Ullrich, K. J. (1973). Phenomenologic description of Na^+, Cl^- and HCO_3^- absorption from proximal tubules of the rat kidney. *Pfluegers Arch. Eur. J. Physiol.*, **343**, 189
2. Ullrich, K. J., Rumrich, G. and Klöss, S. (1976). Active Ca^{2+} reabsorption in the proximal tubule of the rat kidney. Dependence on sodium and buffer transport. *Pfluegers Arch. Eur. J. Physiol.*, **364**, 223
3. Zwiebel, R., Wiechmann, J., Höhmann, B. and Kinne, R. (1970). Das Verhalten der Pyridinnucleotide und einiger Metaboliten in der Nierenrinde der Ratten bei Normoxie und Anoxie. *Hoppe-Seyler's Z. Physiol. Chem.*, **351**, 854.
4. György, A. Z. and Kinne, R. (1971). Energy source for transepithelial sodium transport in rat renal proximal tubules. *Pfluegers Arch. Eur. J. Physiol.*, **327**, 234
5. Brendel, U., György, A. Z. and Kinne, R. (1977). Studies on the binding characteristics of antimycin A and albumin in relation to the inhibitor activity of the complex on rat proximal tubular sodium transport. *Pfluegers Arch. Eur. J. Physiol.*, **372**, 77

6. Kinne, R. and György, A. Z. (1972). *In vivo* and *in vitro* studies on the energy source for transepithelial sodium transport in rat renal proximal tubule. In M. Hohenegger (ed.). *Biochemische Aspekte der Nierenfunktion*, pp. 97–110 (Munich: Goldmann)

7. Heidrich, H. G., Kinne, R., Kinne-Saffran, E. and Hannig, K. (1972). The polarity of the proximal tubule cell in rat kidney: different surface charges for the brush-border microvilli and plasma membranes from the basal infoldings. *J. Cell Biol.*, **54**, 232

8. Kinne, R. and Kirsten, R. (1968). Der Einfluss von Aldosterone auf die Aktivität mitochondrialer and cytoplasmatischer Enzyme in der Rattenniere. *Pfluegers Arch. Eur. J. Physiol.*, **300**, 244

9. Edelman, I. S. (1978). Candidate mediators in the action of aldosterone on Na⁺ transport. In J. Hoffman (ed.). *Membrane Transport Processes*, Vol. 1, p. 125. (New York: Raven Press)

10. Kirsten, R. and Kirsten, E. (1972). Redox state of pyridine nucleotides in renal response to aldosterone. *Am. J. Physiol.*, **223**, 229

11. Ullrich, K. J., Capasso, G., Rumrich, G., Papavassiliou, F. and Klöss, S. (1977). Coupling between proximal tubular transport processes, studied with ouabain, SITS and HCO_3^--free solutions. *Pfluegers Arch. Eur. J. Physiol.*, **368**, 245

12. Katz, A. J. and Epstein, F. H. (1967). The role of sodium–potassium-activated adenosinetriphosphatase in the reabsorption of sodium by the kidney. *J. Clin. Invest.*, **46**, 1999

13. Gmaj, P., Murer, H. and Kinne, R. (1979). Calcium ion transport across plasma membranes isolated from rat kidney cortex. *Biochem. J.*, **178**, 549

14. Murer, H., Hopfer, U. and Kinne, R. (1976). Sodium proton antiport in brush-border-membrane vesicles isolated from rat small intestine and kidney. *Biochem. J.*, **154**, 597

15. Kinne-Saffran, E. and Kinne, R. (1979). Further evidence for the existence of an intrinsic bicarbonate-stimulated Mg^{2+}-ATPase in brush border membranes isolated from rat kidney cortex. *J. Membrane Biol.*, **49**, 235

16. Loeschke, K., Uhlich, E. and Kinne, R. (1974). Stimulation of sodium transport and Na⁺–K⁺–ATPase activity in the hypertrophying rat cecum. *Pfluegers Arch. Eur. J. Physiol.*, **346**, 233.

17. Schiffl, H. and Loeschke, K. (1977). Induction of Na–K-ATPase in plasma membranes of rat cecum mucosa by diet: time course and kinetics. *Pfluegers. Arch. Eur. J. Physiol.*, **372**, 83

18. Ullrich, K. J. (1978). Renal transport of organic solutes. In G. Giebisch, D. C. Tosteson and H. H. Ussing (eds.). *Handbook of Membrane Transport in Biology*, Vol. IV A, *Transport Organs*, pp. 413–448. (Berlin: Springer)

19. Kinne, R. (1978). Metabolic correlates of tubular transport. In G. Giebisch, D. C. Tosteson and H. H. Ussing (eds.). *Handbook of Membrane Transport in Biology*, Vol. IV A, *Transport Organs*, pp. 529–562. (Berlin: Springer)

20. Barac-Nieto, M., Murer, H. and Kinne, R. (1981). Lactate–Sodium cotransport in rat renal brush border membranes. *Am. J. Physiol.* (In press)

21. Eveloff, J., Kinne, R., Kinne-Saffran, E., Murer, H., Silva, P., Epstein, F.

H., Stoff, J. and Kinter, W. B. (1978). Coupled sodium and chloride transport into plasma membrane vesicles prepared from dogfish rectal gland. *Pfluegers Arch. Eur. J. Physiol.*, **378,** 87

22. Evers, C., Murer, H. and Kinne, R. (1978). Effect of parathyrin on the transport properties of isolated renal brush-border vesicles. *Biochem. J.*, **172,** 49

23. Stoll, R., Kinne, R., Murer, H., Fleisch, H. and Bonjour, J.-P. (1979). Phosphate transport by rat renal brush border membrane vesicles: influence of dietary phosphate, thyroparathyroidectomy, and 1,25-dihydroxyvitamin D_3. *Pfluegers Arch. Eur. J. Physiol.*, **380,** 47

SECTION THREE

Transport in Brain

5

The needs of the brain for amino acids and how they are transported across the blood–brain barrier

O. E. Pratt

Introduction

The severe effects of hypoglycaemia on the brain were first observed in 1922 by Mann and Magath[1] who showed that cerebral tissue is dependent for its continued functioning upon a continuous and adequate supply of glucose, as well as of oxygen. Later, Harris[2] reported on the many cases of hypoglycaemia which had been caused by hyperinsulinism. The evidence that the brain needs amino acids is, by comparison, indirect. An important indication of how vital amino acids are to the brain is the mental retardation which is caused by many inborn errors which disturb the metabolism of amino acids in the body as a whole, which have been classified as the aminoacidaemias. Further evidence for the importance of amino acids to the brain has been provided by the discovery of highly specialized transport systems whose function is to carry amino acids across the blood–brain barrier. It is a reasonable supposition that these complex and chemically specific transport systems serve to meet fairly precisely the actual needs of the cerebral cells for amino acids. Further circumstantial evidence is provided by the rapid turnover of much of the protein of the brain. Seta *et al.* and Lajtha have shown that the brain uses amino acids at the rate of some 75 nmol/min per g of tissue just for the resynthesis of cerebral protein[3,4]. A proportion of the amino acids which are used for this resynthesis are provided from the breakdown of cerebral protein, but since much of the protein which is formed in the neuronal cell bodies passes down the axons to be broken down at the periphery[5], further supplies of amino acids have to be brought into the brain from the circulating blood (Figure 5.1). In fact the site of cerebral protein breakdown may often be far removed from that of its synthesis, e.g. some of the protein made in a Betz cell in the human motor-cortex may be broken down in the anterior horn of the spinal cord, perhaps more than 0.5 m away from where it was synthesized in the brain. This is important since protein in the cortical layers of the brain is renewed rapidly with a half-life of 2 or 3 days in contrast to the proteolipid protein of white matter which has a half-life of some months[6,7].

THE SUPPLY OF AMINO ACIDS TO THE BRAIN

Why does the brain need amino acids?

Protein continuously leaves the cerebral nerve cells. The loss of this protein from the cerebral nerve cells is not only due to catabolic activities within these cells, but due to the steady, continuous supply of protein which passes out of the cell body and down the axis cylinder, in the form of axoplasm (Figure 5.1). Axoplasm passes down the axons at a remarkably rapid rate[5] and must be continually replaced by new axoplasm which has to be synthesized from amino acids within the cell body. The brain uses amino acids not only for resynthesis of its proteins but for a number of other specialized metabolic purposes which are summarized in Table 5.1. Some of the more important of these specialized metabolic purposes are: the synthesis of cerebral neurotransmitters, e.g. serotonin which is made from tryptophan; methylation, in which the methyl groups are provided by the amino acid methionine and are used to methylate, for example, the side chain of arginine to make it less lipid-repellant during the formation of myelin[8,9], and the oxidative metabolism of the branched-chain amino acids which occurs actively in the brain, although the major site of their metabolism is muscle[10]. The metabolites of the branched-chain amino acids, isoleucine, leucine and valine, probably provide essential components for the synthesis of cerebral lipids.

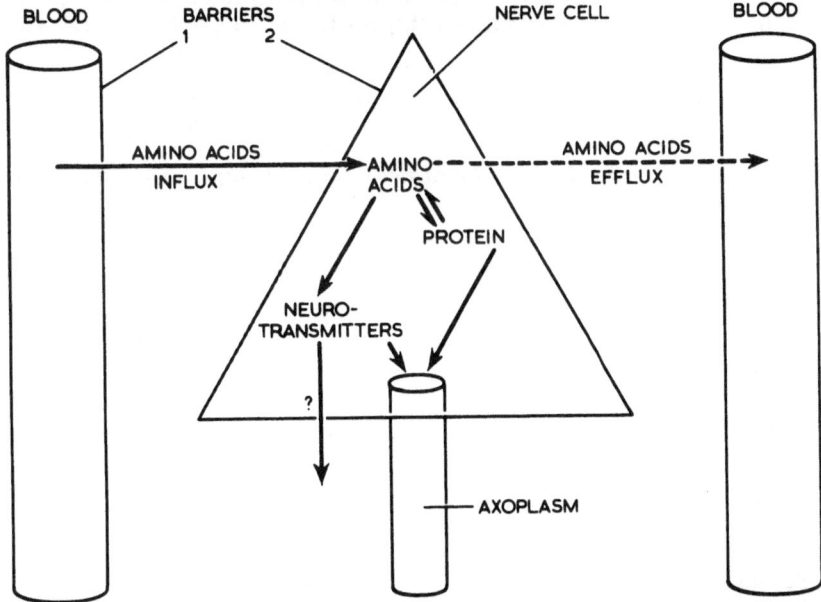

Figure 5.1   The sites of the two blood–brain barriers are shown and the fates of the amino acids which are transported across them are indicated. Under normal conditions a proportion of the amino acids re-enter the blood, so that there is some margin of safety if abnormal conditions develop. Some of the protein which is formed in the nerve cells passes down the axon as axoplasm; some disappears in ways as yet unknown. The quantities of amino acids needed to form neurotransmitters are small

Transport of amino acids across the blood–brain barrier

Recently a valuable technical advance has made it easier to measure the rate of transport of substances into the brain from the circulating blood. This advance is based upon the ability to maintain, by means of a programmed intravenous injection, steady raised levels of one or more substances in the circulating blood (Figure 5.2). Thus, not only can a predetermined level of specific radioactivity of an amino acid be attained very rapidly and maintained in the bloodstream, but also a raised level of the same amino acid, unlabelled, can be maintained in the bloodstream over a period of time[11-15]. This technique yields information which is different from and complementary to that obtained by the indicator dilution method in which intracarotid injections are used[16-18]. These

TABLE 5.1 Classification of amino acids according to whether they enter the brain from the blood or whether they are formed within the cerebral cells

	Protein synthesis	Neurotransmitters or precursors of neurotransmitters	Osmotic regulation	Special functions*
Amino acids entering the brain by carrier-mediated transport across the cerebral capillaries				
Alanine	+			
Arginine	+			
Citrulline				
Glutamate	+	+	+	3
Glutamine				3
Glycine	+	+	+	
Histidine	+	+		
Isoleucine	+			1
Leucine	+			1
Lysine	+			
Methionine	+	+		2
Ornithine				
Phenylalanine	+			
Proline	+			
Serine	+			
Tryptophan	+	+		
Tyrosine	+	+		
Valine	+			1
Amino acids which probably do not enter the brain from the blood under normal conditions				
Aspartate	+	+	+	
Cysteine	+			
Dihydroxyphenyl-alanine		+		
N-Acetylaspartate			+	
γ-Aminobutyrate		+		

*1, Possible source of material for synthesis of cerebral lipids. 2, Source of CH_3–groups for synthesis of special compounds in the brain. 3, Removal of surplus NH_2-groups from the cerebral cells[109, 112].

complementary results are in general agreement[19]. In addition, the steady-state measurements of influx give an indication of the actual rates of transport under *physiological conditions*.

Valuable information about the needs of the brain for amino acids is provided by studying the rates of transport of these nutrients across the blood–brain barrier. Transport across this barrier is highly selective and the results of the work which my colleagues and myself have done not

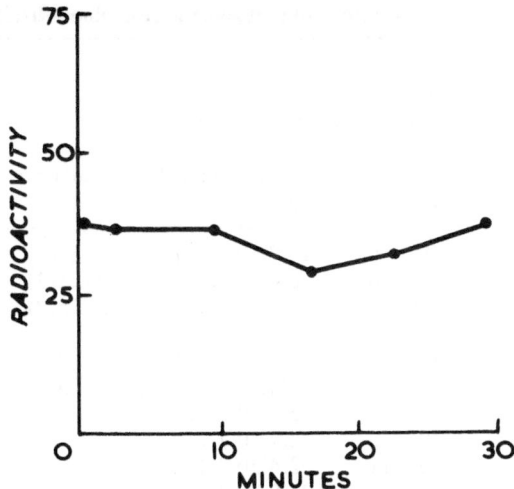

Figure 5.2 Shows how a desired level of radioactivity can be attained rapidly and maintained steadily in the circulating blood of a rat which has been given a programmed intravenous injection of ^{14}C-labelled L-phenylalanine. Abscissa: radioactivity in counts per minute per microlitre of blood plasma. Ordinate: time in minutes

only show which amino acids can cross this barrier in appreciable amounts, but they also indicate what quantities of these substances the brain is likely to be receiving from the blood. Thus, suppose that the brain metabolizes two amino acids, A and B, and can make either one from the other but cannot synthesize them easily from anything else. If amino acid A is rapidly transported into the brain from the blood while the transport of amino acid B across the blood–brain barrier is slow, it seems likely that the brain needs a supply of A equal to the rate at which it uses both amino acids, since amino acid A is also being used to make amino acid B.

How many amino acids does the brain need?

The first question to be answered is which of the amino acids circulating in the blood have to be supplied to the brain? These are the ones which the brain needs but which it cannot make itself. In this respect the major amino acids found in the blood fall into three main groups, two of which comprise amino acids which the brain cells obtain from the blood and a

TABLE 5.2   Amino acid transport across blood–brain barrier*

Amino acid	Concentration in blood plasma§ (μmol/l)	Influx across the blood–brain barrier (nmol/min per g of brain)	Cerebral gain (nmol/min per g of brain)	Efflux (nmol/ min per g of brain)	Efflux / Influx
Leucine†	100±10	11.7±0.9 (4)	2.5 (2)	9.2	0.79
Lysine†	340±10	8.4±1.6(11)	3.0±0.1(3)	5.4	0.64
Phenyl-alanine†	50±2	5.5±0.4 (5)	1.8±0.5(9)	3.7	0.67
Tyrosine	69±3	4.5±0.4 (6)	2.1±0.2(3)	2.4	0.53
Histidine	79±4	4.24±0.32(5)	1.34±0.03(5)	2.90	0.68
Threonine†	188±9	3.3±0.5 (6)	—	—	—
Alanine	405±50	2.7±0.7 (6)	—	—	—
Serine	188±11	2.4±0.3 (8)	—	—	—
Valine†	171±5	2.19±0.2 (9)	—	—	—
Methionine†	33±2	2.04±0.19(6)	—	—	—
Isoleucine†	73±3	1.89±0.2 (8)	—	—	—
Tryptophan†	55±3*	1.8±0.1(10)	—	—	—
Arginine	138±20	1.8±0.2(16)	—	—	—
Cysteine	105±60	1.16±0.2 (5)	—	—	—
Glutamate	160±20	1±0.4 (4)	—	—	—
Glycine	224±22	0.65±0.03(14)	—	—	—
Citrulline	61±10	0.57±0.17 (3)	—	—	—
Proline	163±14	0.31±0.03 (8)	—	—	—
Taurine	46±11	0.13±0.02 (5)	—	—	—
Aspartate	20±4	0.19±0.03 (6)	—	—	—
Thyroxine	0.06	0.036 (2)	—	—	—

* The movement of various amino acids in order of decreasing influx, into the brain across the blood–brain barrier (influx) together with values for the net uptake (cerebral gain) of the amino acid (if known) from which the movement outwards (efflux) across the blood–brain barrier has been calculated. (Means ± SEM with No. of determinations in parentheses)
† Nutritionally essential amino acid
‡ On the assumption that 75% of the tryptophan which is bound to albumin becomes available for transport into the brain
§ Means of 10–12 estimations
Based upon references 24, 27, 29, 57, 59, 60a, 110.

third group of amino acids which can be made by the cerebral cells (Table 5.2).

Nutritionally-essential amino acids which must be supplied from the blood   These amino acids are needed by the brain because, by definition, they cannot be synthesized by any of the cells of the body and therefore cannot be made by the cells of the brain. These eight essential amino acids which the body cannot synthesize[20-22] must be obtained from the diet and delivered to the brain from the blood. The influx of each into the brain is high (Table 5.2).

Other amino acids which the brain needs but which it cannot make
There is a further group of amino acids which the brain almost certainly needs. Like the essential amino acids, the brain cells cannot make, or cannot easily make, these amino acids. They include not only the semi-essential amino acids, histidine and arginine which the body cannot make in adequate amounts, but also a number of non-essential amino acids, e.g. tyrosine, an amino acid which can be made from phenylalanine by the liver but which cannot be made at an appreciable rate in the brain. Even when the brain can make one amino acid from another, one or other of the pair has to be supplied to the cerebral cells. The transformation is usually reversible so that it is only by work *in vivo* that it is possible to find out which amino acid must be supplied to the brain from the blood. Thus, for example, serine and glycine are readily interconvertible by brain cells[23] so that it might appear that the brain could manage quite well if supplied with either one of them. That this is not so is shown by the relative transport rates of these two compounds across the blood–brain barrier. The high rate of transport of serine into the brain compared with the low rate of transport of glycine makes it clear that in life the cerebral cells make glycine from serine, rather than the reverse[24]. Thus, the influx of serine into the brain must meet the combined needs of the cerebral cells both for serine and for glycine. This must be the reason why serine has a high rate of transport across the blood–brain barrier, comparable with that of the essential amino acids (Table 5.2). A similar explanation probably accounts for the high rate of transport of alanine into the brain compared with the lower rates of aspartate and glutamate[24], since it is from alanine that the cerebral cells must be making the other two amino acids[25]. The dibasic amino acids, citrulline and ornithine, which are formed in the liver but cannot readily be made in the cerebral cells[26], also have a high rate of influx into the brain and, although they are not used for cerebral protein synthesis, they must meet some other metabolic need of the brain[24,27].

Amino acids which need not be supplied from the blood because the brain cells can make them This group includes not only aspartate and glutamate (which, as seen above, the brain cells make from alanine), but also a number of other non-essential amino acids such as taurine, which the brain cells can make from other sulphur-containing amino acids. These non-essential amino acids all have quite a low or negligible influx across the blood–brain barrier (Table 5.2). Included in this group also are *N*-acetylaspartic acid and 4-aminobutyric acid, both of which are found abundantly in cerebral tissue but not elsewhere in the body. These are examples of amino acids which are made only by brain cells and do not cross the blood–brain barrier in either direction.

In a special position is glutamine which is formed in the brain and released into the circulation in considerable quantities. This cerebral synthesis of glutamine on a large scale almost certainly provides a means of removing from the brain surplus amino groups which are released, for example, by the metabolic breakdown of the branched-chain amino acids, isoleucine, leucine and valine, or by other catabolic processes which involve amino acids.

The quantities of amino acids needed by the brain

An indication of the quantities of the different amino acids which are needed by the brain is given by their influx, that is the rate of transport from the blood inwards across the blood–brain barrier. The actual rates of net movement of amino acids into the brain may be reduced if efflux occurs at the same time as influx, so that amino acids are simultaneously moving outwards. The net movement inwards, therefore, is given by the influx minus the efflux (Table 5.2). The influx thus represents the maximum rate at which the amino acid can be supplied to the cerebral cells from the blood. Normally, only between a third and a half of the quantity of any amino acid which enters the brain is retained by the cerebral cells (Table 5.2).

The influx varies greatly for different amino acids. Influx of all of the nutritionally essential amino acids into the brain is high[27], ensuring that the brain normally receives an adequate supply to meet its needs for protein synthesis (Table 5.2). The influx of these amino acids is at its highest during the perinatal period[28,29] since this is when the brain is growing and forming new protein as well as breaking down and resynthesizing previously-formed protein.

In the case of six or seven other amino acids which are not nutritionally essential (because they can be made elsewhere in the body, although the brain cells cannot make them), influx across the blood–brain barrier is also high, so high that it falls within the range of those of the nutritionally essential group[24]. These are tyrosine, histidine, alanine, serine, arginine, cysteine and perhaps also glutamate.

How are amino acids supplied to the brain?

It has been known since the last century that dyes injected into the bloodstream do not stain the main bulk of the brain[30,31]. Thus, some sort of barrier prevents the free entry of these dyes into the cerebral substance. It has also been known for a long time that if isolated pieces of brain are suspended in a saline medium, they take up nutrients selectively, including amino acids[32,33].

In this respect it is clear that brain cells resemble many other cells, e.g. erythrocytes or the cells of the kidney's tubules, in that they have a cell membrane which is impermeable to almost all substances except a few small molecules, such as water and oxygen, and also to substances which are soluble in lipids, for example the volatile anaesthetics. Other substances, including amino acids, can only move across cell membranes by making use of specific carrier molecules, located *in* the cell membrane[34].

The activities of these carrier molecules resemble, in many ways, the activities of enzymes[35]. Thus, they handle only one particular group of amino acids[36]. Their capacity to transport an amino acid across the cell membrane is limited, i.e. they can be saturated by a high concentration in the blood of the substance which they transport and in addition the speed of transport cannot be increased beyond a specific rate, however high in the blood the concentration is raised. Carrier molecules are generally able to transport two or more amino acids which compete with one another for the use of the carrier: thus one may monopolize it and act as an inhibitor, partially preventing the others from crossing the barrier.

The transport of amino acids across the cell membranes may either consume energy, or make it available. These transport systems may be linked to those which transport other substances, so that energy derived from the one system can enable the other system to transport amino acids through a membrane against a concentration gradient[37]. Nevertheless, most amino acids are transported across the capillary endothelial barrier of the brain from a high concentration to a lower one so that energy need not be supplied[38].

Although amino acids can be transported in both directions across a membrane, the rates at which they move in each direction are usually quite different. This may be due to the differences in the concentration of the substance on each side of the membrane, to the differences in the concentrations of competitive inhibitors in the blood, or to the differences in the energy couplings of the transport processes. Influx and efflux of substances into or out of a cell may even be mediated by different carriers[37].

Where is the effective blood–brain barrier?

The transport systems of the cerebral cell membranes were studied, especially during the 1960s, in work *in vitro* and usually brain slices were used. It progressively became clear, however, that there was, as suggested by Lajtha[39], a second set of transport systems which take amino acids across a second barrier, located in the cell membranes of the endothelial cells of the cerebral blood capillaries (Figure 5.1). Movement across the capillary wall can best be studied *in vivo*, although Goldstein and co-workers[40] have recently studied the transport of glucose and potassium ions into isolated brain capillaries. It is important to remember that the cerebral capillaries differ from those anywhere else in the body, in that they have tight junctions between the endothelial cells[41], i.e. most substances cannot diffuse through the junctional tissue between the cells.

In life the continuing supplies of amino acids which the brain needs are supplied by the circulating blood, and a proper understanding of the needs of the brain for amino acids and how they are supplied to it can only be obtained by studying the living animal. Comparison of the findings of workers who study the uptake of amino acids by brain slices or brain-cell cultures *in vitro* and those of workers who study transport across the blood–brain interface *in vivo* suggests that there are two sites at which the transport systems that carry amino acids into and out of the brain are found, both of which carry these substances across the blood–brain barrier. The first, and in many ways the most important, site is located in the cell membranes of the endothelial cells of the cerebral capillaries. The second site is found in the membranes of the cerebral cells themselves (Figure 5.1). The carrier mechanisms in this second site are probably able to transport amino acids and to take them up with a higher affinity, as well as more rapidly, than those which are present in the walls of the cerebral capillaries, so that the rate at which the brain capillary systems can carry amino acids determines the speed of influx of these substances into the brain. Both systems are carrier-mediated. However, the systems in the walls of the capillaries may be more selective than those in the membranes of the cerebral cells. For example, even though some amino acids which the cerebral cells are able to synthesize are present at high concentrations in the blood plasma (e.g. proline and glycine) their rates of transport into the brain are low (Table 5.2). The first part of the blood–brain barrier, that on the surfaces of the endothelial cells of the capillaries, also excludes a number of amino acids which the brain does not need, but which nevertheless have been found to be transported into the cerebral cells *in vitro*. Examples of these are some amino acids which are not naturally found in the body, such as 2-aminoadipate and 2-aminoisobutyrate. These amino acids cross the walls of the cerebral capillaries only very slowly and probably do so by diffusion rather than by carrier-mediated transport[24,42]. It may well be that most amino acids which are not needed by the brain only cross the barrier at the cerebral capillaries by diffusion even if some of them enter the brain cells by means of transport systems.

Characteristics of the carrier-mediated transport systems in membranes of the capillary cells and cerebral cells

The specificities of the carrier systems in the membranes which form the walls of the cerebral capillaries differ from those of the carriers in the surface membranes of the cerebral cells. In the latter site some ten or more different carriers have been reported, some of which are highly specific. For example, there is one on the surfaces of neurons which transports the neurotransmitter 4-aminobutyrate into the cells and one on the surfaces of glial cells which takes up taurine. Especially important are systems on the surfaces of glial cells which take up amino acids with a high affinity, even though the concentrations may be low in the extracellular space of the brain. There are such systems for tryptophan[43] and for tyrosine and phenylalanine[44]. In contrast there appear to be only four carriers in the walls of the cerebral capillaries[45]. Of these four, two in particular predominate: the L-system, which transports a wide range of amino acids[46] and a carrier which transports the dibasic amino acids, including arginine, lysine and ornithine[47,48].

Thus the two sets of transport systems, the first located in the membranes which form the walls of the cerebral capillaries and the second in the membranes forming the surfaces of the brain cells, operate in series. It appears that the first stage in the transport process is movement across the wall of the capillary. This is normally the slower transport system and its activity largely determines the overall rate of movement of substances into the brain from the blood. It is because only one barrier, that on the surface of the capillary endothelium, is really important that the curve showing the movement of radioactively labelled amino acids into the brain from the blood always takes a simple monophasic form like that shown in Figure 5.3[49]. Confirmation of this was subsequently obtained by direct measurements *in vivo* which show that alanine moves more slowly across the capillary barrier than it does into the cells[50]. There are probably three reasons why movement into the brain cells is faster than that across the capillary wall. In the membranes of the cerebral cells there is a wider variety of carriers than are present in the membranes of the capillary cells, so that any given substance may be transported by two or more carriers through the walls of the cerebral cells. The second reason is that the cells of the brain have a much larger surface than the capillary endothelium. Thus there are likely to be more carrier molecules on the surfaces of the cerebral cells than on the surfaces of the capillary cells so that the maximum rate of transport (V), (see Table 5.3) will be higher for transport across the surface barrier of the cerebral cells than that across the surface barrier of the endothelial cells. The third reason is that the high affinity of many of the systems on the surfaces of brain cells will enable them to take up amino acids effectively, even if their concentrations are low in the extracellular space. The effect of the difference in the transport systems will be that nutrient substances which are taken up by the cerebral cells will become available for metabolism as fast as they can cross the barrier on the surface of the capillary endothelium. It is this latter barrier which is important for investigation, since it determines the rate at which substances are supplied to the brain. The capillary endothelial barrier is almost certainly double, with two sets of carriers, one on the luminal surfaces and one on the outer surfaces of the endothelial cells of the blood capillaries of the brain[51].

Most of the carrier systems on the membranes of the brain cells derive their energy from the sodium gradient[46], but little is known about how the energy which is released by the transport across the cerebral capillaries from a high to a low concentration is made available for some other purpose. Exceptionally, one of the essential amino acids, threonine, is able to move across the blood–brain barrier into the brain *in vivo* in spite of the fact that it is present at a higher concentration in the cerebral tissue than in circulating blood[27]. Nevertheless it is likely that the concentration in the extracellular space is kept so low that transport across the epithelial barrier does not require energy.

An alternative route by which amino acids can reach the brain is provided by the cerebrospinal fluid (CSF) which is in continuity with the extracellular fluid of the brain. A third set of transport carriers takes amino acids into or out of the CSF[52, 52a]. Unlike transport from the blood into the brain, but like that from the extracellular space into brain cells, transport from the CSF into the brain commonly takes place against a

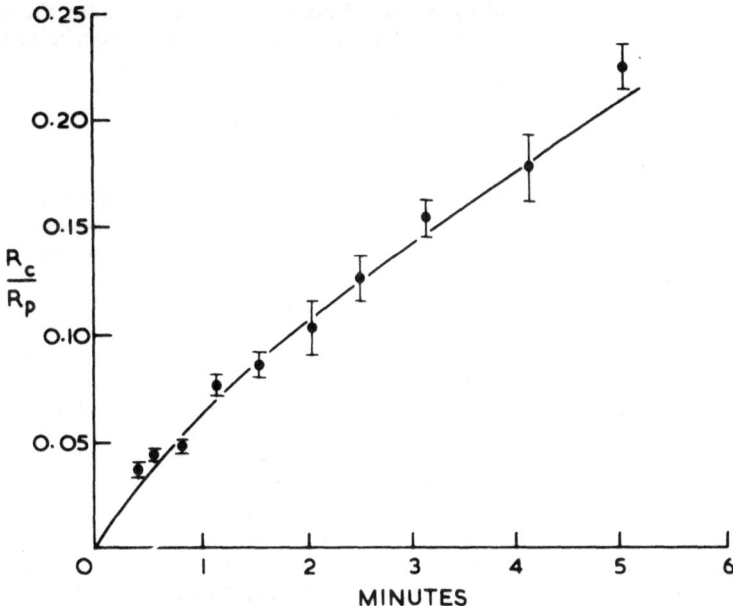

Figure 5.3 The rate at which radioactivity accumulated within the brain in the time during which a steady specific activity of labelling of L-leucine was maintained in the circulating blood. Radioactivity in the cerebrum, R_c, compared with radioactivity in the blood plasma, R_p. Each point represents the mean of 3–6 experiments; bars represent the standard error. (Crockett, Daniel and Pratt, unpublished data)

concentration gradient. This route will be unimportant, however, from a quantitative point of view, since the rate of flow of blood through the brain is greater by an order of magnitude than the rate at which the CSF is formed.

From recent work a picture is emerging of a blood–brain barrier which can only be crossed to any appreciable degree by means of a series of specific, carrier-mediated, interdependent transport systems, whose activity *in vivo* varies in a complex manner, being influenced by a number of factors, most of which have not been properly defined as yet. The highly selective nature of the barrier, as well as the overall rate of transport of amino acids into the brain, appears to be determined mainly by those carrier-mediated systems which are located in the walls of the cerebral capillaries. These capillaries are the main site of the blood–brain barrier, the transport across which can only be studied *in vivo*.

TABLE 5.3   Estimates of the values of the kinetic parameters for the carrier-mediated transport of various amino acids across the blood–brain barrier

Amino acid	Maximum carrier-mediated transport rate V (nmol/min per g of brain)	Equilibrium constant K (mmol/l)	Apparent diffusion coefficient D (nmol/min per g brain per mmol/l in plasma)	
Alanine	39.1	0.72±0.20 (3)	0.8	
Arginine	28±1	0.58±0.20 (4)	<0.3	
Glutamine	290	9.3 (2)	0.8	
Glycine	119	8.9±3.4 (4)	0.8	
Histidine	49±11	0.13±0.03 (5)	2.0±0.2	(9)
Isoleucine	73±21	0.38±0.09 (7)	1.6±0.3	(3)
Leucine	86±7	0.13±0.03 (3)	1.3±0.4	(6)
Lysine	189±13	2.1±0.6 (4)	<0.3	
Methionine	42±2	0.144±0.05 (4)	5.0±0.3	(6)
Phenylalanine	50±3	0.092±0.016(7)	2.5±0.3	(8)
Serine	52±5	4.6±1.1 (3)	0.8	
Threonine	64±17	1.33±0.23 (4)	0.8±0.2	(3)
Tryptophan	47±2	0.15±0.03 (6)	4.9±1.5	(8)
Tyrosine	58±11	0.15±0.03 (3)	3.8±1.6	(6)
Valine	90±10	0.73±0.15 (7)	1.23±0.24	(8)

V – the maximum rate of carrier-mediated transport. K – the equilibrium constant for the combination of the amino acid with the carrier. D – estimate of the apparent diffusion coefficient for the non-saturable component of influx (probably passive diffusion). The numbers of determinations are given in parentheses. Where for some values of V and D a standard error is not given, the value shown is a likely one which is consistent with the other data.
Sources: References 29, 54–56, 66, 72, 72a, 110, 112

Mechanism of transport

As pointed out above, the carrier-mediated transport mechanisms, which are probably located at the surfaces of the cells of the capillary endothelium of the brain capillaries and at the surfaces of cerebral cells, prevent the free diffusion of amino acids and thus form the so-called 'blood–brain barrier'. However, this barrier may not be completely impermeable to the diffusion of amino acids, at least in such localized areas as the hypothalamus or the floor of the fourth ventricle[53]. In addition, there is evidence for a non-saturable component in the transport of some amino acids into the brain[54-56], and a few amino acids appear to enter the brain solely by passive diffusion at a slow rate[24,42]. The quantities of amino acids entering the organ by diffusion are normally very small, though this mechanism may be of some importance in states of disease such as the aminoacidaemias[48,54-56] as well as for large lipid-soluble molecules like the thyroid hormones, i.e. thyroxine (Table 5.2).

Saturation of the transport systems

The way the rate of transport of an amino acid into the brain changes as its concentration in the blood alters is rather complex. Thus, when the concentration of the amino acid is within, or not far from, the normal range, its influx into the brain is usually directly proportional, for all practical purposes, to its concentration in the blood plasma[24,27]. However, if its concentration in the blood is higher than the normal level, the transport system may become saturated[42,48,49,57-59].

If the concentration of an amino acid in the blood is raised artificially to really high levels, the proportion of the total amount of amino acid which is transported into the brain by the carrier becomes smaller until, at very high concentrations, saturation is complete, i.e. the carrier is transporting the maximum amount of the amino acid which it is able to carry into the brain, and further increases in its concentration in the blood do not increase the influx any further (Figure 5.4). As originally suggested by Christensen in 1953[60], in the aminoacidaemias such saturation of the carrier will limit the amount of amino acid reaching the brain[17,28,57,58].

For an understanding of the brain damage that may be caused early in life by one of the aminoacidaemias, it is important to know the concentration of an amino acid in the blood at which saturation of the transport mechanism begins to occur, that is of the equilibrium constant, K, for combination of the amino acid with the transport carrier. As will be seen below, the effective value of K due to competitive inhibition from other amino acids in the blood (the second term in the denominator in equation 1) will be considerably higher than the actual value of K. This increase is the main reason why there is a proportional relation between influx and concentration in the blood over the normal range.

An indication of the values of K for various amino acids needed by the brain is given in Table 5.3. In the immature brain a number of amino acids are transported into the cerebral tissue at a high rate[28]. Despite this finding a permeability barrier is already present in the neonatal period,

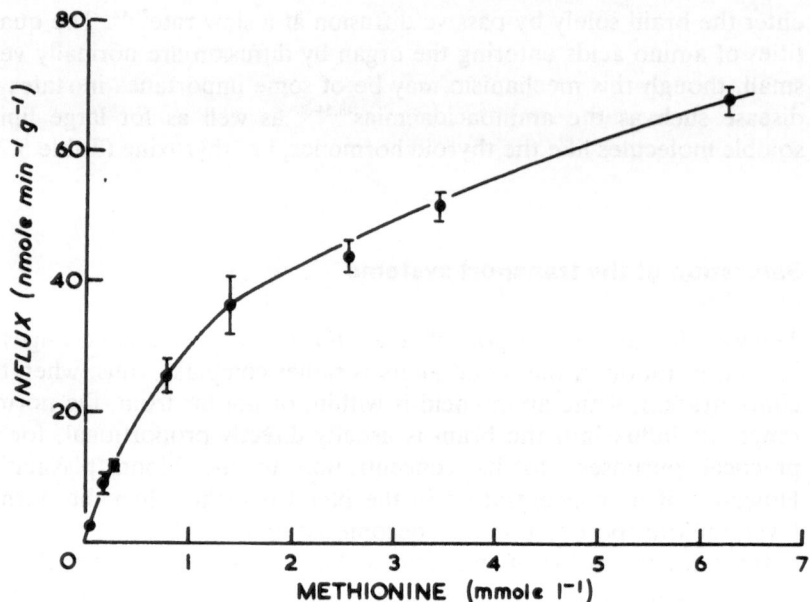

Figure 5.4 The effect of raising the concentration of L-methionine in the circulating blood of adult rats upon its influx into the brain stem. Each point represents the mean of 3–6 experiments; bars represent the standard error. A curve has been fitted statistically to the data. Note that as a result of the saturation of the transport carrier the influx does not increase in proportion to the concentration of the amino acid in the blood. (Crockett, Daniel and Pratt, unpublished data)

since the transport of amino acids into the immature brain shows saturation[29].

Further evidence that a permeability barrier to amino acids already exists between the blood and the brain before adult life is reached is shown by the competitive inhibition by methionine (Figure 5.5) on the transport of phenylalanine, into the brain of the suckling rat[29,60a]. In addition, in the suckling animal there is already a barrier to the entry of glucose[19,61]. Although it has been shown that the transport systems for essential amino acids are already well-developed in the foetal brain[62], there are likely to be changes in the barrier during antenatal development, as well as changes in the transport systems across it. Thus, the preterm infant may have transport systems suitable only for intrauterine life, so that the supply of amino acids to the brain of a premature infant may be inadequate for postnatal needs[19].

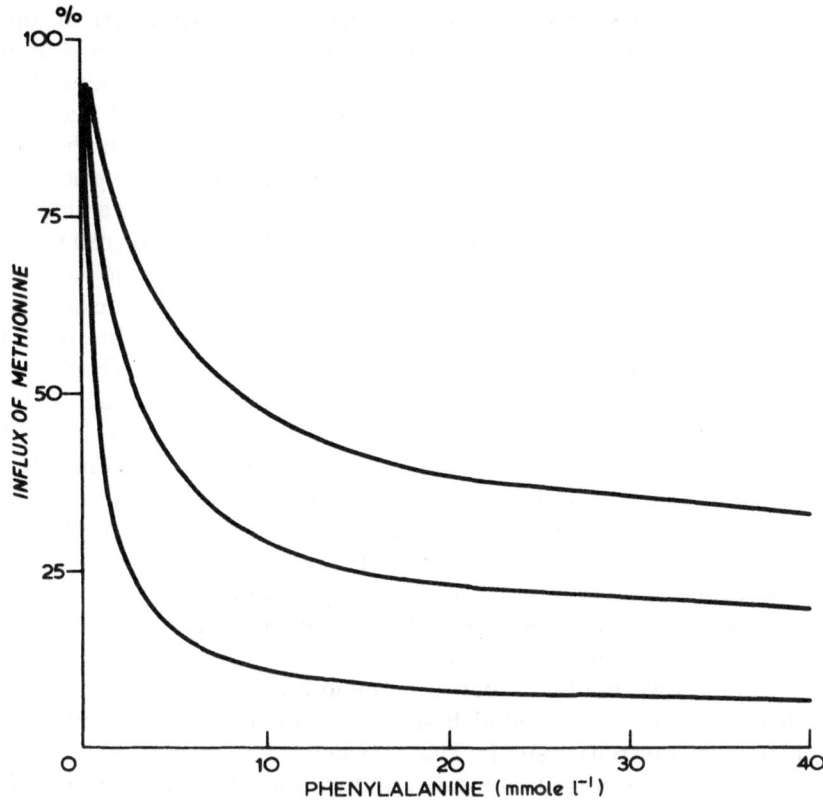

Figure 5.5 To show how an increase in the concentration of L-methionine in the blood can overcome the inhibitory effect of L-phenylalanine upon the transport of methionine across the blood–brain barrier. The curves were drawn by fitting equation (1) (p.104) to unpublished data of Crockett, Daniel and Pratt. The lower curve is one which has been fitted to the data from experiments in which the methionine level was not raised above the normal range of 0.046±0.03 mmol/l of plasma. The middle curve was obtained by fitting this equation to the data from experiments in which the methionine level was raised to 3.6±0.4 mmol/l of plasma and the upper curve from those in which the isoleucine level was raised still further to 8.6±0.5 mmol/l of plasma. It can be seen that the inhibitory effect of a raised level of phenylalanine in the blood is progressively reduced as the methionine level is raised

Competitive inhibition

Competitive inhibition between chemically related substances is a well established phenomenon in both the enzyme and in the transport fields[35,63]. That such inhibition can operate in the transport of amino acids across the blood–brain interface into the brain *in vivo* was first shown for the chemically-related dibasic amino acids, arginine, lysine and ornithine[47] and for various neutral amino acids[17,47]. If one of the dibasic amino acids is present at a high concentration in the blood plasma, it tends to monopolize the transport-carrier operating across the blood–brain barrier and largely prevents the other dibasic amino acids from being transported into the brain. This partial exclusion can be over-come if the concentration of the excluded amino acid in the circulating blood is simultaneously increased[48]. A well documented example of competitive inhibition is provided by the interaction between the branched-chain amino acids, isoleucine, leucine or valine. When any one of these is present in the circulating blood at a high concentration, of the order of 10 nmol/l, not only does it saturate its own transport system, but it partially excludes the other branched-chain amino acids from entering the brain. For example, the influx of isoleucine into the brain can be reduced progressively by raising the concentration of valine in the blood plasma to successively higher levels. However, this exclusion of isoleu-cine from the brain can be overcome by simultaneously increasing its concentration in the circulating blood[56]. Another example of this sort of competition is shown in Figure 5.5.

Competitive inhibition between amino acids occurs because most of them pass across the blood–brain barrier by means of shared carrier-mediated transport systems. The branched-chain amino acids and many others are transported into the brain by a carrier system referred to as the L-system[65]. There is thus competition between the amino acids for the shared transport carrier and this causes a marked congestion, one amino acid crowding another out from the carrier which transports them across the blood–brain barrier. The rate at which one amino acid, A, is transported will be reduced as the levels in the blood of competing amino acids are raised. Thus transport of A across the blood–brain barrier, i.e. the influx, v, will be given by

$$v = \frac{sV}{s + K_0 \left(1 + \frac{i_1}{K_1} + \frac{i_2}{K_2} + \cdots + \frac{i_n}{K_n}\right)} \tag{1}$$

where V is the maximum rate at which A can be transported across the barrier, K_0 is the affinity constant for A combining with the carrier, s is the concentration of A in the blood plasma and i_1, i_2, i_n and K_1, K_2, K_n are the levels in the blood and the affinity constants, respectively, of a series of other neutral amino acids (e.g. valine) which compete with A for the shared transport carrier[66].

It follows from equation (1) that if the level of A in the blood is raised the effect of competitive inhibitors will be overcome, and this is what we have observed for all the pairs of amino acids which we have studied. This can be seen, for example, in Figure 5.5 which shows that raising the level of phenylalanine in the blood has little effect upon the influx of methionine into the brain if the level of the latter is first raised to about 8 mmol/l of plasma.

The amino acids which are present in the highest concentrations in the blood tend to monopolize the carrier molecules, which are thus unable to carry the other amino acids across the blood–brain barrier. Another group of chemically-related amino acids which compete with one another for transport across the brain–blood interface are the aromatic amino acids phenylalanine, tyrosine, tryptophan and histidine[67]. This group also includes the aromatic amino acid L-dihydroxyphenylalanine (levadopa) which is present in the brain, but not normally present in the blood. This amino acid is widely used to treat Parkinsonism and, at a blood concentration of less than 1 mM, levadopa considerably reduces the influx of other aromatic amino acids into the brain [57,67].

When levadopa is used to treat patients with Parkinson's disease, the reduction in rigidity achieved is closely related to the changes in the concentration of the drug in the blood[68], and it must be borne in mind by the clinician that levadopa is likely to cross the cerebral barrier as easily as phenylalanine.

An important aromatic amino acid is tryptophan, since it is needed by the brain not only for protein synthesis, but also to make the cerebral neurotransmitter serotonin; an adequate supply of tryptophan to the brain is, therefore, likely to be a critical factor in cerebral nutrition. The concentration of free tryptophan in the blood, and also that which is free in the brain itself, is low, since the major part of the tryptophan in the blood is bound to the serum albumin. Thus, the extent to which other amino acids interfere with the transport of tryptophan from the blood into the brain will be a matter of great importance[66,67,69–72].

Most of the other amino acids which are normally present in the circulation have been tested as potential inhibitors of tryptophan transport and it has been found that there is a wide variation in the blood concentrations at which they are effective as inhibitors[66,67]. Exclusion of an amino acid from the brain is more likely to be severe and to be of practical importance if it takes place when the concentration of the inhibitor in the blood is low. Thus, the transport of tryptophan into the brain is easily susceptible to inhibition by raised concentrations in the blood of other aromatic amino acids[66,69,72]. The aromatic amino acids are also highly effective inhibitors of the transport across the blood–brain barrier of leucine, an amino acid which is not an aromatic amino acid. The aromatic amino acids inhibit the transport of leucine into the brain at concentrations in the blood which are lower than those at which other neutral amino acids (including even the other two branched-chain amino acids, isoleucine and valine, which are so similar chemically to leucine) inhibit its transport[72a]. The aromatic amino acids are such effective inhibitors of the transport of many other amino acids into the brain because they have an unusually high affinity for the transport carrier[66,67] as indicated by the low values of the equilibrium constant, K, shown in Table 5.3.

It must be concluded that, especially during the perinatal period, abnormally high levels in the blood of any of the aromatic amino acids are especially likely to interfere with the nutrition of the brain by restricting its supply of other amino acids. It is not surprising that inborn errors in the metabolism of these aromatic amino acids are generally associated with varying degrees of mental retardation and other abnormalities of development.

THE EFFECT OF INBORN ERRORS OF METABOLISM UPON THE SUPPLY OF AMINO ACIDS TO THE BRAIN

There is a considerable number of inborn errors of metabolism, in each of which one particular enzyme is lacking[73]. This block in metabolism causes one or more amino acids, which cannot be metabolized in the normal manner, to accumulate in the blood. The levels of these amino acids in the blood may reach 20–40 times the normal level. This imbalance in the blood will alter the supply of amino acids to the brain. Large quantities of the accumulating amino acids will enter the brain, while the quantities of some other amino acids entering the brain will be reduced by competitive inhibition.

Phenylketonuria (PKU), the first aminoacidaemia to be thoroughly investigated

The progress which has been made during the last 15 years in the diagnosis and treatment of a number of inborn errors affecting amino acid metabolism is based, to a large extent, upon the experience gained in the treatment of one disease, phenylketonuria (PKU). Over the years a general strategy for the treatment of this disease has been worked out. The success of treatment depends greatly upon detecting the affected babies very early in life and the institution of suitable screening methods has dramatically increased the numbers which are found. Fortunately, if treatment is started really early in life the biochemical changes which would interfere with the normal development not only of the brain, but also of the body, can be prevented.

In the untreated phenylketonuric, phenylalanine accumulates in the blood because there is a metabolic defect in the initial step in its catabolism (i.e. in its conversion into tyrosine), so that levels of 1–1.2 nmol/l of phenylalanine in the blood plasma may be reached. The normal level is 0.04–0.12 nmol/l of plasma. Ideally, an infant should be given no more phenylalanine than the body needs for growth, which is about 50–100 mg/kg daily during the first year. If such a correctly regulated intake could be attained, phenylalanine should not accumulate in the blood. Thus, the original aim of the treatment of PKU was to restrict the intake of phenylalanine in the diet to such an extent as to bring its level in the blood back to within the normal range[74-76].

It was found that the treatment of a child suffering from PKU by means of a diet very low in phenylalanine was extremely effective: in a matter of days the general condition and mental awareness improved. However, it was soon realized that a diet which achieved a blood level of phenylalanine below the normal range could be dangerous (and placed an impossible burden upon biochemical monitoring resources) if the reduction in the level of phenylalanine in the blood was all too easily carried too far, as this led to a deficiency of phenylalanine. Not only does a deficiency restrict growth, but it can also cause other serious effects. The ill-effects of excessively low levels of phenylalanine in the blood have been described in children who have been wrongly diagnosed as having PKU[77] and also in children suffering from PKU whose blood level of phenylalanine has been excessively reduced[78,79]. A common feature of phenylalanine deficiency is a bright red rash, refractory to local treatment. Even if a severe deficiency does not prove to be fatal, prolonged low blood levels of phenylalanine impair mental development[80]. Despite the problem posed by the difficulty in maintaining the optimum level of phenylalanine in the blood, there is no longer any question that restriction of phenylalanine in the diet has proved highly effective as a treatment for PKU. It has led to the prevention of the brain damage which is seen in untreated PKU, especially now that improvement in screening methods has made it possible to begin giving the diet early in life. It is, however, a difficult undertaking to maintain a patient upon a strictly controlled diet from the neonatal period until late adolescence and Clayton[81] has drawn attention to some of the problems which may arise:

1. 'The diet, although as satisfactory as present knowledge permits, may nonetheless not be ideal for the growth and development of the infant and the child.'

2. 'Phenylalanine deficiency can of itself lead to intellectual impairment and must be avoided'.

3. 'A strict diet causes emotional problems in the patient and his family'.

The evolving strategy of dietary treatment for maintaining a satisfactory blood level of phenylalanine

In order to meet the difficulties in maintaining a satisfactory level of phenylalanine in the blood, there has been, over the last 20 years or so, a change in the strategy adopted. As knowledge has increased the recommended level of phenylalanine in the blood has been raised. Thus, in the early 1960s a range of 0.06–0.33 mmol/l of plasma was commonly recommended, whereas during the last 15 years higher ranges have been allowed, e.g. 0.12–0.24 mmol/l of plasma[82]; 0.18–0.42[83]; 0.30–0.91[84]; 0.24–0.48[85]; 0.18–0.48[81]. Important evidence about the treatment of PKU was provided by the American 8-year collaborative study which showed that there were no differences in IQ or in mental performance between two groups of patients suffering from PKU, both groups having received treatment from an early age. In one group the aim was to keep the level of phenylalanine in the blood between 0.06 and 0.30 mmol/l of plasma; in the other group a higher range was allowed, 0.33–0.61 mmol/l[86]. The advantages of using the diet which gave the higher range of blood levels are that dietary control can be less strict and that the danger of a deficiency of phenylalanine is more remote than when the diet giving the lower range is used.

What causes the damage in PKU?

In PKU the most severe organic damage to the brain occurs early in life and is associated with high levels of phenylalanine in the blood. That cerebral damage occurs is indicated by a low brain weight, defects in myelination and sponginess of the white matter[87]. Although blood levels of phenylalanine of over 1.2 mmol/l are associated with brain damage in PKU, it is not clear how dangerous are levels between 0.6 and 1.2 mmol/l of plasma[81,85].

One of the difficulties experienced in keeping the phenylalanine levels within tolerable limits in treated cases is that unforeseen fluctuations may occur in the blood concentration, so that levels may be reduced excessively or raised to a dangerous extent. Vomiting or refusal to take the diet would lead to the phenylalanine in the blood dropping to too low a level. On the other hand, an infection or other illness may lead to breakdown of body protein which will release phenylalanine; or the child may take more food than is allowed and thus cause the blood phenylalanine to rise to too high a level for safety.

It is becoming clear that damage to the brain in PKU is largely, if not entirely, a direct consequence of the raised level of phenylalanine in the blood. It seems likely that the abnormalities which are found in the structure of the brain in PKU, such as the reduced myelination of tracts and the gliosis and spongy degeneration of the cerebral white matter, occur because the brain is being deprived of one or more amino acids. This is caused by the high level of phenylalanine in the blood which interferes with the transport of other amino acids across the blood–brain barrier. In addition, it seems likely that the more easily reversible changes in the brain which cause children with PKU to develop behavioural problems or to become psychotic[88,89] are due to abnormalities in the metabolism of neurotransmitters within the brain. Such abnormalities may be due either to a lack of tyrosine or tryptophan or to an excess of phenylalanine within the brain cells.

The danger that the brain will be deprived of certain amino acids in PKU

There are about a dozen or more amino acids which the brain obtains from the blood in order to make cerebral protein or for other synthetic purposes. These amino acids normally enter the brain only a little faster (some 2 to 3 times) than they are being used by the cerebral cells (Table 5.2). The surplus, which returns to the bloodstream by efflux, provides a margin of safety. When the level of phenylalanine in the blood is high it will interfere with the transport of these other amino acids into the brain by competing for the transport carrier on the surface membrane of the endothelial cells of the cerebral capillaries. Under certain conditions this interference will be severe (Table 5.4) and the brain will be partially deprived of some of the amino acids that it needs. If the brain cells were not using amino acids, this competitive inhibition would not matter as amino acid levels in the brain would eventually follow changes in the blood, even if delayed. It is particularly when the brain cells are rapidly using amino acids, e.g. to make protein, that the danger of deprivation by inhibition of transport is severe. We now know enough about the transport of neutral amino acids across the blood–brain barrier to assess whether such deprivation is likely to play a part in causing the defective brain development which is seen in untreated cases of PKU, and in increasing the degree of mental retardation which is seen in older children. Although it is not possible to measure the kinetic parameters of transport across the blood–brain barrier in children with PKU, the similarity between the parameters found in various mammals, e.g. the rat, mouse and rabbit[19,66,69] make it reasonable to assume that they will not be very different from those given in Table 5.3, which have been calculated for the human. On this basis it is clear that the influx into the brain of several amino acids, especially methionine, tryptophan and histidine, will be reduced much below the normal in children with PKU (Figure 5.6).

TABLE 5.4   Conditions in which competitive inhibition of the carrier-mediated transport of one particular amino acid across the blood–brain barrier may endanger the brain through deprivation of an important nutrient

	Concentration in the blood	Affinity for the carrier*	Rate of use by the brain	Rate of diffusion across blood–brain barrier
Amino acid	low	low	high	low
Inhibitor	high	high	—	—

* A low affinity for the carrier means a high value of the affinity constant, K, and vice versa, see equation (1)

Some problems in the dietary treatment of PKU

It is difficult to know how long a child should be compelled to keep to a strict diet. Although most of the cerebral nerve cells are formed soon

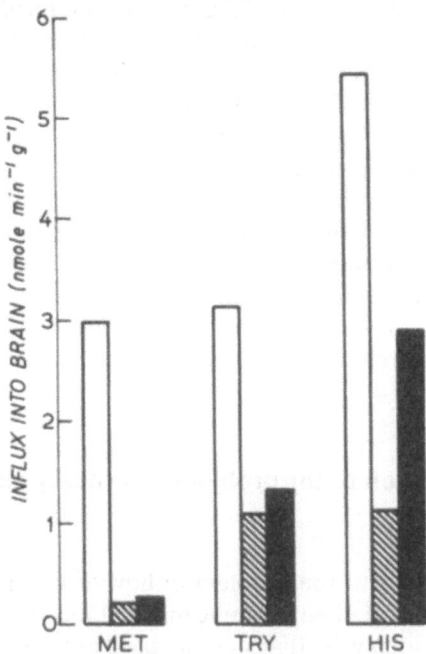

Figure 5.6 The estimated influx into the brain of the three amino acids, methionine, MET, tryptophan, TRY, and histidine, HIS, in normal children, ▭, in children with phenylketonuria who are on a normal diet,▨ and in children with phenylketonuria who are on a diet low in phenylalanine, ▬

after birth[90], myelination continues until the age of 15–20 years[8]. In practice a strictly controlled diet is usually abandoned well before adolescence because of the severe psychological difficulties of keeping to it, but Clayton[81] advises that older patients should limit their intake of first class protein to prevent excessive rises in the blood phenylalanine level. It is possible that some sort of controlled diet (e.g. like that suggested below) should be maintained for much longer than the strict diets of the past.

A further problem has now been added to the question of the dietary treatment of PKU by the very success of the screening programmes and dietary control from about 1955 onwards. This is that girls born with PKU who were treated in childhood are now adult women of fairly normal intelligence, and are reaching child-bearing age[91]. These women pose a new and more serious therapeutic problem, for there is amongst the offspring of mothers with PKU a very high incidence of severe congenital abnormalities, including microcephaly and growth retardation with an IQ commonly of below 80[91–93]. This damage to the metabolically normal foetus is caused by the high level of phenylalanine which crosses the placental barrier[94] and it can be prevented by maintaining the mother on a strict diet during pregnancy.

Practically all the difficulties in the dietary treatment of PKU arise because the range of the safe level of phenylalanine in the blood is so narrow. Because of natural fluctuations in the level of phenylalanine in the circulation, the safety margin is too small. The dietary treatment of any other metabolic defect in which one or more amino acids tend to accumulate in the circulation is equally difficult, for similar reasons.

A possible solution to the problem of an acceptable and safe diet in PKU

A possible solution to the problem of how to obtain a wider margin of safety for the level of phenylalanine in the blood was first suggested by us in 1974[57,58]. The idea was, that since a raised level of phenylalanine in the blood caused the partial exclusion of other amino acids from the brain, supplements of these excluded amino acids should be added to the diet, so as to raise their levels in the circulation. Thus the monopolization of the carrier by phenylalanine is overcome, the margin of safety of the phenylalanine level is widened considerably, and the diet need not be so strictly controlled. That such an approach is likely to be effective, is shown by the findings of Snyderman et al.[95] who found that feeding a specially devised amino-acid mixture to patients lacking the enzyme arginase, gave better results than did simple restriction, while Anderson and Avins[96] found that supplementing the diet of rats made phenylketonuric with other large neutral amino acids prevented the phenylalanine content of the brain from rising to high levels. Following our suggestion, supplements of the branched-chain amino acids, isoleucine, leucine and valine have been given to PKU patients by Berry et al.[97]. Brouwer et al.[98] have reported that a high dietary intake of tyrosine (one of the amino acids most likely to be excluded from the brain by a high level of phenylalanine in the blood) is desirable in the treatment of PKU. Ways in which such supplementation can be carried out have been considered by Kaufman[99] and Christensen[65]. Recently-developed methods for assessing the competition between amino acids for transport across the blood–

brain barrier[49,66,100] have made more precise recommendations for improved treatment possible[101].

The advantages of maintaining a high intake of amino acids other than phenylalanine in the treatment of PKU

A raised level of phenylalanine in the blood deprives the brain of its normal supplies of various essential amino acids, e.g. methionine. This deprivation is brought about in different ways.

Firstly, the absorption from the gut of these amino acids is impeded since the high levels of phenylalanine in the bile and the digestive juices are likely to monopolize the transport carrier in the intestinal wall; this transport is largely carrier-mediated[102,103]. The competitive inhibition caused by the high level of phenylalanine will slow down the absorption of other netural amino acids from the gut, especially tryptophan and tyrosine[104]. Low levels of methionine, tryptophan, histidine and tyrosine in the blood of patients with PKU have been reported by Effron et al.[105] and Smith et al.[80]. The low levels of these amino acids are dangerous for various reasons. The lack of a sufficient quantity of even one single essential amino acid in the blood will not only interfere with the normal growth of both brain and body, but also cause protein catabolism, especially in muscles[64,106,106a], which will lead to a sharp rise in the level of phenylalanine in the blood. However, if there is an adequate, or raised, intake of the amino acids listed in Table 5.5, their increased level in the gut contents will overcome the competitive inhibition caused by phenylalanine, of their transport across the intestinal wall. In this way a better supply of these amino acids will enter the bloodstream and thus the dangerously low levels which are found in PKU, will be avoided.

A further advantage of a high intake of the amino acids listed in Table 5.5 is that they will compete with phenylalanine for transport by the carrier in the intestinal wall and thus will slow down the absorption of phenylalanine. This slowing down of the absorption of phenylalanine will be especially advantageous when there is an uncontrolled intake of this amino acid such as will occur when an unprescribed meat meal is eaten. The slowed absorption of phenylalanine will reduce the size of the transient peak in the level of phenylalanine in the blood which has been found 1–4 h after an oral load of this amino acid[107].

If a high level of the amino acids listed in Table 5.5 is maintained in the blood, their rate of transport across the blood–brain barrier will be increased, since they will partially overcome the inhibitory effect,

TABLE 5.5   **Proposed supplements to a low phenylalanine diet for patients with phenylketonuria***

Amino acid	Desirable levels in the circulation (μmol/l of plasma)	Suggested supplement to low phenylalanine diet (mg/kg body weight daily)
Threonine	200–400	—
Serine	150–300	—
Glycine	400–800	—
Alanine	400–800	—
Valine	200–400	25–50
Methionine	75–150	50–100
Isoleucine	100–200	25–50
Leucine	150–300	25–50
Tyrosine	100–200	50–100
Phenylalanine	250–900	—
Histidine	125–250	50–100
Tryptophan	80–160†	50–100
Lysine	200–400	—
Arginine	100–200	25–50

* The approximate levels at which each of the nutritionally important amino acids should be maintained in the blood are given, as are the supplements of each amino acid which should be added to a diet low in phenylalanine, based on commercial amino acid mixtures such as those suggested in reference 80.
† Total tryptophan, i.e. free tryptophan plus that which is bound to blood albumin

equation (1), of the high level of phenylalanine in the circulation (Figure 5.5). This will eliminate the risk that the brain will be deprived of any of these amino acids.

Again, as in the case of the gut, the inhibitory effect of the amino acids listed in Table 5.5 on the transport of phenylalanine across the blood–brain barrier, equation (1), will slow down the entry of phenylalanine into the brain, and will prevent the level of this amino acid in the brain from rising to too high a level when there are unexpected rises in the blood level, as with an uncontrolled intake of protein, rich in phenylalanine.

In cases of maternal PKU, it is likely that a diet which supplied a high intake of the amino acids listed in Table 5.5 will be most successful in preventing damage to the foetus and allowing the production of a normal child. There will be beneficial effects upon the absorption of the essential amino acids, and the better balance of amino acids in the mother's circulation will give the foetus a more balanced supply across the placenta. Here again, the passage of amino acids across the placenta takes place[108] by carrier-mediated processes, like those which are found in the blood–brain barrier and in the intestinal wall. The effect of a diet with supplements should be to avoid any deficiencies in the foetal circulation of the amino acids listed in Table 5.5. It should also limit any increase in the phenylalanine level in the foetal circulation after any abnormal rise in the level of this amino acid in the mother's bloodstream. Thus, the foetus and its brain should develop normally.

In summary, there is a series of four consecutive processes: transport across the intestinal wall, transport across each of the two parts of the blood–brain barrier, the endothelial cell and the surface membranes of the brain cells, and a final process in which amino acids enter into cerebral metabolism, e.g. protein synthesis. In maternal PKU an additional process is interposed, namely, transport across the placental barrier. In each of these processes competition between neutral amino acids for a shared carrier operates and the effects of any imbalance of amino acids will be cumulative. Increasing the amounts of the amino acids listed in Table 5.5 in the food intake will redress the amino acid imbalance at the starting point of this series of processes and will have a normalizing action because of its cumulative effect throughout the series.

Evidence for the advantages of maintaining as normal as possible a ratio of other amino acids to phenylalanine in the intestinal lumen at the start of this series is provided by the general experience of those treating PKU, that a protein-free diet, which would produce an abnormally high ratio of phenylalanine to other amino acids, has no place in treatment and is almost always ill-advised[111]. Failure to achieve improvement by increasing the intake of tyrosine alone or even of two or three amino acids is not unexpected, since brain damage will occur if only one amino acid is excluded. It is absolutely essential that the intake of all amino acids likely to be excluded should be raised (Table 5.5).

Acknowledgements

The work reported here was carried out with the aid of grants from the Wellcome and Kennedy Trusts and the National Fund for Research into Crippling Diseases.

References

1. Mann, F. C. and Magath, T. B. (1922). Studies on the physiology of the liver. III The effect of administration of glucose in the condition following total extirpation of the liver. *Arch. Intern. Med.*, **30**, 171

2. Harris, S. (1936). The diagnosis and treatment of hyperinsulinism. *Ann. Intern. Med.*, **19**, 514

3. Seta, K., Sansur, M. and Lajtha, A. (1973). The rate of incorporation of amino acids into brain protein during infusion in the rat. *Biochim. Biophys. Acta*, **294**, 472

4. Lajtha, A. (1974). Amino acid transport in the brain *in vivo* and *in vitro*. In G. E. W. Wolstenholme and D. W. Fitzsimons (eds), *Aromatic Amino Acids in the Brain*, pp. 25–41. Ciba Foundation Symposium (new series). (Amsterdam: Elsevier)

5. Ochs, S. and Worth, R. M. (1978). Axoplasmic transport in normal and pathological systems. In S. G. Waxman (ed.), *Physiology and Pathobiology of Axons*, pp. 251–264. (New York: Raven Press)

6. Lajtha, A., Marks, N. and Teller, D. (1973). In S. Bogoch (ed.), *Biological Diagnosis of Brain Disorders*, pp. 103–118. (New York: Spectrum)

7. Benjamins, J. A. and Morrell, P. (1978). Proteins of myelin and their metabolism. *Neurochem. Res.*, **3**, 137

8. Davison, A. N. (1970). *Myelination*. (Illinois: Thomas)

9. Aspillaga, M. O. and McDermott, J. R. (1977). The N^G-methylated arginine content of rat myelin during development. *J. Neurochem.*, **28**, 1147

10. Odessey, R. and Goldberg, A. L. (1972). Oxidation of leucine by rat skeletal muscle. *Am. J. Physiol.*, **223**, 1376

11. Daniel, P. M., Donaldson, J. and Pratt, O. E. (1974). The rapid achievement and maintenance of a steady level of an injected substance in the blood plasma. *J. Physiol.*, **237**, 8P

12. Daniel, P. M., Donaldson, J. and Pratt, O. E. (1975). A method for injecting substances into the circulation to reach rapidly and to maintain a steady level. *Med. Biol. Eng.*, **13**, 214

13. Daniel, P. M., Donaldson, J. and Pratt, O. E. (1976). Infusion schedules for prescribed blood concentration time courses. *J. Appl. Physiol.*, **41**, 608

14. Donaldson, J. and Pratt, O. E. (1975). A method for displaying the effect of altering the constants of a function and an application to the problem of maintaining steady blood concentrations. *J. Physiol.*, **252**, 5P.

15. Pratt, O. E. (1974). An electronically controlled syringe drive for giving an injection at a variable rate according to a preset programme. *J. Physiol.*, **237**, 5P

16. Oldendorf, W. H. (1971). Brain uptake of radiolabeled amino acids, amines and hexoses after arterial injection. *Am. J. Physiol.*, **221**, 1629

17. Oldendorf, W. H. (1973). Saturation of blood–brain barrier transport of amino acids in phenylketonuria. *Arch. Neurol.*, **28**, 45

18. Yudilevich, D. L., de Rose, N. and Sepúlveda, F. V. (1972). Facilitated transport of amino acids through the blood–brain barrier of the dog studied in a single capillary circulation. *Brain Res.*, **44**, 569

19. Pratt, O. E. (1979). Adequate nutrition of the developing brain. In R. Korobkin and C. Guilleminault (eds), *Advances in Perinatal Neurology*, Vol. 1, pp. 21–55. (New York: Spectrum)

20. Borman, A., Wood, T. R., Black, H. C., Anderson, E. G., Oesterling, M. J., Womack, M. and Rose, W. C. (1946). The role of arginine in

growth with some observations on the effects of argininic acid. *J. Biol. Chem.*, **166**, 585

21. Rose, W. C. and Cox, G. J. (1924). The relation of arginine and histidine to growth. *J. Biol. Chem.*, **61**, 747

22. Rose, W. C., Oesterling, M. J. and Womack, M. (1948). Comparative growth on diets containing ten and nineteen amino acids with further observations upon the role of glutamic and aspartic acids. *J. Biol. Chem.*, **176**, 753

23. Shank, R. P. and Aprison, M. H. (1970). The metabolism *in vivo* of glycine and serine in eight areas of rat central nervous system. *J. Neurochem.*, **17**, 1461

24. Baños, G., Daniel, P. M., Moorhouse, S. R. and Pratt, O. E. (1975). The requirements of the brain for some amino acids. *J. Physiol.*, **246**, 539

25. Balász, R. (1965). Control of glutamate metabolism. The effect of pyruvate. *J. Neurochem.*, **12**, 63

26. Levin, B. (1971). Hereditary metabolic disorders of the urea cycle. In O. Bodansky and A. L. Latner (eds), *Advances in Clinical Chemistry*, pp. 65–143. (New York: Academic Press)

27. Baños, G., Daniel, P. M., Moorhouse, S. R. and Pratt, O. E. (1973). The influx of amino acids into the brain of the rat *in vivo:* the essential compared with some non-essential amino acids. *Proc. R. Soc. Lond.*, **B183**, 59

28. Baños, G., Daniel, P. M., Moorhouse, S. R. and Pratt, O. E. (1971). The entry of amino acids into the brain of the rat during the post-natal period. *J. Physiol.*, **213**, 45P.

29. Baños, G., Daniel, P. M. and Pratt, O. E. (1978). The effect of age upon the entry of some amino acids into the brain, and their incorporation into cerebral protein. *Devel. Med. Child Neurol.*, **20**, 335

30. Ehrlich, P. (1885). *Das Sauerstoff- Bedurfnis des Organismus – Eine Farbendanalytische Studie.*, p. 69. (Berlin: Hirshwald)

31. Goldmann, E. E. (1909). Die aussere und innere Sekretion des gesunden und kranken Organismus in Lichte der 'vitalen Farbung'. *Beitr. Klin. Chirurg.*, **64**, 192

32. Quastel, J. H., Tennenbaum, M. and Wheatley, A. H. M. (1936). Choline esterase formation in, and choline esterase activities of tissues *in vitro*. *Biochem. J.*, **30**, 1668

33. Rafaelson, M. E., Winzler, R. J. and Pearson, H. E. (1949). The effects of Theiler's GDVII virus on the incorporation of radioactive carbon from glucose into minced one-day-old mouse brain. *J. Biol. Chem.*, **181**, 595

34. Widdas, W. F. (1952). Inability of diffusion to account for placental glucose transfer in the sheep and consideration of the kinetics of a possible carrier transfer. *J. Physiol.*, **118**, 23

35. Dixon, M. and Webb, E. C. (1964). *Enzymes*, 2nd Edn., pp. 318–320. (London: Longmans).

36. Christensen, H. N. (1977). Implications of the cellular transport step for amino acid metabolism. *Nutr. Rev.*, **35**, 129

37. Christensen, H. N. (1976). Metabolite transport at cell membranes. In G. Levi, L. Battistin and A. Lajtha (eds), *Transport Phenomena in the*

Nervous System: Physiological and Pathological Aspects, pp. 3–12. (New York: Plenum)

38. Rapoport, S. I. (1976). Blood–Brain Barrier in Physiology and Medicine. (New York: Raven Press)

39. Lajtha, A. (1964). Protein metabolism of the nervous system. Int. Rev. Neurobiol., 6, 1

40. Goldstein, G. W., Wolinsky, J. S. and Csejtey, J. (1977). Isolated brain capillaries: a model for the study of lead encephalopathy. Ann. Neurol., 1, 235

41. Brightman, M. W. and Reese, T. S. (1969). Junctions between intimately apposed cell membranes in the vertebrate brain. J. Cell Biol., 40, 648

42. Baños, G., Daniel, P. M., Moorhouse, S. R. and Pratt, O. E. (1970). The passage of amino acids into the rat's brain. J. Physiol., 210, 149P

43. Bauman, A., Bourgoin, S., Benda, P., Glowinski, J. and Hamon, M. (1974). Characteristics of tryptophan accumulation by glial cells. Brain Res., 66, 253

44. Archer, E. G. and Breakefield, X. (1974). Transport of tyrosine and phenylalanine in cultured neuroblastoma cells. Trans. Am. Soc. Neurochem., 5, 98

45. Sershen, H. and Lajtha, A. (1979). Inhibition pattern by analogs indicates the presence of ten or more transport systems for amino acids in brain cells. J. Neurochem., 32, 719

46. Christensen, H. N. (1975). Biological Transport.(New York: Benjamin)

47. Baños, G., Daniel, P. M. and Pratt, O. E. (1971). Inhibition of entry of L-arginine into the brain of the rat, in vivo, by L-lysine or L-ornithine. J. Physiol., 214, 24P.

48. Baños, G., Daniel, P. M. and Pratt, O. E. (1974). Saturation of a shared mechanism which transports L-arginine and L-lysine into the brain of the living rat. J. Physiol., 236, 29

49. Pratt, O. E. (1976). The transport of metabolizable substances into the living brain. In G. Levi, L. Battistin and A. Lajtha (eds), Transport Phenomena in the Nervous System: Physiological and Pathological Aspects, pp. 55–75. (New York: Plenum Press)

50. Daniel, P. M., Love, E. R., and Pratt, O.E. (1979). Insulin-sensitive transport of alanine across the blood–retinal barrier. J. Physiol., 291, 41P

51. Pappenheimer, J. R. and Setchell, B. P. (1973). Cerebral glucose transport and oxygen consumption in sheep and rabbits. J. Physiol., 233, 529

52. Rodriguez, E. M. (1976). The cerebrospinal fluid as a pathway in neuroendocrine integration. J. Endocrinol., 71, 407

52a. Bradbury, M. (1979) The Concept of a Blood–Brain Barrier. (Chichester, New York, Brisbane, Toronto: John Wiley)

53. Wislocki, G. B., and Leduc, E. H. (1952). Vital staining of the hematoencephalic barrier by silver nitrate and trypan blue, and cytological comparisons of the neurohypophysis, pineal body, area postrema, intercolumnar tubercle and supraoptic crest. J. Comp. Neurol., 96, 371

54. Daniel, P. M., Pratt, O. E. and Wilson, P. A. (1977). The influx of isoleucine into the cerebral hemispheres and cerebellum: carrier-mediated transport and diffusion. Q. J. Exp. Physiol., 62, 163

55. Daniel, P. M., Pratt, O. E. and Wilson, P. A. (1977). The transport of

L-leucine into the brain of the rat *in vivo* – saturable and non-saturable components of influx. *Proc. R. Soc. Lond.*, **B196**, 333

56. Daniel, P. M., Pratt, O. E. and Wilson, P. A. (1977). The exclusion of L-isoleucine or L-leucine from the brain of the rat, caused by raised levels of L-valine in the circulation, and the manner in which this exclusion can be partially overcome. *J. Neurol. Sci.*, **31**, 421

57. Baños, G., Daniel, P. M., Moorhouse, S. R. and Pratt, O. E. (1974). Inhibition of entry of some amino acids into the brain, with observations on mental retardation in the aminoacidurias. *Psychol. Med.*, **4**, 262

58. Baños, G., Daniel, P. M., Moorhouse, S. R. and Pratt, O. E. (1974). Inhibition of neutral amino acid entry into the ·brain of the rat *in vivo*. *J. Physiol.*, **237**, 22P

59. Crockett, M. E., Daniel, P. M., Love, E. R., Moorhouse, S. R. and Pratt, O. E. (1977). Exchange of nutritional substances between blood and brain. *J. Physiol.* **27**, 24P

60. Christensen, H. N. (1953). Metabolism of amino acids and proteins, *Ann. Rev. Biochem.*, **22**, 235

60a. Daniel, P. M., Moorhouse, S. R. and Pratt, O. E. (1978). Post-natal changes in the transport of aromatic amino acids into the brain. *J. Physiol.*, **284**, 42P

61. Love, E. R., (1981). This volume, chapter 6

62. Sershen, H. and Lajtha, A. (1976). Perinatal changes of transport systems for amino acids in slices of mouse brain. *Neurochem. Res.*, **1**, 417

63. Neame, K. D. (1968). A comparison of the transport systems for amino acids in the brain, intestine, kidney and tumour. *Prog. Brain Res.*, **29**, 188

64. Daniel, P. M., Pratt, O. E. and Spargo, E. (1977). The metabolic homoeostatic role of muscle and its function as a store of protein. *Lancet*, **ii**, 446

65. Christensen, H. N. (1979). Developments in amino acid transport, illustrated for the blood–brain barrier. *Biochem. Pharmacol.*, **28**, 1989

66. Pratt, O. E. (1979). Kinetics of tryptophan transport across the blood–brain barrier. *J. Neural Trans. Supplement* **15**, 29

67. Daniel, P. M., Moorhouse, S. R. and Pratt, O. E. (1976). Amino acid precursors of monoamine neurotransmitters and some factors influencing their supply to the brain. *Psychol. Med.*, **6**, 277

68. Marsden, C. D. and Parkes, J. D. (1976). "On–off" effects in patients with Parkinson's disease on chronic levadopa therapy. *Lancet*, **i**, 292

69. Daniel, P. M., Love, E. R., Moorhouse, S. R. and Pratt, O. E. (1981). The effect of insulin upon the influx of tryptophan into the brain of the rabbit. *J. Physiol.*, **312**, 551

70. Munro, H. N., Fernstrom, J. D. and Wurtman, R. J. (1975). Insulin plasma amino acid imbalance and hepatic coma. *Lancet*, **i**, 722

71. Wurtman, R. J. and Fernstrom, J. D. (1972). L-tryptophan, L-tyrosine, and the control of brain monoamine biosynthesis. In S. N. Snyder (ed.), *Perspectives in Neuropharmacology*, pp. 143–193. (New York: Oxford University Press)

72. Daniel, P. M., Moorhouse, S. R. and Pratt, O. E. (1978). Partial exclusion of tryptophan from the brain due to saturation of the transport carrier. *J. Physiol.*, **282**, 9P

72a. Crockett, M. E., Daniel, P. M. and Pratt, O. E. (1976). Competition between some neutral amino acids for carrier-mediated transport into the brain *in vivo*. *J. Physiol.*, **263**, 206P

73. Stanbury, J. B., Wyngaarten, J. B. and Fredrickson, D. S. (1978). *The Metabolic Basis of Inherited Disease*, 4th edn. (New York: McGraw Hill)

74. Bickel, H., Gerrard, J. and Hickmans, E. M. (1953). Influence of phenylalanine intake on phenylketonuria. *Lancet*, **ii**, 812

75. Hsia, D. Y-Y. (1959) *Inborn Errors of Metabolism*, p. 111. (Chicago: Yearbook Publishers)

76. Woolf, L. I., Griffiths, R. and Moncrieff, A. (1955). Treatment of phenylketonuria with a diet low in phenylalanine. *Br. Med. J.*, **i**, 57

77. Rouse, B. M. (1966). Phenylalanine deficiency syndrome. *J. Pediatr.*, **69**, 246

78. Fisch, R. O., Walerk, W. A. and Anderson, J. A. (1966). Prenatal and postnatal developmental consequences of maternal phenylketonuria. *Pediatrics*, **37**, 979

79. Pitt, D. (1971). "Normal" untreated PKUs. In Cohen, B. E., M. I. Rubin and A. Szeinberg (eds), *Proc. Internat. Symp. on Phenylketonuria and Allied Disorders*, p. 287. (Tel-Aviv: Translators Pool)

80. Smith, I., Francis, D. E. M., Clayton, B. E. and Wolff, O. H. (1975). Comparison of an amino acid mixure and protein hydrolysates in treatment of infants with phenylketonuria. *Arch. Dis. Child.*, **50**, 864

81. Clayton, B. M. (1975). The principles of treatment by dietary restriction as illustrated by phenylketonuria. In D. N. Raine (ed.) *The Treatment of Inherited Metabolic Disease*, pp. 1–32. (Lancaster: MTP Press)

82. Clayton, B., Francis, D. and Moncrieff, A. (1965). A method for feeding the phenylketonuric infant. *Br. Med. J.*, **i**, 54

83. Bickel, H. (1970). Phenylalaninaemia or classical phenylketonuria (PKU). *Neuropädiatrie*, **1**, 379

84. Hanley W. B. Linsao, L., Davidson, W, and Moes, C. A. F. (1970). Malnutrition with early treatment of phenylketonuria. *Paediatr. Res.*, **4**, 318

85. Blaskovics, M. E. (1974). Phenylketonuria and other phenylalaninemias. In H. Bickel (ed.), *Congenital and Acquired Diseases of Amino Acid Metabolism*, pp. 87–105. (London: Saunders)

86. Williamson, M., Koch, R. and Dobson, J. C. (1973). *PKU Collaborative Study – Current Status*. A report presented at the 3rd IASSMD Congress, The Hague, The Netherlands

87. Crome, L. and Pare, C. M. B. (1960). Phenylketonuria: a review and a report of the pathological findings in four cases. *J. Ment. Sci.*, **106**, 862.

88. Knox, W. E. (1978). Phenylketonuria. In J. B. Stanbury, J. B. Wyngaarden and D. S. Fredrickson (eds), *The Metabolic Basis of Inherited Disease*, 4th Edn, Chap. 11, pp. 266–295. (New York: McGraw-Hill)

89. Crome, L. and Stern, J. (1972). *Pathology of Mental Retardation*, 2nd Edn. (Edinburgh: Churchill Livingstone)

90. Dobbing, J. (1974). The later development of the central nervous system and its vulnerability. In J. A. Davis and J. Dobbing (eds), *Scientific Foundations of Pediatrics*, pp. 565–577. (London: Heinemann).

91. Komrower, G. M., Sardharwalla, I. B., Coutts, J. M. J. and Ingham, D.

(1979). Management of maternal phenylketonuria: an emerging clinical problem. *Br. Med. J.*, **i**, 1383

92. Hsia, D. Y-Y. (1970). Phenylketonuria and its variants. *Prog. Med. Genet.*, **7**, 29

93. Angeli, E., Denman, A. R., Harris, R. F., Kirman, B. H. and Stern, J. (1974). Maternal phenylketonuria: a family with seven mentally retarded siblings. *Devel. Med. Child Neurol.*, **16**, 800

94. Kerr, G. R., Chamore, A. S., Harlow, A. S. and Waisman, H. A. (1968). Fetal PKU: the effect of maternal hyperphenylalanemia during pregnancy in the rhesus monkey (*Macaca mulatta*). *Pediatrics*, **42**, 27

95. Snyderman, S. E., Sansaricq, C., Chen, W. J., Norton, P. M. and Phansalkar, S. V. (1977). Argininemia. *J. Pediatr.*, **90**, 563

96. Anderson, A. E. and Avins, L. (1976). Lowering brain phenylalanine levels by giving other large neutral amino acids. A new experimental therapeutic approach to phenylketonuria. *Arch. Neurol.*, **33**, 684

97. Berry, H. K., Butcher, R. E., Brunner, R. L., Bray, N. W., Hunt, M. M. and Wharton, C. H. (1977). New approaches to treatment of phenylketonuria. In P. Mittler (ed.) *Research to Practice in Mental Retardation.*, *Vol. III, Biomedical Aspects*, p. 229. (Baltimore, London, Tokyo: University Park Press)

98. Brouwer, M., de Bree, P. K., van Sprang, F. J. and Wadman, S. K. (1977). Low serum-tyrosine in patients with phenylketonuria on dietary treatment. *Lancet*, **i**, 1162

99. Kaufman, S. (1977). Properties of pterin-dependent aromatic amino acid hydroxylases. In G. E. W. Wolstenholme and D. W. Fitzsimons (eds), *Aromatic Amino Acids in the Brain*, p. 85. (Amsterdam: Elsevier)

100. Pardridge, W. M. (1977). Regulation of amino acid availability to the brain. In R. Wurtman and J. J. Wurtman (eds), *Nutrition and the Brain*, p. 141 (New York: Raven Press)

101. Pratt, O. E. (1980). A new approach to the treatment of phenylketonuria. *J. Ment. Defic. Res.*, **24**, 203

102. Matthews, D. M. and Laster, L. (1965). Competition for intestinal transport among five neutral amino acids. *Am. J. Physiol.*, **208**, 601

103. Schultz, S. G. and Frizzell, R. A. (1975). Amino acid transport by the small intestine. In T. Z. Csáky (ed.), *Intestinal Absorption and Malabsorption*, pp. 77–93. (New York: Raven Press)

104. Yarbro, M. T. and Anderson, J. A. (1966). L-Tryptophan metabolism in phenylketonuria. *J. Pediatr.*, **68**, 895

105. Efron, M. L., Kang, E. S., Visakorpi, J. and Fellers, F. X. (1969). Effect of elevated plasma phenylalanine levels on other amino acids in phenylketonuric and normal subjects. *J. Pediatr.*, **74**, 399

106. Daniel, P. M., Pratt, O. E. and Spargo, E. (1977). The mechanism by which glucagon induces the release of amino acids from muscle and its relevance to fasting. *Proc. R. Soc. Lond.*, **B196**, 347

106a. Spargo, E., Pratt, O. E. and Daniel, P. M. (1979). Metabolic functions of skeletal muscles of man, mammals, birds and fishes. *J. R. Soc. Med.*, **72**, 921

107. Güttler, F. and Wamberg, E. (1977). Fasting serum phenylalanine in

untreated institutionalised patients with phenylketonuria. *J. Ment. Def. Res.*, **21**, 55

108. Young, M. (1979). Transfer of amino acids. In G. V. P. Chamberlain and A. W. Wilkinson (eds), *Placental Transfer*, pp. 142–158. (Tunbridge Wells: Pitman Medical Publishing)

109. Weiser, M., Riederer, P. and Kleinberger, G. (1978). Human cerebral free amino acids in hepatic coma. *J. Neural Trans., Supplement* 14, 95

110. Crockett, M. E., Daniel, P. M. and Pratt, O. E. (1978). A comparison of the transport systems which carry L-methionine across the blood–retinal and blood–brain barriers. *J. Physiol.*, **280**, 39P.

111. Francis, D. E. M. (1974). *Diets for Sick Children*. 3rd Edn. (Oxford: Blackwell Scientific Publications)

112. Pratt, O. E. (1980). The transport of nutrients into the brain: the effect of alcohol on their supply and utilisation. In D. Richter (ed.), *Addiction and Brain Damage*, pp. 94–128. (Croom Helm: London)

6

Some aspects of the transport of glucose and ketone bodies into the brain and retina

E. R. Love

This chapter, based on work *in vivo*, is restricted essentially to transport at the blood–tissue interface. The kinetic characteristics of transport at the blood–brain and blood–retinal interfaces will determine the quantities of the metabolites (in this case glucose or ketone bodies) which become available to the cells of the tissue and will therefore play an important role in the regulation of metabolism. Indeed, experimental evidence suggests that, at least for the brain, metabolism can be restricted by the activity of the transport process. This particularly applies to the ketone bodies[1,2] and also under certain circumstances e.g. hypoglycaemia, to glucose[3-5].

THE NATURE OF THE BARRIER

The physical nature of the capillary wall in most tissues of the body[6] is such that small molecules, present in the bloodstream, are able to diffuse without appreciable restriction into the extracellular, extravascular space of the tissue[7,8]. In such tissues, therefore, the only functional barrier, to small molecules, between the bloodstream and the metabolic machinery of the cell is the cell membrane[9]. In the brain and the retina, however, two barriers are present, the first of which lies in the capillary wall and the second in the membranes of the cerebral cells.

The endothelial cells of the capillaries in both the brain and the retina are joined by 'tight junctions'[10,11]. These junctions restrict the movement of even small molecules into the tissue and constitute, it is now believed, the physical sites of the so-called 'blood–brain' and 'blood–retinal' barriers. The retina also receives blood from a second source, via capillaries in the choroid. These capillaries do not possess tight junctions and are freely permeable to blood-borne molecules[11]. The movement of these molecules into the retina is restricted, however, by the retinal pigmented epithelium, the external layer of the retina nearest to the choroid. This restriction is due to the presence between the epithelial cells of junctions which are similar to the tight junctions between the capillary endothelial cells in both brain and retina[12-15]. Thus the blood–retinal barrier is a composite structure and any measurement of transport into the retina *in vivo* will include transport at both the retinal capillaries and the pigment epithelium. A second potential route for the supply of nutrients to the cerebral cells also exists, namely via the choroid plexus, cerebrospinal fluid (CSF) and ependyma into the cerebral extracellular space. However, although the choroid plexus and CSF have many important functions[16,17] it seems unlikely that they play a major role in the supply of glucose and ketone bodies to the cerebral cells[18,19].

THE METABOLISM OF GLUCOSE AND KETONE BODIES IN THE BRAIN AND RETINA

In the normally fed adult both the brain and the retina are almost exclusively dependent upon glucose as a source of energy[20-22]. Indeed the brain, which constitutes only some 2% of the body weight, consumes roughly 20% of the total supply of glucose to the whole body[23,24]. The retina, on a weight for weight basis, metabolizes glucose at a similar rate to the brain[25]. However, the bulk of the retina is so small that it will not contribute significantly to the overall bodily consumption of glucose.

For many years it was thought that glucose was the only source of energy available to the brain, since the other substances which the brain was capable of utilizing *in vitro*, e.g. mannose, lactate, pyruvate and glutamate[23] were either not present in sufficient quantities in the circulating blood or traversed the blood–brain interface only at a very slow rate. However, Owen et al.[26] found that in fasting obese humans a considerable quantity of the ketone bodies, 3-hydroxybutyrate and acetoacetate, were utilized by the brain. These findings have been amply confirmed[1,2,27,28] and it is now accepted that under certain conditions, e.g. during fasting and in suckling babies when the concentrations of ketone bodies in the circulation are high, these substances act as important alternative sources of energy to glucose. Recent work upon the transport of ketone bodies into the retina during fasting indicate that these substances may be even more important for the energy requirements of the retina than they are for those of the brain[29]. Apart from this work nothing appears to be known about the metabolism of ketone bodies in the retina.

In addition to their role in energy metabolism, glucose and the ketone bodies are incorporated, both in the brain and also probably in the retina, into non-essential amino acids, e.g. glutamic acid, alanine, γ–aminobutyric acid and aspartic acid[30–37]. This synthesis of the non-essential amino acids is of quantitative importance in the brain since these substances traverse the blood–brain barrier only very slowly[38,39]. The importance of glucose in the metabolism of cerebral amino acids is illustrated by the profound changes which occur in the levels of amino acids in the brain during insulin-induced hypoglycaemia[40]. Glucose and, to a lesser extent, ketone bodies also act as precursors of cerebral lipids during the development of the brain[41].

In conclusion then, it appears that under special circumstances the metabolism of ketone bodies can supplement that of glucose in the brain and also probably in the retina. It must be stressed, however, that glucose is an essential substance upon which both brain and retina are mainly dependent for their energy requirements.

THE TRANSPORT OF GLUCOSE AND KETONE BODIES INTO THE BRAIN AND RETINA

Definition of terms

There is a continuous movement of molecules between the blood and the brain or the retina. The term influx is used to denote unidirectional movement of molecules into the tissues, while efflux denotes unidirectional movement of molecules out of the tissues and into the blood. Net flux defines the difference between influx and efflux, thus:

$$\text{net flux} = \text{influx} - \text{efflux}$$

When influx is greater than efflux, the net flux is in the direction blood to brain (or retina) and when efflux is greater than influx there is a net flux out of the tissues into the blood. For glucose and ketone bodies the net flux is always into the brain or retina and usually represents the rate at which these substances are utilized by the tissue. For lactate, which is not normally utilized to any great extent and is formed in the tissue, the net flux is usually outwards from the brain into the bloodstream[1,28,42].

Transport into brain

Although the presence of a carrier-mediated process for the transport of glucose into the brain had been indicated by previous work[43,44], the first

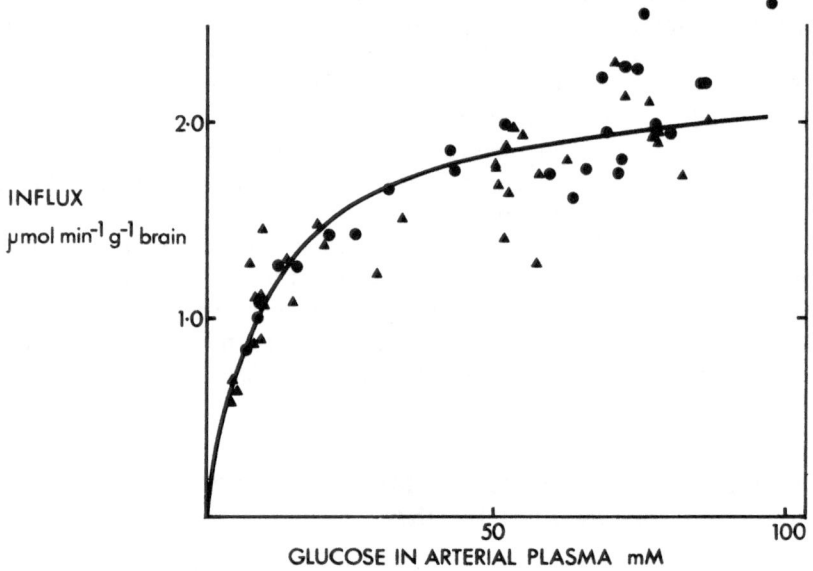

Figure 6.1 The effect of increasing the concentration of glucose in the circulation upon its influx into the brain. ●, animals which had been fasted for 24 h and in which a steady raised level of insulin (2–5 U/ml of plasma) was maintained in the circulation for a period of 17 min prior to and during the measurement of influx. ▲, controls, fasted for 24 h but not given insulin. The curve was fitted to the data by the method of Wilkinson[46] on the assumption that the influx conformed to simple Michaelis–Menten kinetics. (From reference 4)

quantitative study of the influx of glucose into the brain was made by Crone[45]. Crone demonstrated that at high concentrations of glucose in the plasma, the influx of glucose into the brain displayed saturation kinetics. Subsequent work confirmed that saturation of glucose transport occurs (Figure 6.1) and the kinetic constants for the carrier-mediated transport process were calculated. It is not relevant here to discuss the various techniques used to study glucose transport *in vivo*; suffice it to say that the kinetic parameters derived were all in fairly good agreement (Table 6.1).

In addition to the phenomenon of saturation, other characteristics which distinguish the transport of glucose into the brain as a carrier-mediated process have been demonstrated, for example, stereospecificity[54-56]; competitive inhibition[38,53,57-59] and finally transport counterflow[47,60].

TABLE 6.1 **Values of the kinetic constants for the transport of glucose into the brain** *in vivo*

Species	Technique of measurement	K_t^* (mmol/l ± SE)	V† (μmol/min per g of brain ± SE)	Reference
Rat } Mouse }	Tracer distribution between brain and serum	7 6	1.5 (approx) 2.1	47 48
Rat	Controlled intravenous injection	7.1 ± 2.2	1.21 ± 0.15	49
Dog	Indicator dilution (bolus injection)	8.3 ± 1.7	1.75 ± 0.11	50
Rabbit } Sheep }	Cerebral arterio-venous difference	5.5 6.0	2.8 2.6	51 51
Rat	Controlled intravenous injection	10.5 ± 1.2	2.2 ± 0.1	4
Rat } Rat }	Tritiated water reference (bolus injection)	11.0 9.0	1.6 1.56	52 53

* Michaelis constant for transport
† Maximum influx

The transport of ketone bodies into the brain has not been studied as extensively as the transport of glucose, since their importance in cerebral metabolism has only been realized fairly recently. Daniel et al.[2] found that the influx of ketone bodies into the brain was similar to their net flux over a wide range of concentrations in the plasma. Thus there is a negligible efflux of ketone bodies from the brain, and hence the rate at which these substances are transported into the cerebral tissue is the major factor which regulates their metabolism. Subsequent work has indicated that ketone bodies enter the brain by a saturable transport process[61] although saturation was not readily demonstrated when a different *in vivo* technique was used[62] (Figure 6.2). This apparent discrepancy may be due to the fact that, in the latter study, the ketone bodies were injected into the general circulation instead of being presented to the brain as a bolus containing Ringer–HEPES solution. Any substance present in the blood which competes with the ketone body for transport into the brain, e.g. lactate and pyruvate[63] will increase the apparent K_t (Michaelis constant) of the transport process with regard to the ketone body and as a result saturation will become more difficult to demonstrate. This effect of competition upon K_t was present in the study of Daniel et al.[62] in which normal blood (carrying ketone bodies and their natural competitors) was presented to the cerebral transport system but was not present when the bolus technique was employed[61]. Stereospecificity of the transport process has also been demonstrated, the D-isomer of hydroxybutyrate entering the brain more rapidly than the L form[62,64].

Perhaps the most important finding obtained so far with regard to the transport of ketone bodies into the brain is that the activity of the carrier appears to be modified by the nutritional status of the animal and also by the stage of cerebral development which has been reached[61,62,64]. These interesting observations are discussed in a subsequent section.

Transport into retina

Because of methodological difficulties, studies of the transport of substances across the blood–retinal interfaces are sparse. Dollery et al.[55] measured the distribution of D and L-glucose between the blood and the retina after the injection of ^{14}C-labelled tracers. They found a much higher retina/blood ratio for the D-isomer compared with the L-form, indicating the presence of a stereospecific transport process. Later, Daniel et al.[29] showed that glucose transport into the retina exhibits saturation kinetics (Figure 6.3). The kinetic constants of the transport process are significantly different from those in the brain (Table 6.2). This results in a lower influx of glucose into the retina compared with the

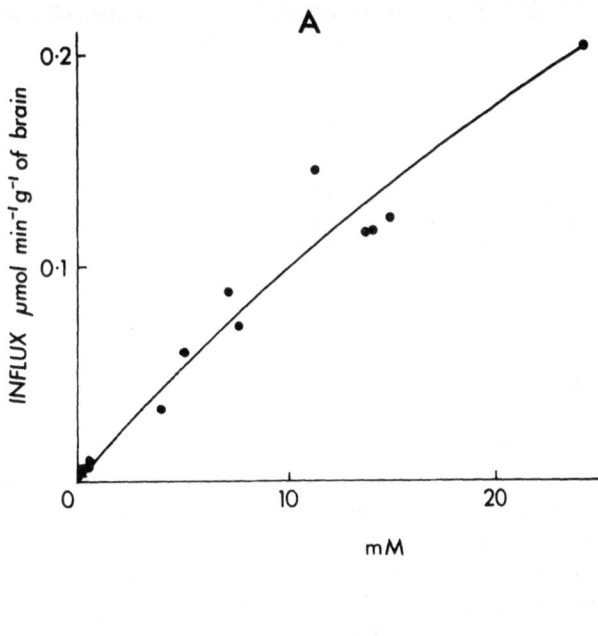

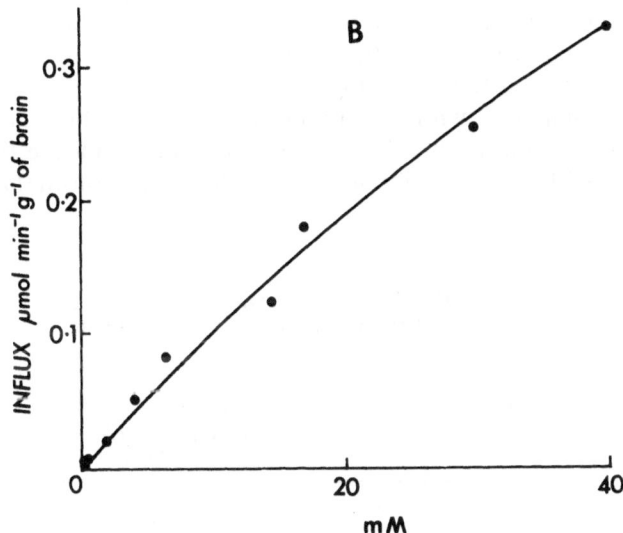

Figure 6.2 The effect of raising the concentration of a ketone body in the circulation upon its influx into the brain. A: 3-hydroxybutyrate; B: acetoacetate. Lines were fitted to the data by eye. (From reference 62)

TABLE 6.2   Kinetic constants for the transport of glucose into brain and retina

Tissue	K_t^* (mmol/l of plasma ± SE)	V (μmol/min per g of tissue ± SE)
Brain	10.5 ± 1.2	2.2 ± 0.1
Retina	$84 \pm 18^*$	$5.3 \pm 0.8^*$

* Significantly different from the values for the brain ($p<0.001$, normal deviate test)

brain at normal endogenous concentrations of glucose in the plasma (Figure 6.3 and Table 6.3).

In contrast to the transport of glucose, the transport of 3-hydroxybutyrate into the retina shows no evidence of saturation (Figure 6.4). However, the influx of hydroxybutyrate into the retina is some 5–6 times higher than its influx into the brain over a wide range of concentrations in the plasma (Figure 6.4). The most likely explanation for this higher influx is that there is a more efficient transport process in the retina. The alternative possibility that there is a higher rate of simple diffusion seems less likely, since such a higher rate of diffusion should also apply to glucose. However, the influx of glucose into the retina is lower than its influx into the brain (Figure 6.3, Table 6.3).

Thus, compared with the brain, more hydroxybutyrate but less glucose enters the retina. These transport studies indicate that ketone bodies may be of greater importance in retinal metabolism than they are in the brain.

TABLE 6.3   The influx of glucose into the brain and the retina of normally fed adult rats

Tissue	Influx (μmol/min per g of tissue ± SEM)
Brain	0.97 ± 0.13 (10)
Retina	0.46 ± 0.05 (8)*

Number of experiments in parentheses
* Significantly lower than values for the brain ($p < 0.001$, t-test)

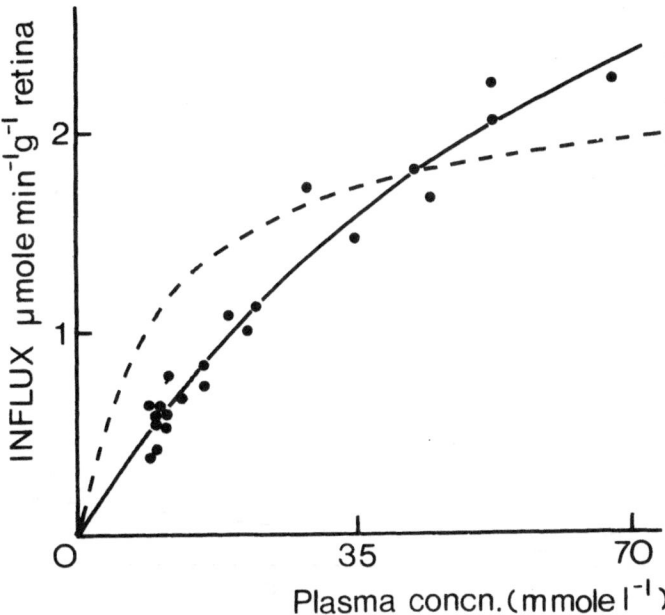

Figure 6.3 The effect of increasing the concentration of glucose in the circulation upon its influx into the retina.

For comparison the dashed curve is that fitted to the data for the influx of glucose into the brain (see Figure 6.1). The solid curve was fitted to the points by the method of Wilkinson[46] on the assumption that, like the brain, influx occurred by a saturable carrier-mediated transport process which conforms to Michaelis–Menten kinetics (Daniel, Love and Pratt, unpublished)

THE FUNCTIONAL SIGNIFICANCE OF TRANSPORT PROCESSES

It is all very well to state that glucose and ketone bodies enter the brain and the retina by carrier-mediated transport processes with definable characteristics. What does this actually mean with regard to the supply of these substances to the cells for their metabolism, and what are the functions of carrier-mediated transport?

The most important function is well illustrated by studies on the erythrocyte. It has been shown that glucose enters the red cell at a rate some 10 000 times that at which it can diffuse across the cell membrane[65]. Thus for substances like glucose and ketone bodies, which diffuse only slowly across membranes, the presence of carrier processes are essential if sufficient substrate is to be transported into the cell to support its metab-

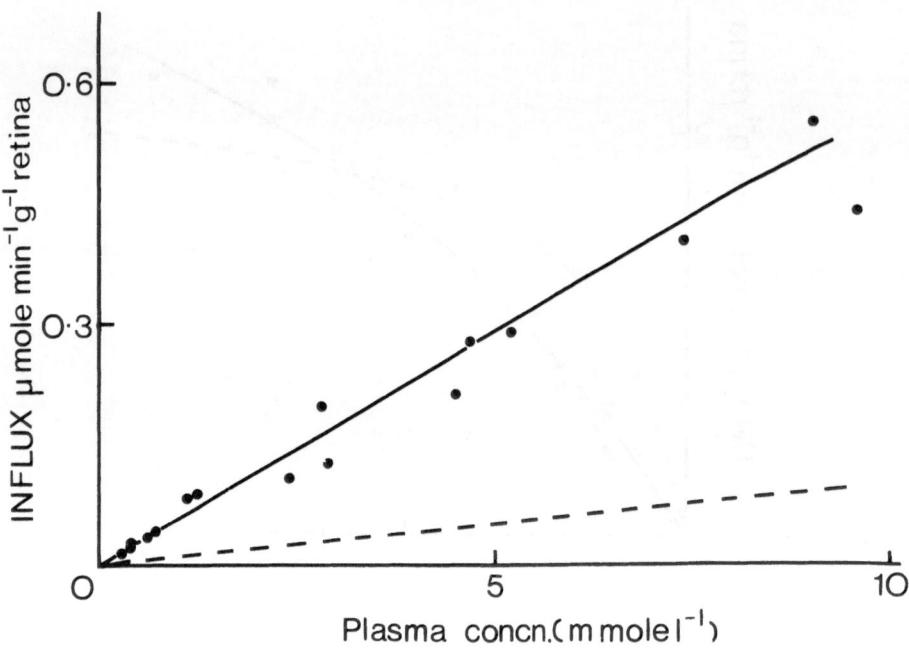

Figure 6.4 The influx of 3-hydroxybutyrate into the retina at raised concentrations of the ketone body in the circulation. The solid line was fitted to the points by linear regression. The dashed line represents linear regression analysis of the data for the influx of 3-hydroxybutyrate into the brain (Daniel, Love and Pratt, unpublished)

olism. Carrier mechanisms are of the utmost importance in the brain and retina where passive diffusion is negligible[19,49].

As a result of carrier-mediated transport the influx of glucose into the brain of the normally-fed adult rat is about 1 μmol/min per g of brain[4], which compares with a rate of utilization by the cerebral cells of about 0.3–0.7 μmol/min per g of brain[4,22,66,67]. Thus only some 30–70% of the glucose entering the brain is used and the rest must pass back into the blood by the process of efflux. Under normal circumstances the brain is therefore provided with a 'margin of safety' in its supply of glucose, thereby buffering it against modest fluctuations in blood glucose levels. The kinetic characteristics for transport (with a K_t approaching the normal concentration of glucose in the plasma) ensure a highly efficient transfer of glucose into the brain when the concentration of glucose in the blood is in the normal range. However, in hypoglycaemic conditions the influx falls sharply (Figure 6.1) and a point will be reached where insufficient glucose enters the brain to sustain metabolism. At this point, the energy reserves of the brain will rapidly be exhausted and cerebral dysfunction will start to occur. The efficiency of the carrier mechanism for glucose is such, however, that these symptoms do not appear until values as low as 1–2 mmol/l of glucose in the plasma are reached[3,47]. It is interesting that in the retina, the kinetic characteristics of transport do not ensure such an efficient transfer of glucose into the tissue (Figure 6.3; Table 6.3) and yet the retina has a very high rate of glucose utilization[20]. On this basis, it could be expected that the retina would suffer in hypoglycaemia at an earlier stage than the brain and indeed one of the very first symptoms in this condition is visual disturbances[23].

In the opposite condition, hyperglycaemia, we obtain a clear illustration of the important homeostatic role that the glucose transport

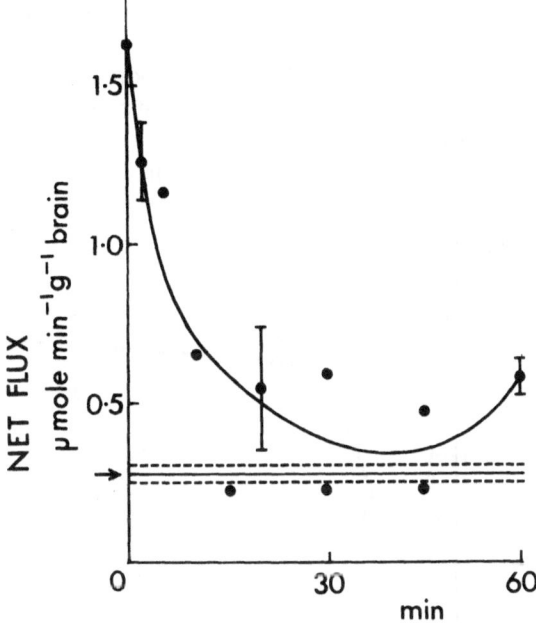

Figure 6.5 The curve shows the net flux (influx minus efflux) of glucose into the brain during hyperglycaemia. The points with bars represent the mean ± SEM of from 4 to 19 experiments. The hyperglycaemia was rapidly induced (10 s) by the intravenous injection of glucose and sustained at a steady concentration (a mean concentration of 36 mmol/l of plasma) for periods of up to 60 min[68]. The arrow (solid and dashed horizontal lines) represents the net flux (± SEM) of glucose into the brains of animals with normal concentrations of glucose in the plasma

process can play at the blood–brain interface. This function is biphasic. At the onset of hyperglycaemia, saturation of the transport process limits the rise in influx of glucose into the brain (Figure 6.1). However, if the hyperglycaemia continues and the concentration of glucose in the brain rises, there is a concomitant rise in the efflux of glucose from the brain. Thus the net flux of glucose into the brain (influx minus efflux) falls to values approaching those found in animals with normal concentrations of glucose in the plasma (Figure 6.5, see also reference 68). The efflux mechanism is so beautifully co-ordinated with the concentration of glucose in the brain that the ratio of the concentration of glucose in the brain to that in the plasma (G_b/G_p), soon returns to values approaching those found in normoglycaemic animals (Figure 6.6). In this way, the transport mechanism not only restricts the rise in the concentration of glucose within the brain, but also ensures that osmotic equilibrium between the brain and the blood is maintained during prolonged hyperglycaemia.

Thus, using the example of glucose transport into the brain, we can obtain some idea of the important roles played by transport mechanisms, not only in regulating cerebral metabolism but also in helping to maintain a constant environment within the brain.

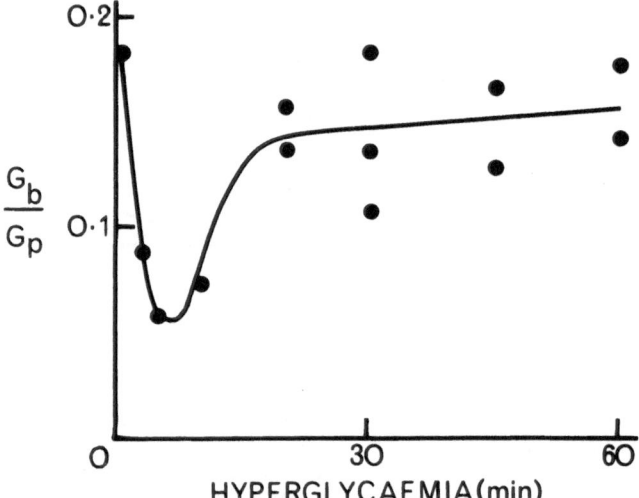

Figure 6.6   The effect of increasing periods of hyperglycaemia ($> 20\,mmol/l$ of plasma) upon the ratio of the concentration of glucose in the brain compared with that in the plasma, G_b/G_p. The point at zero time represents the G_b/G_p ratio in animals with normal concentrations of glucose in the plasma[68]

TRANSPORT IN THE DEVELOPING BRAIN

Tight junctions are already present between cerebral capillary endothelial cells in the foetuses of several species of animals, including man[69-73]. Although the presence of these tight junctions is not necessarily correlated with a fully functional blood–brain barrier[17] it appears that by the time the 'critical period' of development of the cerebral cortex occurs the barrier is relatively 'tight'. Flexner[74] first put forward the concept of the critical period of brain development as being associated with rapid changes in morphological and metabolic parameters in the cerebral cortex. Later Dawes[75] correlated these changes with the development of the cerebral cortical activity which occurs at different times in different species (Table 6.4).

TABLE 6.4   The onset of cortical activity in the developing brain of various species

Man	12–16 weeks gestation
Pig	80 days gestation
Sheep	80–100 days gestation
Cat	2–4 weeks after birth
Rat	10 days after birth

Data from Dawes[75]

Thus it appears that a functional blood–brain barrier is present at an early stage in the development of the central nervous system. The question therefore arises as to how closely any changes in the characteristics of transport at the blood–brain interface during development are correlated to changes in the metabolic activity of the growing brain. The metabolism of glucose alters considerably during development[76,77], so too does that of the ketone bodies[41]; are there concomitant changes in transport?

It has been found that the influx of glucose into the brain of suckling rats is lower than that into the brain of the young adult[5,63] (Figure 6.7). This decreased influx of glucose is due to the fact that the maximum influx (V) in the suckling animal is only some 50% of the adult value, while K_t remains unaltered[5,78] (Table 6.5). The lower value of V in suckling animals means that at normal concentrations of glucose in the plasma, the influx is reduced from the value of about 1 μmol/min per g of brain which is found in young adults to approximately 0.5 μmol/min per g of brain. This lower influx is associated with only a slightly reduced rate of utilization of glucose in the suckling animal[1]. Thus in the young animal the margin of safety between the influx of glucose and its rate of utilization is much less than that in the adult. On the basis of these results the brain of the young animal should be more sensitive to a fall in blood glucose than that of the adult. This is not the case[79]. The reason for the resistance of the brain of the young animal to hypoglycaemia is clarified when the influx of ketone bodies into the brain is considered.

TABLE 6.5 A comparison of the kinetic parameters for glucose transport into the brain of suckling rats and of fed adult rats

Group	Age (weeks)	K_t (mmol/l of plasma ± SE)	V (µmol/min per g of brain ± SE)
Suckling	2.4	11.8 ± 6.3	0.9 ± 0.16*
Adult	7.9	10.5 ± 1.2	2.2 ± 0.1

Data from Daniel et al.[5]
* Significantly lower than the value in the young adult ($p < 0.001$, t-test)

In contrast to glucose, the influx of ketone bodies into the brain is higher during the suckling period than at any other time[62,63]. This higher

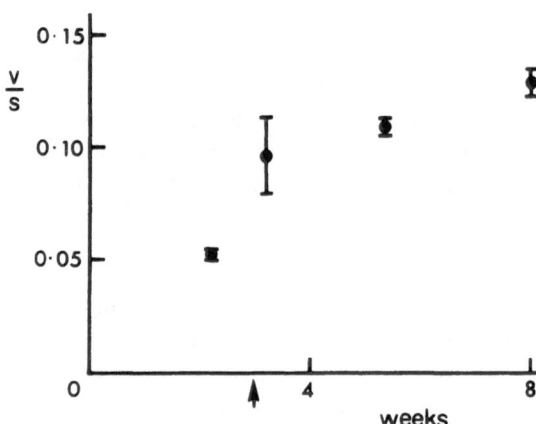

Figure 6.7 The change with age in the ratio of the influx of glucose into the brain compared with its concentration in the blood plasma, v/s. The arrow indicates the age at which animals were weaned. Each point represents the mean of 3–10 experiments. Bars represent SEM. (From Daniel et al.[5])

influx is due only in part to the higher concentrations of ketone bodies in the blood of the young animal. Thus when variations in the concentrations of ketone bodies in the blood during development are eliminated by calculation of the ratio of the influx to the concentration of ketone bodies in the blood (*v/s*), this ratio is higher in suckling animals compared with adults (Figure 6.8). These results indicate that there is a more efficient transfer of ketone bodies into the brain of the young animal than into the brain of the adult. The kinetic basis of this increased efficiency has not yet been elucidated.

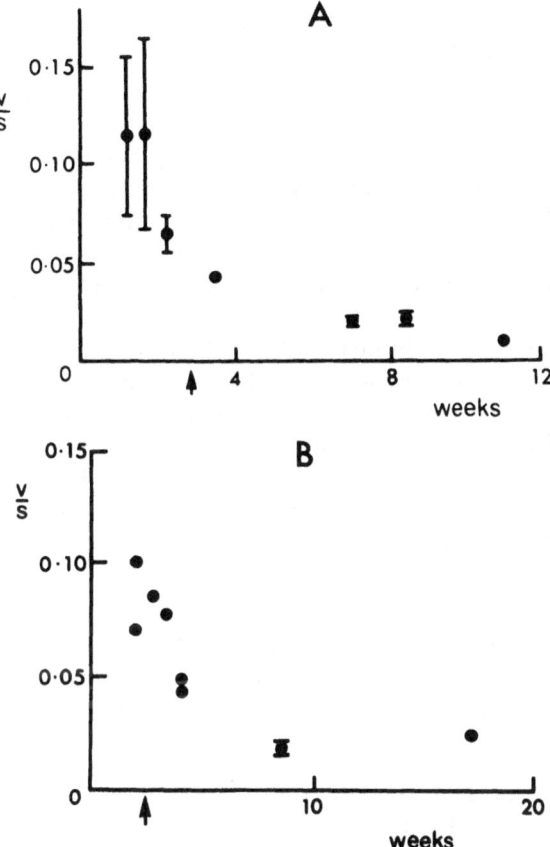

Figure 6.8 The effect of age upon the ratio of the influx of a ketone body into the brain compared with its concentration in the blood plasma, *v/s*. A: 3-hydroxybutyrate; B: acetoacetate. The arrows indicate the age at which animals were weaned. Each point represents a separate experiment or the mean of from 3 to 6 experiments (in which case the bars represent SEM)

In terms of influx, therefore, the growing brain, when compared with that of the adult, receives a lower, but adequate supply of glucose and an increased supply of ketone bodies. This results in a decreased dependence of the brain upon glucose which imparts a greater metabolic flexibility to the growing brain. Such flexibility must be of the utmost importance during the development of the brain, since it ensures that there are adequate supplies of alternative nutrients in the face of adverse conditions, e.g. hypoglycaemia.

The changes in the influx into the brain of glucose and ketone bodies during development are closely paralleled by changes in the activities of many of the enzymes associated with the metabolism of these substrates[77,80]. Some of these changes may be induced by the availability of the substrates in the blood. Thus the prolonged ketonaemia which occurs during the suckling period and also during fasting, induces an increased activity of the carrier-mediated transport process[61,62,64]. This inducible nature of the carrier-protein lends support to the possibility of an enzymatic basis to the blood–brain barrier[81]. Severe hyperketonaemia in the young animal also produces changes in the developmental pattern of some of the enzymes in the cerebral cells which are associated with glutamate metabolism[82].

The capacity of the brain to utilize ketone bodies is species dependent. The sheep, for example, does not utilize ketone bodies, even when very high levels of these substances are present in the blood[83]. The important thing, however, in the present context, is that in the human the ketone bodies act as significant sources of energy for the brain during development and as in the rat[1], their rate of utilization by the brain is proportional to their concentrations in the blood[28,83a].

THE CONSIDERATION OF TRANSPORT INTO THE BRAIN IN RELATION TO SOME INBORN ERRORS OF METABOLISM

Because of the lack of basic information upon both the transport of nutrients into and their metabolism by the retina, particularly during development, the speculations in this section are restricted to considerations of the brain. However, since carrier-mediated processes have been shown to exist at the blood–retinal interface (see earlier) the general principles of the arguments presented must also apply to the retina.

The preceding sections have shown how glucose and the ketone bodies enter the brain by carrier-mediated mechanisms. The characteristics of these transport processes are such that the influx of a substance into the brain is susceptible to alteration. For example, the presence in the blood of a raised level of a second substance which competes for transport by the carrier molecule will reduce the quantity of the first substance being transported. The severity of the reduction will, of course, depend upon the relative affinities of the carrier for each substance. Such competitive effects can reduce the entry of nutrients into the brain to the detriment of cerebral metabolism and function. A good illustration of this is provided by the amino acid phenylalanine. This amino acid is transported into the brain by a carrier which it shares with the other essential neutral amino acids[38, 84, 85]. In phenylketonuria, the high concentrations of phenylalanine in the blood will competitively inhibit the transport of the other neutral amino acids into the brain. The imbalance in the supply of these various amino acids to the developing brain causes the mental deficiency which is so often seen[86]. Do similar situations exist with regard to the transport of glucose and ketone bodies into the brain?

Sugars which could compete with glucose for transport into the brain are normally present in the blood only at very low concentrations. One of these sugars is galactose, which has been shown to reduce the influx of glucose into the brain by competitive inhibition[53]. Thus in galactosaemia, the raised levels of galactose in the blood as a result of the genetic enzymatic defect in galactose metabolism[87], will partially inhibit the transport of glucose into the brain. Since the influx of glucose into the baby's brain is low (Figure 6.7) the inhibitory effect of galactose will be heightened. The situation will be further exacerbated by the hypoglycaemia which is commonly present in galactosaemic patients[88]. The partial exclusion of glucose from the developing brain could well be a contributing factor to the mental retardation found in galactosaemia. That this is not the only factor, however, is shown by the finding that in patients suffering from the form of the disease which is due to a deficiency of the enzyme galactokinase, mental retardation is not usually present, despite raised levels of galactose in the blood[87]. The severity of the effects of raised levels of galactose in the blood upon glucose transport into the brain will, of course, vary from patient to patient, depending upon the concentration of galactose in the blood and upon the presence and degree of hypoglycaemia.

The ketone bodies are transported into the brain by a carrier-mediated mechanism which they share with lactate and pyruvate[42, 63]. Since the carrier displays relatively high affinities (low K_i) for both lactate and pyruvate[78], these substances will strongly inhibit the transport of ketone bodies into the brain. There are a number of metabolic disorders associated with raised levels of lactate and pyruvate in the blood, e.g. hyperlacticacidaemia, hyperpyruvic acidaemia and hyperalalinaemia, and it can be expected that in these conditions the influx of ketone bodies into the brain will be reduced by competition. It seems unlikely, however, that the partial exclusion of ketone bodies from the growing brain *per se* would be detrimental to cerebral development in cases in which there are adequate levels of glucose in the blood. However, should hypoglycaemia also be present, then normal cerebral development may well be at risk. That is to say, in some disorders of metabolism, as a result of competition, the normal flexibility of the brain with regard to its source of energy may be removed and in the face of a further metabolic insult, e.g. hypoglycaemia, cerebral damage may occur.

The production of carrier-molecules, like that of enzymes, is under genetic control[89]. Genetic aberrations result in the enzyme defects which produce the group of diseases categorized as the inborn errors of metabolism[90]. It is reasonable to expect that genetic aberrations will also result in defects in the production of carrier molecules. Such defects may often be fatal, but one can envisage situations in which survival may be possible. Thus, for example, a defect in the transport of ketone bodies may have little detectable effect until hypoglycaemia occurs. In this situation the organs for which glucose is essential, in particular the brain, would suffer to the greatest extent. The possibility remains, therefore, that defects in the production of carrier molecules as a result of genetic aberrations may contribute to the large group of diseases regarded as unclassified mental retardation.

CONCLUSIONS

It is hoped that the work presented in this chapter illustrates the important functions of carrier-mediated transport processes, both in ensuring adequate supplies of vital nutrients to the brain and the retina and in regulating the internal environment of the central nervous system. It is suggested that the metabolic abnormalities found in the inborn errors associated with carbohydrate metabolism might produce deficiencies in the supply of energy-yielding substrates to the developing brain. Such deficiencies could contribute to the mental retardation found in these conditions.

On a wider basis, it must be stressed that in any metabolic disorder in which an abnormally high concentration of a substance is present in the blood, then the effects of this high concentration upon cerebral transport processes must be considered with regard to the adequate nutrition of the brain. These comments apply especially to the developing brain when adverse conditions elicit their greatest effect upon eventual intellectual performance.

Acknowledgements

I would like to thank the Medical Research Council for a grant and also the Wellcome Trust and the Research Fund of the Bethlem Royal and Maudsley Hospitals for grants to my colleague, Dr O. E. Pratt, which helped to support this work.

References

1. Hawkins, R. A., Williamson, D. H. and Krebs, H. A. (1971). Ketone body utilization by adult and suckling rat brain *in vivo*. *Biochem. J.*, **122**, 13
2. Daniel, P. M., Love, E. R., Moorhouse, S. R., Pratt, O. E. and Wilson, P. (1971). Factors influencing utilization of ketone bodies in normal rats and rats with ketoacidosis. *Lancet*, **2**, 637
3. Bachelard, H. S. (1971). Glucose transport and phosphorylation in the control of carbohydrate metabolism in the brain. In J. B. Brierley and B. S. Meldrum (eds.). *Brain Hypoxia*, pp. 251–260. (London: Heinemann)
4. Daniel, P. M., Love, E. R. and Pratt, O. E. (1975). Insulin and the way the brain handles glucose. *J. Neurochem.*, **25**, 471
5. Daniel, P. M., Love, E. R. and Pratt, O. E. (1978). The effect of age upon the influx of glucose into the brain. *J. Physiol.*, **274**, 141
6. Karnovsky, M. J. (1967). The ultrastructural basis of capillary permeability studied with peroxidase as a tracer. *J. Cell Biol.*, **35**, 213
7. Crone, C. (1963). The permeability of capillaries in various organs as determined by use of the indicator diffusion method. *Acta Physiol. Scand.*, **58**, 292
8. Alvarez, O. A. and Yudilevich, D. L. (1969). Heart capillary permeability to lipid-insoluble molecules. *J. Physiol.*, **202**, 45
9. Elbrink, J. and Bihler, I. (1975). Membrane transport: its relation to cellular metabolic rates. *Science NY*, **188**, 1177
10. Brightman, M. W. (1977). Morphology of blood–brain interfaces. *Exp. Eye Res.*, **25**, Suppl., 1–25
11, Cunha-Vaz, J. G. (1976). The blood-retinal barriers. *Doc. Ophthalmol.*, **41**, 287
12. Shiose, Y. (1968). Electron microscopic changes and early changes of in-

herited dystrophic mouse retina. *J. Ophthalmol.*, **12**, 181
13. Peyman, G. A., Spitznas, M. and Straatsma, B. R. (1971). Peroxidase diffusion in the normal and photocoagulated retina. *Invest. Ophthalmol.*, **10**, 181
14. Shakib, M., Rutkowski, P. and Wise, G. E. (1972). Fluorescein angiography and the retinal pigment epithelium. *Am. J. Ophthalmol.*, **74**, 206
15. Raviola, G. (1977). The structural basis of the blood–ocular barriers. *Exp. Eye Res.*, **25**, Suppl. 27–63
16. Davson, H. (1976). The blood–brain barrier. *J. Physiol.*, **255**, 1
17. Bradbury, M. (1979). *The Concept of a Blood–brain Barrier*, pp. 289–322. (Chichester: Wiley)
18. Wolff, P. H. and Tschirgi, R. D. (1956). Inability of cerebrospinal fluid to nourish the spinal cord. *Am. J. Physiol.*, **184**, 220
19. Lund-Andersen, H. (1979). Transport of glucose from blood to brain. *Physiol. Rev.*, **59**, 305
20. Lolley, R. N. (1969). Metabolic and anatomical specialization within the retina. In A. Lajtha (ed.). *Handbook of Neurochemistry*, Vol. 2, pp. 473–504. (New York: Plenum Press)
21. Graymore, C. N. (1970). Biochemistry of the retina. In C. N. Graymore (ed.). *Biochemistry of the Eye*, pp. 645–735. (London: Academic Press)
22. Siesjö, B. K. (1978). *Brain Energy Metabolism*, pp. 101–130. (Chichester: Wiley)
23. Himwich, H. E. (1951). *Brain Metabolism and Cerebral Disorder*, pp. 257–302. (Baltimore: Williams and Wilkins)
24. Kety, S. S. (1957). General metabolism of the brain *in vivo*. In D. Richter (ed.). *Metabolism of the Nervous System*, pp. 221–237. (London: Pergamon Press)
25. Törnquist, P. and Alm, A. (1979). Retinal and choroidal contribution to retinal metabolism *in vivo*. A study in pigs. *Acta Physiol. Scand.*, **106**, 351
26. Owen, O. E., Morgan, A. P., Kemp, H. G., Sullivan, J. M., Herrera, M. G. and Cahill, G. F. Jr. (1967). Brain metabolism during fasting. *J. Clin. Invest.*, **46**, 1589
27. Ruderman, N. B., Ross, P. S., Berger, M. and Goodman, M. N. (1974). Regulation of glucose and ketone-body metabolism in brain of anaesthetized rats. *Biochem. J.*, **138**, 1
28. Kraus, H., Schlenker, S. and Schwedesky, D. (1974). Developmental changes of cerebral ketone body utilization in human infants. *Hoppe-Seylers Z. Physiol. Chem.*, **355**, 164
29. Daniel, P. M., Love, E. R. and Pratt, O. E. (1979). The influx of glucose and hydroxybutyrate into the retina of the rat *in vivo*. *J. Physiol.* (In press)
30. Roberts, R. B., Flexner, J. B. and Flexner, L. B. (1959). Biochemical and physiological differentiation during morphogenesis. XXIII: Further observations relating to the synthesis of amino acids and proteins by the cerebral cortex and liver of the mouse. *J. Neurochem.*, **4**, 78
31. Gaitonde, M. K., Dahl, D. R. and Elliott, K. A. C. (1965). Entry of glucose carbon into amino acids of rat brain and liver *in vivo* after injection of uniformly ^{14}C-labelled glucose. *Biochem. J.*, **94**, 345
32. O'Neal, R. M. and Koeppe, R. E. (1966). Precursors *in vivo* of glutamate, aspartate and their derivatives of rat brain. *J. Neurochem.*, **13**, 835

33. Lindsay, J. R. and Bachelard, H. S. (1966). Incorporation of [^{14}C] from glucose into α-ketoacids and amino acids in rat brain and liver *in vivo*. *Biochem. Pharmacol.*, **15**, 1045

34. Flock, E. V., Tyce, G. M. and Owen, C. A. (1966). Utilization of [U-^{14}C] glucose in brain after total hepatectomy in the rat. *J. Neurochem.*, **13**, 1389

35. Cremer, J. E. (1964). Amino acid metabolism in rat brain studied with [^{14}C]-labelled glucose. *J. Neurochem.*, **11**, 165

36. Cremer, J. E. (1971). Incorporation of label from D-β-hydroxy [^{14}C] butyrate and [3-^{14}C] acetoacetate into amino acids in rat brain *in vivo*. *Biochem. J.*, **122**, 135

37. Morjaria, B. and Voaden, M. J. (1979). The formation of glutamate, aspartate and GABA in the rat retina; glucose and glutamine as precursors. *J. Neurochem.*, **33**, 541

38. Oldendorf, W. H. (1971). Brain uptake of radiolabelled amino acids, amines and hexoses after arterial injection. *Am. J. Physiol.*, **221**, 1629

39. Baños, G., Daniel, P. M., Moorhouse, S. R. and Pratt, O. E. (1973). The influx of amino acids into the brain of the rat *in vivo*: the essential compared with some non-essential amino acids. *Proc. R. Soc. London B*, **183**, 59

40. Lewis, L. D., Ljunggren, B., Norberg, K. and Siesjö, B. K. (1974). Changes in carbohydrate substrates, amino acids and ammonia in the brain during insulin-induced hypoglycaemia. *J. Neurochem.*, **23**, 659

41. Cremer, J. E., Teal, H. M. and Heath, D. F. (1975). Regulatory factors in glucose and ketone body utilization by the developing brain. In F. A. Hommes and C. J. Van den Berg (eds.). *Normal and Pathological Development of Energy Metabolism*, pp. 133–142. (London: Academic Press)

42. Daniel, P. M., Love, E. R., Moorhouse, S. R., Pratt, O. E. and Wilson, P. (1972). The movement of ketone bodies, glucose, pyruvate and lactate between the blood and the brain of rats. *J. Physiol.*, **221**, 22P

43. Geiger, A., Magnes, J., Taylor, R. M. and Veralli, M. (1954). Effect of blood constituents on uptake of glucose and on metabolic rate of the brain in perfusion experiments. *Am. J. Physiol.*, **177**, 138

44. Fishman, R. A. (1964). Carrier transport of glucose between blood and cerebrospinal fluid. *Am. J. Physiol.*, **206**, 836

45. Crone, C. (1965). Facilitated transfer of glucose from blood into brain tissues. *J. Physiol.*, **181**, 103

46. Wilkinson, G. N. (1961). Statistical estimations in enzyme kinetics. *Biochem. J.*, **80**, 324

47. Buschiazzo, P. M., Terrell, E. B. and Regen, D. M. (1970). Sugar transport across the blood–brain barrier. *Am. J. Physiol.*, **219**, 1505

48. Growdon, W. A., Bratton, T. S., Houston, M. C., Tarpley, H. L. and Regen, D. M. (1971). Brain glucose metabolism in the intact mouse. *Am. J. Physiol.*, **221**, 1738

49. Bachelard, H. S., Daniel, P. M., Love, E. R. and Pratt, O. E. (1973). The transport of glucose into the brain of the rat *in vivo*. *Proc. R. Soc. London B*, **183**, 71

50. Betz, A. L., Gilboe, D. D., Yudilevich, D. L. and Drewes, L. R. (1973). Kinetics of unidirectional glucose transport into the isolated dog brain. *Am. J. Physiol.*, **225**, 586

51. Pappenheimer, J. R. and Setchell, B. P. (1973). Cerebral glucose transport and oxygen consumption in sheep and rabbits. *J. Physiol.*, **233**, 529

52. Brender, J., Andersen, P. E. and Rafaelsen, O. J. (1975). Blood–brain transfer of D-glucose, L-leucine and L-tryptophan in the rat. *Acta Physiol. Scand.*, **93**, 490

53. Pardridge, W. M. and Oldendorf, W. H. (1975). Kinetics of blood–brain barrier transport of hexoses. *Biochim. Biophys. Acta*, **382**, 377

54. Crone, C. and Thompson, A. M. (1970). Permeability of brain capillaries. In C. Crone and N. A. Lassen (eds.). Alfred Benzon Symp. II. *Capillary Permeability*, pp. 447–453. (Copenhagen: Munksgaard)

55. Dollery, C. T., Henkind, P. and Orme, M. L'E. (1971). Assimilation of D and L1-C-14 glucose into the retina, brain and other tissues. *Diabetes*, **20**, 519

56. De Rose, N. and Yudilevich, D. L. (1971). Blood–brain transfer of glucose and other molecules measured by rapid indicator dilution. *Am. J. Physiol.*, **220**, 841

57. Betz, A. L. and Gilboe, D. D. (1974). Kinetics of cerebral glucose transport *in vivo*: inhibition by 3-*O*-methylglucose. *Brain Res.*, **65**, 368

58. Betz. A. L., Drewes, L. R. and Gilboe, D. D. (1975). Inhibition of glucose transport into brain by phlorizin, phloretin and glucose analogues. *Biochim. Biophys. Acta*, **406**, 505

59. Yudilevich, D. L. and Sépulveda, F. V. (1976). The specificity of amino acid and sugar carriers in the capillaries of the dog brain studied *in vivo* by rapid indicator dilution. *Adv. Exp. Med. Biol.*, **69**, 77

60. Cutler, R. W. P. and Sipe, J. C. (1971). Mediated transport of glucose between blood and brain in the cat. *Am. J. Physiol.*, **220**, 1182

61. Gjedde, A. and Crone, C. (1975). Induction processes in blood–brain transfer of ketone bodies during starvation. *Am. J. Physiol.*, **229**, 1165

62. Daniel. P. M., Love, E. R., Moorhouse, S. R. and Pratt, O. E. (1977). The transport of ketone bodies into the brain of the rat (*in vivo*). *J. Neurol. Sci.*, **34**, 1

63. Cremer, J. E., Braun, L. D. and Oldendorf, W. H. (1976). Changes during development in transport processes of the blood–brain barrier. *Biochim. Biophys. Acta*, **448**, 633

64. Moore, T. J., Lione, A. P., Sugden, M. C. and Regen, D. M. (1976). β-Hydroxybutyrate transport in rat brain: developmental and dietary modulations. *Am. J. Physiol.*, **230**, 619

65. Stein, W. D. (1967). *The Movement of Molecules Across Cell Membranes*, p. 126. (New York: Academic Press)

66. McIlwain, H. and Bachelard, H. S. (1971). *Biochemistry of the Central Nervous System*, p. 100. (London: Churchill)

67. Hawkins, R. A., Miller, A. L., Cremer, J. E. and Veech, R. L. (1974). Measurement of the rate of glucose utilization by rat brain *in vivo*. *J. Neurochem.*, **23**, 917

68. Daniel, P. M., Love, E. R. and Pratt, O. E. (1977). The influence of insulin upon the metabolism of glucose by the brain. *Proc. R. Soc. London B,* **196**, 85

69. Donahue, S. and Pappas, G. D. (1961). The fine structure of capillaries in

the cerebral cortex of the rat at various stages of development. *Am. J. Anat.*, **108**, 331

70. Peterson, R. G. (1968). The fine structure of vascular–neural relationships in the brain of the developing chick. *J. Cell Biol.*, **39**, 105A

71. Bärr, T. and Wolff, J. R. (1972). The formation of capillary basement membranes during internal vascularization of the rat's cerebral cortex. *Z. Zellforsch. Mikrosk. Anat.*, **133**, 231

72. Møllgård, K. and Saunders, N. R. (1975). Complex tight junctions of epithelial and of endothelial cells in early foetal brain. *J. Neurocytol.*, **4**, 453

73. Saunders, N. R. (1977). Ontogeny of the blood–brain barrier. *Exp. Eye Res.*, **25**, Suppl. 523–550

74. Flexner, L. B. (1951–52). The development of the cerebral cortex: a cytological, functional and biochemical approach. *Harvey Lect.*, **47**, 156

75. Dawes, G. S. (1968). *Foetal and Neonatal Physiology*, pp. 225–226. (Chicago: Year Book Medical Publisher)

76. O'Neall, J. (1974). Carbohydrate metabolism in the developing nervous system. In W. Himwich (ed.). *Biochemistry of the Developing Brain*, Vol. 2, pp. 69–121. (New York: Dekker)

77. Baquer, N. Z., Hothersall, J. S., McLean, P. and Greenbaum, A. L. (1977). Aspects of carbohydrate metabolism in developing brain. *Devel. Med. Child Neurol.*, **19**, 81

78. Cremer, J. E., Cunningham, V. J., Pardridge, W. M., Braun, L. D. and Oldendorf, W. H. (1979). Kinetics of blood–brain barrier transport of pyruvate, lactate and glucose in suckling, weanling and adult rats. *J. Neurochem.*, **33**, 439

79. Marks, V. and Rose, C. F. (1965). *Hypoglycaemia*, p. 208. (Oxford: Blackwell)

80. Williamson, D. H. (1973). Tissue-specific direction of blood metabolites. In: *Rate Control of Biological Processes*. Symposia of the Society for Experimental Biology. Symposium XXVII, pp. 283–298. (Cambridge: Cambridge University Press)

81. Meister, A. (1974). An enzymatic basis for a blood–brain barrier? The γ-glutamyl cycle – background and considerations relating to amino acid transport in the brain. In F. Plumb (ed.). *Brain Dysfunction in Metabolic Disorders*, pp. 273–291. (New York: Raven Press)

82. Tildon, J. T., Ozand, P. T. and Cornblath, M. (1975). The effects of hyperketonaemia on brain metabolism. In F. A. Hommes and C. J. Van den Berg (eds.). *Normal and Pathological Development of Energy Metabolism*, pp. 143–154. (London: Academic Press)

83. Lindsay, D. B. and Setchell, B. P. (1976). The oxidation of glucose, ketone bodies and acetate by the brain of normal and ketonaemic sheep. *J. Physiol.*, **259**, 801

83a. Persson, B., Settergren G. and Dahlquist, G. (1972). Cerebral arterio-venous differences of acetoacetate and D-β-hydroxybutyrate in children. *Acta Paediatr. Scand.*, **61**, 273

84. Daniel, P. M., Moorhouse, S. R. and Pratt, O. E. (1976). Amino acid precursors of monoamine neurotransmitters and some factors influencing their supply to the brain. *Psychol. Med.*, **6**, 277

85. Pardridge, W. M. (1977). Kinetics of competitive inhibition of neutral

amino acid transport across the blood–brain barrier. *J. Neurochem.*, **28,** 103

86. Pratt, O. E. (1980). This volume, Chapter 5.
87. Kalckar, H. M., Kinoshita, J. H. and Donnell, G. N. (1973). Galactose-mia: biochemistry, genetics, patho-physiology and developmental aspects. In G. E. Gaull (ed.). *Biology of Brain Dysfunction*, Vol. 1, pp. 31–88. (New York: Plenum Press)
88. Crome, L. and Stern, J. (1972). *Pathology of Mental Retardation*, 2nd Edn., pp. 402–406. (Edinburgh: Churchill Livingstone)
89. Pardee, A. B. and Palmer, L. M. (1973). Regulation of transport systems: a means of controlling metabolic rates. In: *Rate Control of Biological Processes*. Symposia of the Society for Experimental Biology. Symposium XXVII, pp. 133–144. (Cambridge: Cambridge University Press).
90. Garrod, A. E. (1909). *Inborn Errors of Metabolism*. (London: Frowde, Hodder and Stoughton. Reprinted by OUP in 1963)

SECTION FOUR

Renal Transport

7

The function and organization of kidney microvillar proteins

A. J. Kenny

Inborn errors of amino-acid transport in the kidney proximal tubule have been recognized for many years. Indeed, much of our understanding of the group-specific transport systems was gained from investigations of these defects. In recent years our knowledge of the molecular architecture of the brush border in which the transport systems are located has increased rapidly. But the transport proteins in the membrane have yet to be characterized in molecular terms. Transport in the kidney tubule is predominantly a physiological study, its promotion to the realm of molecular biology is something to be contemplated for the future. In this chapter, I shall attempt to review some of the current knowledge of the proteins which, together with lipids and glycolipids, make up the microvillus. A more extensive review of the ultrastructure, enzymology and molecular organization of microvilli, including those of the intestinal brush border, has recently appeared[1].

ULTRASTRUCTURE OF MICROVILLI

The brush borders that line the kidney proximal tubule and those lining the small intestine have many structural features in common. The microvilli of both membranes serve the same type of function in hydrolysis and transport, have many enzymes and structural proteins in common and seem to differ in only relatively few details. Kidney microvilli are 1–2 μm in length and about 0.1 μm in diameter – just at the limit of resolution by light microscopy. They are a specialization of the epithelial-cell plasma membrane which is thus polarized into two functionally and morphologically distinct regions: the luminal (brush border) membrane and the basolateral membrane (Figure 7.1). The structural feature that delineates the luminal from the basolateral region is the *tight junction* – a belt-like feature surrounding the cell just below the brush border in which the membranes of adjacent cells fuse, thereby restricting diffusional movement and preventing exchange of the proteins that are characteristic of each pole. Just beneath the tight junction is another membrane junctional structure – a belt desmosome from which intermediate filaments arise, contributing to a zone of the cytoplasm rich in intermingling filaments and small vesicles.

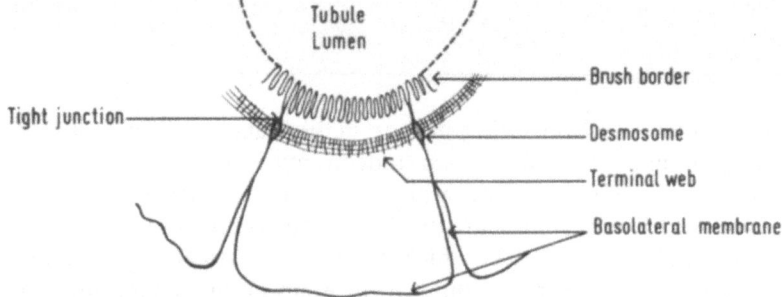

Figure 7.1   Tight junctions separate the apical (luminal) membrane from the basolateral membrane

The microvillar core

Figure 7.2 illustrates some of the detailed features that can be revealed by electron microscopy. The microvillus is maintained in its cylindrical shape by a cytoskeletal system, referred to as the *core*. From the tip, apparently arising from a densely staining protein, as yet uncharacterized, are seven microfilaments running lengthwise and braced laterally by regular crossbridges that join the filaments to the membrane. The microfilaments are composed of F-actin, a polymer of G-actin (subunit molecular weight of 42 000). The cross-bridge protein has a subunit molecular weight of 95 000. Its length and properties led workers to assume that it was identical with α-actinin, the protein of the Z-line in striated muscle. However some recent immunological studies have shown that, while the terminal web region reacts positively, microvilli react negatively when intestinal cells are treated with antisera raised to α-actinin[2]. Bretscher and Weber[3] have isolated the cross-bridge protein from intestinal microvilli, which they have named villin, and shown it to be distinct from α-actinin. Villin has the ability to bind to actin subunits with a periodicity of about 35 nm between each cross-bridge, but the identity of the membrane component to which the other end of this elongated protein attaches is unknown. In isolated preparations of brush borders and microvilli the cross-bridges readily become detached from the membrane and the microvilli quickly lose their original shape and vesiculate[4].

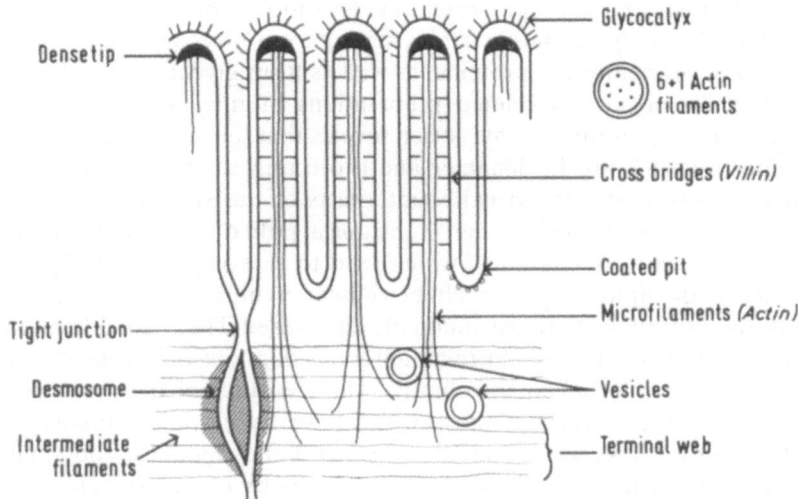

Figure 7.2 Details of the structure of kidney microvilli and the apical region of the cytoplasm

The microvilli do not possess a contractile system. No myosin has been identified in the core, though it has been postulated to be present in the terminal web[5]. Here actin filaments mix with intermediate filaments of the desmosomal complex and it is possible to visualize how microvilli might be retracted downwards towards the terminal web by actin–myosin interaction. Isolated brush borders (which include some of the terminal web region in their midst) do change shape when ATP is added to the medium in which they are suspended[6]. Mooseker[7] has shown that retraction of the cores can be induced by ATP in brush border preparations from which much of the membrane has been removed by detergent treatment. Such movement may subserve two useful functions. First, stirring of the fluid layer between microvilli may aid transport of small solutes; secondly, pinocytosis of macromolecules depends on such motility in the formation of a pit between microvilli which can pinch off to form a small apical vesicle. Filtered proteins are reabsorbed by this latter route[8].

The microvillar membrane

The membrane surface is characterized by a fuzzy layer, the glycocalyx. Although it is very prominent around intestinal microvilli, it can usually be demonstrated in preparations of kidney too[9]. It indicates the presence of complex polysaccharide chains arising from glycosylated amino-acid residues of membrane proteins, as well as from glycolipids in the membrane. In negatively-stained preparations of microvilli, the contrast medium, e.g. uranyl acetate, often reveals that the surface is covered by knobs about 8 nm in diameter and projecting slightly above the lipid bilayer. These are the visual counterparts of the stalked proteins (see below) that seem to characterize the apical pole of some epithelial cells. Freeze–fracture techniques, which tend to cleave preferentially in the plane of the lipid bilayers of all the cellular membranes, invariably show intramembranous particles randomly distributed. These are taken to represent the hydrophobic, intramembranous domains of the intrinsic proteins of the microvillar membrane. The identities of the proteins thus visualized are uncertain: those which have been studied topologically (see below) have rather small transmembrane domains, too small to appear as particles 8–10 nm in diameter seen by freeze fracture[10].

ENZYMOLOGY OF KIDNEY MICROVILLAR MEMBRANE

The kidney microvillar membrane is very rich in hydrolases, comparable in their diversity to the lysosomal hydrolases. However the comparison should not be taken too far: the enzymes of the microvillar membrane are best able to hydrolyse small substrates, e.g. oligosaccharides and oligopeptides, and are unable to degrade macromolecules which lysosomes readily attack. The glycosidases and phosphatases shown to be present in kidney microvilli are listed in Table 7.1. The list immediately poses a question (one that arises again in relation to the peptidases):

what is the function of these enzymes and what are their normal substrates? Trehalose is a constitutent of the haemolymph of insects and is present in mushrooms, but if either source were a major constituent of the diet, the disaccharide would be expected to be hydrolysed by the same enzyme in the intestine.Similarly maltose is not normally a constituent of plasma. The same uncertainties exist in relation to the phosphatases.

TABLE 7.1   Glycosidases and phosphatases in kidney microvilli

Trehalase	(hydrolyses trehalose to glucose)
Maltase	(hydrolyses maltose to glucose)
Alkaline phosphatase	(non-specific monoesterase)
5'-Nucleotidase	(AMP to adenosine)
Phosphodiesterase I	(hydrolyses oligonucleotides)
D-inositol 1:2 cyclic phosphate 2-phosphohydrolase	(product is inositol 1-phosphate)

The microvillar peptidases are listed in Table 7.2. They are a group which is capable of a concerted digestion of peptides to form free amino acids. Only one is an endopeptidase[11,12] capable of cleaving simple peptides of up to 30 or 40 residues in length at bonds involving the amino group of hydrophobic amino acids. It is of enzymological interest in being (together with a similar, if not identical enzyme in the intestinal brush border) the only mammalian representative so far discovered of a class otherwise known only in microbial species, e.g. thermolysin in thermophilic bacteria. Like other enzymes in this group, it contains Zn^{2+} at the active site and is very sensitive to a specific inhibitor, phosphoramidon[13]. The endopeptidase is the logical starting point for the hydrolysis of peptides, since it can generate a family of smaller peptides each with a hydrophobic N-terminal amino-acid residue; these are, in turn, ideal substrates for the rather non-specific aminopeptidase M. However, the endopeptidase is limited in its ability to initiate degradation of larger substrates. Insulin, for example, is wholly resistant, although its two reduced chains are readily attacked. The other enzymes have more clearly defined substrate specificities. One, aminopeptidase A, removes N-terminal aspartyl or glutamyl residues, which are only slowly hydrolysed by aminopeptidase M. A pair of enzymes remove terminal residues that are adjacent to proline, referred to as aminopeptidase P and carboxypeptidase P. Another pair of enzymes remove dipeptides from either end of a peptide chain: dipeptidyl peptidase IV is specific for proline or alanine as the second amino acid residue, while peptidyl dipeptidase attacks at the C-terminus in a more non-specific manner. This latter enzyme is sometimes referred to as angiotensin I-converting enzyme, since it is capable of removing His-Leu from the C-terminus of angiotensin I. However, the product, angiotensin II, would be equally susceptible to attack by other peptidases in the group, and it is unlikely that kidney microvillar peptidyl dipeptidase plays this particular role *in vivo*. The level of activity of the peptidases is extraordinarily high. The least active one is the endopeptidase (about 1% of the activity of aminopeptidase M). Even if we assume that hydrolysis by this enzyme is the rate-limiting step in degrading peptide hormones and that rates determined *in vitro* bear some relation to *in vivo* activity, it appears that 1 g of kidney cortex could initiate the hydrolysis of about 1 mg/min of a peptide of 3500 molecular weight (e.g. glucagon). Such a rate seems to be three or more orders of magnitude greater than the expected load of such substrates in the glomerular filtrate. Once again we see that the functional role of a group of microvillar enzymes is very obscure.

TABLE 7.2   Kidney microvillar peptidases

Enzyme	Active site	Specificity	
Neutral endopeptidase	Zn^{2+}	⎯⎯○⎯↓⎯●⎯⎯	(hydrophobic)
Aminopeptidase M	Zn^{2+}	●⎯↓⎯○⎯⎯⎯	(non-specific)
Aminopeptidase A	Ca^{2+}	●⎯↓⎯○⎯⎯⎯	(Asp, Glu)
Dipeptidyl peptidase IV	Serine	○⎯⎯●⎯↓⎯○⎯	(Pro, Ala)
Peptidyl dipeptidase	Zn^{2+}	⎯○⎯●⎯↓⎯●	(non-specific)
Aminopeptidase P	—	○⎯↓⎯●⎯⎯⎯	(Pro)
Carboxypeptidase P	—	⎯⎯●⎯↓⎯○⎯	(Pro)
γ-Glutamyl transferase	—	●⎯↓⎯○⎯⎯⎯	(γ-Glu)

MICROVILLAR PROTEINS

The core proteins, actin and villin, have already been discussed. These two proteins and a glycoprotein of 180 000 subunit molecular weight, but of unknown function, are the only major constituents to be extracted by solutions of sodium chloride and EDTA[14]. The other microvillar proteins are all intrinsic membrane proteins, each anchored to the hydrophobic interior of the lipid bilayer. Such proteins are released only by detergents or by proteinases capable of clipping the polypeptide chain at a point between the anchor and rest of the molecule exposed at the luminal surface. Many enzymes can be released in an active state by papain, trypsin or elastase. Such enzymes belong to the class of proteins that constitute the knobs on the microvillar surface. Some enzymes are wholly resistant, while others are only slowly released by proteinases. Whether this difference in response derives from a different type of association with the membrane, e.g. one in which the bulk of the protein is within the membrane, or whether it simply indicates the lack of a suitably exposed loop of the polypeptide chain available to proteinase attack, is not known. However, the enzymes released by proteinase action differ from the native forms by the loss of the anchoring peptides. Insofar as the anchor may cross the membrane giving the protein a cytoplasmic domain, this part of the peptide chain, too, would be absent in the 'proteinase' form of the enzyme. Non-ionic detergents, such a Triton X-100, are effective in extracting membrane proteins in their native forms. It follows that a comparison of proteinase and detergent forms of a microvillar enzyme can tell us about the size and other properties of the hydrophobic anchor. Another aspect of the topology of an enzyme, whether or not it is transmembrane, can only be investigated by labelling the enzyme protein in separate experiments at the luminal and cytoplasmic surfaces of the membrane.

Principal proteins of kidney microvilli

Table 7.3 summarizes the current state of knowledge on the microvillar proteins. The quantitative information is partly derived from estimates of the amount of protein in stained bands seen in SDS–polyacrylamide gel electrophoresis and partly on comparisons of specific activities of enzymes in the membrane with those in the purified forms. Such estimates are very approximate, but it is clear that two proteins predominate in microvilli: aminopeptidase M in the membrane and actin in the core. Most of the membrane proteins investigated so far have rather large subunits and, typically, they are dimeric when purified. The enzymes in the membrane are all glycoproteins, in contrast to the proteins of the core. This conforms to the general rule that the glycosylated domain of a plasma-membrane protein is at the external (luminal) surface.

The hydrophobic anchor of microvillar membrane proteins

We have recently attempted to study the way in which dipeptidyl pepti-

TABLE 7.3   Principal proteins of kidney microvilli

Protein	Subunit mol. wt. ($\times 10^{-3}$)	Subunits	Glycosylation	Approx. proportion of microvillus protein (%)
Aminopeptidase M	160	2	+++	8
Aminopeptidase A	140 (110, 95, 45)	?	++	1
Dipeptidyl peptidase IV	130	2	+	4
Carboxypeptidase P	130	?	+	1
Neutral endopeptidase	95	? 1 or 2	+	4
Alkaline phosphatase	80	2	+	0.04
γ-Glutamyl transferase	54, 27	2	+	4
Villin	95	1	0	? 1
Actin	42	many	0	9

Data from Booth and Kenny[14] and unpublished work

dase IV is anchored to the membrane[15]. This is one of the enzymes readily freed from the membrane by proteinases, and it was possible to compare the properties of two purified forms, one released by autolysis (by proteinases) and the other by a detergent (Triton X-100). There was no difference in catalytic activity or in susceptibility to serine inhibitors. Hence the active site is uninfluenced by the association of the hydrophobic anchor with a lipid environment. The only differences detected were structural. Both forms were dimeric, but the polypeptide chain was about 30–40 residues longer in the detergent form. The subunit molecular weight was therefore only slightly increased, but the native molecule was enlarged more substantially by the presence of detergent bound to the hydrophobic domain. The two polypeptide chains differed in sequence at the N-termini, but so far as could be determined, the C-termini were similar (Table 7.4.). Treatment of the detergent form with papain generated a form of the enzyme indistinguishable in properties from the autolysis form. In so doing, a fragment was released, and isolated; this was leucine N-terminal, about 3500 molecular weight and with hydrophobic properties. This fragment therefore had the properties of the hydrophobic anchor. These results, as a whole, support the view that each monomer of the enzyme is anchored to the membrane by a relatively small length of polypeptide chain (3% of the total) located at or near the N-terminus. The rest of the molecule protrudes from the membrane surface and includes the active site and glycosylated domains. This type of assembly of plasma membrane protein contrasts with others, such as glycophorin in the erythrocyte membrane (for examples see reference 16) in which the anchoring domain is nearer the C-terminus. Since other microvillar enzymes have provided similar results to those obtained with dipeptidyl peptidase IV[17] it is possible that those studied so far exemplify a special class of membrane proteins anchored near the N-terminus.

TABLE 7.4 **Structural differences between the detergent and proteinase forms of dipeptidyl peptidase IV**

	Detergent form	*Proteinase form*
Subunit mol. wt.	Slightly > 130 000	130 000
Mol. wt. (native dimeric forms)	304 000	266 000
N-terminal amino acid sequence	Leu-Gly-Phe-Ala-	Ser-Thr-Ser-Thr
	Leu-Ala-(Phe)-Ile-	(Tyr)-(Thr)-(Leu)-Thr-

From Macnair and Kenny[15]

Do microvillar enzymes cross the membrane?

This question extends the point discussed in the previous section. Does the anchoring domain extend as far and possibly beyond the cytoplasmic surface of the membrane? We have recently attempted to answer this question by means of two different experimental approaches[18]. When isolated, microvilli form sealed right-side-out vesicles. To answer the question involves methods for covalently labelling proteins unambiguously at the external and internal surfaces. The method used should not produce artifacts due to contramembrane or intramembrane labelling of proteins. It must also enable the labelled proteins to be identified. We first used lactoperoxidase-catalysed radio-iodination of proteins, which were then resolved by SDS–polyacrylamide gel electrophoresis. Although this revealed asymmetric labelling patterns in the radio-autographs of the gels, much of the radioactivity was present in the fatty-acid chains of the membrane phospholipids. This indicated that intramembrane labelling was also taking place. Hence an alternative strategy was sought. A novel photolabelling reagent was synthesized,

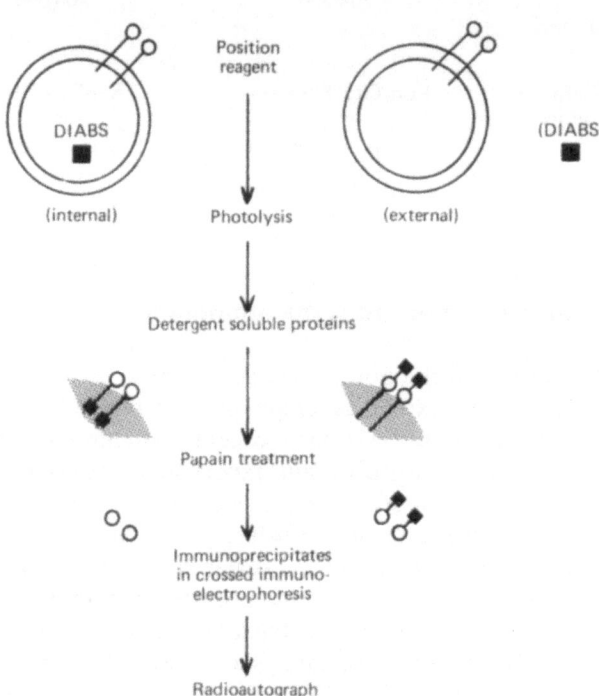

Figure 7.3 The labelling strategy for demonstrating transmembrane proteins in microvillar vesicles using a photolabel

3,5-di[^{125}I]iodo-4-azidobenzene sulphonic acid which, when photolysed, generated a reactive nitrene capable of adding across any C—H bond. It proved possible to position the reagent within the vesicles, by virtue of a transport system which was fortuitously present in the membrane. External labelling was performed at 0°C, a temperature at which the transport system was inactive. The method is summarized in Figure 7.3. The labelled proteins were analysed by crossed immunoelectrophoresis. When a monospecific antibody which recognizes only those determinants on the luminal part of the enzyme was used, a single immunoprecipitate was formed. Other labelled components were not precipitated and were lost during the electrophoresis. A radio-autograph showed that the precipitate from the detergent-solubilized proteins was radioactive from either internal or external labelling. However, papain treatment removed the internal label from the antigenic determinants, and hence that precipitate was no longer radioactive. The experiment was also done with an antiserum raised to the whole membrane, which yielded a complex pattern of immunoprecipitates, but permitted the identification of several antigens by histochemical staining[19].

TABLE 7.5 Enzymes shown to be transmembrane proteins in kidney microvilli

Aminopeptidase M
Aminopeptidase A
Dipeptidyl peptidase IV
Neutral endopeptidase

From Booth and Kenny[18]. Aminopeptidase M has also been shown by Louvard et al.[20], using a different approach, to be transmembrane in intestinal microvilli

This type of labelling experiment was free from the disadvantages noted with lactoperoxidase iodination. It produced neither intra- nor contramembrane labelling and enabled several major microvillar enzymes to be characterized as transmembrane. The list of such proteins characterized so far is shown in Table 7.5. No enzymes which it has been possible to see in radio-autographs have been shown *not* to be transmembrane. It may well be that all intrinsic membrane proteins have at least some part of the polypeptide chain exposed at the cytoplasmic surface.

SUMMARY AND CONCLUSIONS

Figure 7.4 summarizes the structural and topological features of kidney microvilli discussed above. The enzyme molecules are shown typically as dimeric proteins protruding from the luminal surface. At this surface, the stalks are accessible to attack by proteinases, which thereby release enzymes from the membrane. The stalks provide anchors for the proteins in the membrane, which they fully traverse so as to be exposed at the cytoplasmic surface. Our knowledge of the microvillar enzymes is fairly detailed in respect of protein structure, topology and enzymology.

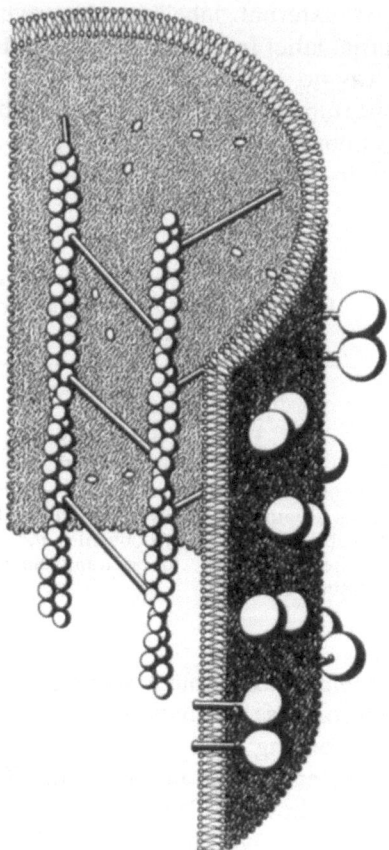

Figure 7.4 The organization of the core and membrane proteins in kidney microvilli

In contrast, our understanding of their physiological roles is rudimentary and little is known in molecular terms about the proteins responsible for the transport functions of the membrane.

References

1. Kenny, A. J. and Booth, A. G. (1978). Microvilli: their ultrastructure, enzymology and molecular organization. *Essays Biochem.*, **14**, 1
2. Geiger, B., Tokuyasu, K. T. and Singer, S. J. (1979). Immunocytochemical localization of α-actinin in intestinal epithelial cells. *Proc. Natl. Acad. Sci. USA*, **76**, 2833
3. Bretscher, A. and Weber, K. (1979). Villin: the major microfilament-associated protein of the intestinal microvillus. *Proc. Natl. Acad. Sci. USA*, **76**, 2321
4. Booth, A. G. and Kenny, A. J. (1976). A morphometric and biochemical investigation of the vesiculation of kidney microvilli. *J. Cell. Sci.*, **21**, 449
5. Mooseker, M. S. and Tilney, L. G. (1975). Organization of an actin filament–membrane complex. Filament polarity and membrane attachment in the microvilli of intestinal epithelial cells. *J. Cell. Biol.*, **67**, 725
6. Rodwald, R., Newman, S. B. and Karnovsky, M. J. (1976). Contraction of isolated brush borders from the intestinal epithelium. *J. Cell. Biol.*, **70**, 541
7. Mooseker, M. S. (1976). Brush border motility: microvillar contraction in triton treated brush borders isolated from intestinal epithelium. *J. Cell. Biol.* **71**, 417
8. Maunsbach, A. B. (1966). Absorption of ^{125}I-labelled homologous albumin by rat kidney proximal tubule cells: a study of microperfused single proximal tubules by electron microscopic autoradiography and histochemistry. *J. Ultrastr. Res.*, **15**, 197
9. Groniowski, J., Biczyskowa, W. and Walski, M. (1969). Electron microscopic studies on the surface coat of the nephron. *J. Cell. Biol.*, **40**, 585
10. Friederici, H. H. R. (1969). The surface structure of some renal cell membranes. *Lab. Invest.*, **21**, 459
11. Kerr, M. A. and Kenny, A. J. (1974). The purification and specificity of a neutral endopeptidase from rabbit kidney brush border. *Biochem. J.*, **137**, 477
12. Kerr, M. A. and Kenny, A. J. (1974). The molecular weight and properties of a neutral metallo-endopeptidase from rabbit kidney brush border. *Biochem. J.*, **137**, 489
13. Kenny, A. J. (1977). Proteinases associated with cell membranes. In A. J. Barrett (ed.). *Proteinases in Mammalian Cells and Tissues*. (Amsterdam: Elsevier/North Holland Biomedical Press)
14. Booth, A. G. and Kenny, A. J. (1976). Proteins of the kidney microvillus membrane. Identification of subunits after sodium dodecyl sulphate/polyacrylamide gel electrophoresis. *Biochem. J.*, **159**, 395
15. Macnair, R. D. C. and Kenny, A. J. (1979). Proteins of the kidney microvillar membrane. The amphipathic form of dipeptidyl peptidase IV. *Biochem. J.*, **179**, 379
16. Rothman, J. E. and Lenard, J. (1977). Membrane asymmetry: the nature

of membrane asymmetry provides clues to the puzzle of how membranes are assembled. *Science*, **195**, 743

17. Brunner, J., Hauser, H., Braun, H., Wilson, K. J., Wacker, H., O'Neill, B. and Semenza, G. (1979). The mode of association of the enzyme complex sucrase–isomaltase with the intestinal brush border membrane. *J. Biol. Chem.*, **254**, 1821

18. Booth, A. G. and Kenny, A. J. (1980). Proteins of the kidney microvillar membrane. Asymmetric labelling of the membrane by lactoperoxidase-catalysed radio-iodination and by photolysis of 3,5-di[^{125}I]iodo-4-azido-benzene sulphonate. *Biochem. J.*, **187**, 31

19. Booth, A., Hubbard, L. M. L. and Kenny, A. J. (1979). Proteins of the kidney microvillar membrane. Immunoelectrophoretic analysis of the membrane hydrolases: identification and resolution of the detergent- and proteinase-solubilized forms. *Biochem. J.*, **179**, 397

20. Louvard, D., Semeriva, M. and Maroux, S. (1976). The brush border intestinal aminopeptidase, a transmembrane protein as probed by macro-molecular photolabelling. *J. Molec. Biol.*, **106**, 1023

8

Cyclic nucleotides and the regulation of water and electrolyte transport
C. L. Browne and A. L. Steiner

**INTRODUCTION TO
CYCLIC NUCLEOTIDE METABOLISM**

Cyclic 3′,5′-adenosine monophosphate (cAMP) is often referred to as a 'second messenger' because of its role as a mediator of nonsteroid hormonal responses. Catecholamines and many peptide hormones act at the level of the plasma membrane by binding to specific cell-surface receptors coupled to the enzyme adenylate cyclase. Interaction of a hormone with its specific adenylate-cyclase-coupled receptor leads to either an increase or a decrease in the intracellular levels of cAMP, depending on the relative activity of stimulated adenylate cyclase and the rate of cAMP degradation by specific phosphodiesterases. The effects of cAMP are mediated through cAMP-dependent protein kinases. Activation of the protein kinases by cyclic AMP results in the phosphorylation of specific regulatory proteins in the cell, the final expression of the original hormonal message.

The exact role of cyclic 3′,5′-guanosine monophosphate (cGMP) in biological regulation is still uncertain, although it too apparently acts as a second messenger in some cases. In many biological systems cyclic AMP and cyclic GMP seem to have opposing regulatory influences, but in others they appear to work in a co-operative fashion. Intracellular cGMP production is the result of the stimulation of the enzyme guanylate cyclase; however, the agents responsible for activation of the enzyme *in vivo* are not known. Hormones which are known to increase cGMP levels *in vivo* have generally not been shown to activate guanylate cyclase *in vitro*. Thus it seems likely that any effect of membrane agents on guanylate-cyclase activity is the result of an indirect mechanism. Like cAMP, intracellular cGMP is degraded by specific phosphodiesterases, and its regulatory effects are mediated by cGMP-dependent protein kinases.

ADENYLATE AND GUANYLATE CYCLASES

Adenylate cyclase has primarily a plasma membrane localization, but has also been reported in nuclei from prostate, liver, and brain, and in the mitochondrial and/or microsomal fractions of brain and cardiac and skeletal muscles[1-7]. Activation of adenylate cyclase results in the intracellular formation of cyclic 3',5'-AMP and inorganic pyrophosphate from ATP[8]. This reaction has an absolute requirement for magnesium[9]. In fact, the true substrate of adenylate cyclase is Mg–ATP and free ATP is inhibitory to the reaction[10,11].

The adenylate-cyclase system is composed of a number of functional components, including not only the specific hormone receptor and catalytic unit, but also independent regulatory sites for guanine nucleotides and Mg^{2+}. Until recently, it was not known whether the receptor and the catalytic unit were separate molecular entities. However, Orly and Schramm fused cells lacking a functional β-adrenergic receptor with cells lacking a functional catalytic unit and showed that the hybrids had a functional hormonally-responsive adenylate cyclase, establishing the independence of the two[12,13]. Subsequently, biochemical purification, component resolution and reconstitution have been used to identify the ligands involved in the adenylate cyclase system and to investigate their physiological roles. Limbird and Lefkowitz and Haga *et al.* succeeded in separating the β-adrenergic receptor from adenylate-cyclase activity using gel filtration and sucrose gradients of detergent solubilized membranes[14,15]. Ross and Gilman have shown that it is possible to reconstitute hormone-stimulated adenylate-cyclase activity by combining detergent extracts of adenylate cyclase from a cell type which lacks β-adrenergic receptors with adenylate-cyclase-deficient membranes containing receptors from another cell type[16]. It is generally believed that the receptors of the adenylate-cyclase system are oriented towards the outer surface of the plasma membrane, while the catalytic components are directed toward the inner surface[17]. The manner in which receptor binding is coupled to adenylate-cyclase stimulation is not yet clear.

Free magnesium in excess of substrate ATP enhances enzyme catalytic activity[11]. Apparently Mg^{2+} binds to a second allosteric site on the adenylate-cyclase receptor complex. In the case of β-adrenergic receptors, this leads to an increased affinity of agonists for the receptor which is believed to enhance the coupling of the hormone receptor to the adenylate cyclase, leading in turn to increased catalytic activity[11,18,19]. The effect of Mg^{2+} on agonist binding is opposite that observed with guanine nucleotides. Rodbell et al. observed that in rat-liver plasma membranes very low concentrations of GTP enhanced glucagon stimulation of adenylate cyclase activity, while at the same time decreased the affinity of hormone binding to the receptor[20,21]. The activation of adenylate cyclase by guanine nucleotides (GTP in particular) is consistent irrespective of the hormone or tissue, leading to the hypothesis that the nucleotide is a required factor in hormonal stimulation of the enzyme[20,22-24].

Guanine nucleotides act through proteins known as guanylnucleotide-binding proteins, which are distinct from both the receptor and catalytic units of the adenylate cyclase[25,26]. It is not yet fully understood how decreased affinity of receptor for agonists and stimulation of enzyme activation are related, or whether these seemingly opposing effects are due to only one, or to two, guanine nucleotide regulatory sites[27,28]. There is some evidence that suggests that the catalytic unit may exist as an Mg–ATP-dependent enzyme which is converted to an Mg–ATP-dependent enzyme upon its association with guanylnucleotide binding proteins[26,29]. It has also been hypothesized that the guanylnucleotide binding proteins may play a role in the regulation of coupling of the receptor to the enzyme[28,30]. The nature of the interaction, if any, between the regulatory functions of the guanine nucleotides and Mg^{2+} is not yet clear.

Adenylate cyclase is also known to be universally activated by sodium fluoride and cholera toxin. The mechanism of stimulation by NaF is not known, but it is believed to act through the guanylnucleotide regulatory proteins[31]. In turkey erythrocyte membranes, cholera toxin has been shown to act by inhibition of a hormonally stimulated GTPase activity at the site of guanylnucleotide binding proteins. In the absence of cholera toxin, the hydrolysis of GTP is believed to play a part in the termination of adenylate cyclase activation[32]. This suggests a dual role for the guanylnucleotide binding component of the adenylate cyclase system: activation in the presence of nucleotide plus hormone, and termination of activation by hydrolysis of bound GTP.

Although guanylate cyclase catalyses a virtually identical reaction to that of adenylate cyclase, i.e. the production of cGMP and inorganic phosphate from GTP, the two enzymes exhibit a number of different properties. Whereas adenylate cyclase is predominantly localized in the plasma membrane, guanylate cyclase can be found in both the soluble and particulate fractions of broken-cell preparations, and the ratio of soluble to particulate guanylate cyclase varies from tissue to tissue[33]. The optional substrate for guanylate cyclase is Mn–GTP and the requirement for Mn^{2+} in excess of substrate for maximum cyclase activity has led to the proposal that guanylate cyclase, like adenylate cyclase, has an additional binding site for divalent cations[34]. The possibility of a second regulatory binding site for nucleotides has also been proposed, based on the ability of ATP to activate the particulate form of uterine guanylate cyclase[35].

The mechanisms regulating guanylate-cyclase activity are not understood. A number of substances have been reported to affect guanylate cyclase activity, such as secretin, lipids, fatty acids, nitrosamines and nucleophiles[36]. Based on observations that oxidants were capable of activating splenic-cell guanylate cyclase, Goldberg et al.[37] have suggested that a general mechanism underlying the activation of the enzyme by all of the above agents may be specific oxidation–reduction events in the cell, which result in sulphydryl–disulphide interconversions on either the enzyme or an associated regulatory component.

CYCLIC NUCLEOTIDE PHOSPHODIESTERASES

Cyclic nucleotide phosphodiesterases convert cyclic AMP and cyclic GMP to their corresponding 5′ monophosphates, thus terminating their actions in the cell[38]. Most tissues appear to contain multiple forms of phosphodiesterases which differ in their tissue distribution, subcellular localization, substrate specificity, kinetic properties, sensitivity to various inhibitors, and regulation by a calcium-dependent modulator protein. Three forms of phosphodiesterase (PDE) first described by Russell et al.[39] in rat-liver preparations, but since reported in other tissues are, in the order in which they elute from DEAE ion exchange chromatography: (1) an enzyme with a four times higher affinity for cGMP than cAMP which is stimulated by calcium-dependent modulator protein, (2) a calcium-independent enzyme with low affinity for both cAMP and cGMP, which at low substrate concentrations hydrolyses cGMP more rapidly than cAMP, but by which the hydrolysis of cAMP is stimulated by cGMP, (3) a calcium-independent enzyme with a high affinity for cAMP. A separate phosphodiesterase with a high affinity for both cAMP and cyclic GMP, which is also stimulated by the calcium-dependent modulator protein, has been reported in human lung tissue[40].

The calcium-dependent stimulation of certain forms of PDE was discovered in early works in which attempts at purification of PDE gave low yields with great loss of activity. Cheung[41] and Kakiuchi[42] independently isolated from rat brain an endogenous protein activator that had been dissociated from the PDE during the purification process. The active form of the protein activator, known now as either the calcium-dependent regulator protein or calmodulin, is a calcium–activator complex[43]. The calcium-dependent regulator protein is structurally very similar to, although distinct from, skeletal muscle troponin-C[44]. When bound to calcium, troponin C modulates the actin–myosin interaction which leads to muscle contraction. To some extent troponin C and the calcium-dependent regulator protein will substitute for one another in their respective biological systems[45].

After the discovery of a calcium-dependent activation of cyclic nucleotide phosphodiesterases, it was subsequently reported by Dedman *et al.*[45] that the calcium-dependent regulator protein also activates brain adenylate cyclase. The mechanism of activation of both phosphodiesterase and adenylate cyclase appears to be the same. In the presence of Ca^{2+}, a calcium–activator complex forms; this alters the helical conformation of the activator in such a way that it can interact with the inactive phosphodiesterase or adenylate cyclase apoenzyme to form an active holoenzyme[45]. This is demonstrated for PDE in the equation below. Lowering the calcium concentration results in the dissociation of the holoenzyme and a return to the basal level of enzyme activity.

$$Ca^{2+} + \text{calmodulin} \rightleftharpoons Ca^{2+}\text{-calmodulin}$$
$$\text{(inactive)} \qquad\qquad \text{(active)}$$

$$Ca^{2+}\text{-calmodulin} + PDE \rightarrow Ca^{2+}\text{-calmodulin-PDE}$$
$$\text{(inactive)} \qquad\qquad \text{(active)}$$

It has been proposed that the activation of both adenylate cyclase, which synthesizes cAMP, and PDE, which degrades it, by the same protein provides a mechanism for the production of transient increases in intracellular cAMP concentration[46]. Stimuli causing an influx of Ca^{2+} through the plasma membrane could result in the activation of adenylate cyclase and an increase in intracellular cAMP. The Ca^{2+} arriving in the cytoplasm shortly thereafter would cause the activation of PDE and the degradation of the short-lived cAMP. It has also been suggested that since the Ca^{2+}-dependent PDE hydrolyses cGMP at a greater rate than cAMP, an influx of Ca^{2+} might result in a simultaneous increase in cAMP and decrease in cGMP concentrations[46].

The activation of phosphodiesterase by the calcium-dependent regulator protein is in some way regulated by two inhibitory proteins which have been isolated from bovine brain and retina[47-49]. The inhibitory proteins bind to the regulator protein in a calcium-dependent manner, preventing its interaction with, and thus stimulation of, the enzyme. The physiological significance of these inhibitory factors is not known.

CYCLIC NUCLEOTIDE-DEPENDENT PROTEIN KINASES

The phosphorylation of cell-specific substrate proteins by cyclic-nucleotide-dependent protein kinases provides a mechanism by which cAMP and cGMP can evoke a wide variety of physiological responses. The cAMP and cGMP-dependent protein kinases are very similar, but there are some notable differences between them. Cyclic AMP-dependent protein kinases exist as a tetramer containing one regulatory subunit dimer, which binds cAMP, and two catalytic subunit monomers which carry out the phosphorylation reaction[50-52]. There are two kinds of cAMP-dependent protein kinases, type I and type II, which differ in their regulatory subunits but have the same catalytic subunit[50]. The ratio of type I to type II varies from tissue to tissue. Type I generally predominates in embryonic tissues, whereas type II is found mostly in well-differentiated tissues[53]. Also, the levels of type I and type II fluctuate throughout the cell cycle of cultured cells[54]. Based on this evidence it has been suggested that the two isozymes have different functions in growth and differentiation[55].

When bound to the regulatory subunit, the activity of the catalytic subunit is inhibited. The holoenzyme is unable to catalyse the phosphorylation of exogenous protein substrate, although under these conditions there is a limited self-phosphorylation of the regulatory subunit by the catalytic subunit[56]. Binding of cAMP to the regulatory subunits releases the catalytic subunits as in the following equation:

$$R_2C_2 + 2\ cAMP \rightarrow R_2(cAMP)_2 + 2C$$

In the dissociated form, the catalytic subunit is fully active and catalyses the transfer of the terminal phosphate of ATP to a serine or threonine hydroxyl group of a substrate protein.

Like cyclic-AMP-dependent protein kinase, cyclic-GMP-dependent protein kinase (G-kinase) also functions by transferring the terminal phosphate of ATP to a serine hydroxyl group of a substrate protein. It, too, can self-phosphorylate, the significance of which is not known[57]. However, G-kinase differs from A-kinase in a number of ways. G-Kinase is a dimer composed of two identical subunits, each of which binds cGMP and possesses catalytic activity[58,59]. It has not been observed to dissociate into catalytic and regulatory subunits upon interaction with cGMP or substrate under normal conditions, although catalytic and cGMP-binding activity can be dissociated in the presence of very high concentrations of cGMP and histones[60,61]. What alternative mechanism is used by cGMP to bring about the activation of its kinase is not known.

Cyclic-GMP-dependent protein kinase is unique in its requirement of a high concentration of Mg^{2+} and the apparent requirement in some systems for a stimulatory protein modulator for activity[62]. Crude preparations of the protein modulator not only stimulate G-kinase, but can also inhibit A-kinase. The stimulatory and inhibitory activities of most tissues can be separated, indicating that they are actually the result of two separate proteins, but purified lobster tail muscle contains both activities as a single entity[62]. The A-kinase inhibitory activity is the result of an interaction of the modulator with the catalytic subunit, but the stimulatory modulator does not appear to interact directly with G-kinase and its mechanism of action is unknown[63]. A second inhibitor protein has been found which inhibits not only cAMP and cGMP-dependent but also cyclic nucleotide-independent protein kinases[63].

Many of the substrates of cyclic-nucleotide-dependent protein kinases can also be phosphorylated by a cyclic-nucleotide-independent protein kinase which is regulated by the calcium-dependent regulator protein of adenylate cyclase and cyclic nucleotide phosphodiesterase[59,60]. This kinase, known as the modulator-dependent protein kinase, is believed to mediate many of the actions of Ca^{2+} in cellular processes. At this point, it is important to emphasize the obviously close relationship between cyclic nucleotides and Ca^{2+} as regulators of intracellular events. Although the evidence is not as clear as it is for the cyclic nucleotides, it is apparent that Ca^{2+} also acts as a second messenger, the intermediary between a stimulus and the appropriate intracellular response. While calcium has profound influence on cyclic nucleotide metabolism by its regulation of cyclases and phosphodiesterases, cyclic nucleotides are also involved in the regulation of calcium metabolism, and the two often act in sequence as co-messengers[64,65]. In considering the role played by cyclic nucleotides in any physiological process, it is often impossible not to consider also the role of calcium.

CYCLIC NUCLEOTIDES AND TRANSPORT

Kidney

There is now considerable evidence that cyclic nucleotides play a role in the regulation of the transport of water and electrolytes across membranes. However, the exact mechanisms by which cyclic nucleotides affect transport are not yet clear. The first demonstration that cyclic AMP affected transport was in the kidney. Vasopressin (anti-diuretic hormone) is a posterior pituitary hormone that stimulates water reabsorption by the renal cortical tubules and medullary collecting ducts, and increases active sodium transport and water permeability of the skin and urinary bladder in amphibia[66]. Evidence that the effects of vasopressin on transport are mediated by cyclic AMP are as follows: (1) Cyclic AMP and theophylline (a phosphodiesterase inhibitor) can reproduce the effects of vasopressin on the urinary bladder of the toad and collecting tubules of the rabbit kidney[67-69]. (2) Cyclic AMP concentrations increase in the epithelial cells of the toad bladder and in the renal medulla following exposure to physiological concentrations of vasopressin[69-71]. (3) Vasopressin also increases adenylate cyclase activity in the toad bladder and renal cortical and medullary collecting tubules[72-75].

A number of hormones which interact with vasopressin in the regulation of water permeability and sodium transport may also act through cyclic nucleotides. Aldosterone increases sodium transport and stimulates vasopressin-initiated increases in water permeability in the toad bladder[76]. It also increases cAMP levels in the presence of vasopressin, possibly a result of its inhibition of cAMP phosphodiesterase activity[77,78]. Prostaglandins and catecholamines, whose effects are known to be mediated through cyclic nucleotides[79,80], also alter the water permeability and sodium-transport responses to vasopressin. Prostaglandins, which are produced by the renal medulla after vasopressin stimulation, decrease the magnitude of water-permeability response to vasopressin of the toad bladder[81]. The water permeability and sodium-transport response to vasopressin of the toad bladder are also inhibited by α-adrenergic agents, but β-adrenergic agents appear to potentiate this response[81].

TABLE 8.1 Cyclic nucleotides and water and electrolyte transport

Tissue	Hormone	Cyclic nucleotides	Transport
Kidney tubules and toad bladder	vasopressin	↑ cAMP ↑ adenylate cyclase	↑ H_2O permeability ↑ Na^+ transport
Kidney tubules	parathyroid hormone	↑ cAMP ↑ adenylate cyclase activity	↑ Ca^{2+} reabsorption ↓ PO_4^-, Na^+, HCO_3^- reabsorption
Intestine	parathyroid hormone	↑ cAMP	↑ Ca^{2+} absorption
	calcitonin	↑ cAMP	↓ Ca^{2+} absorption
	epinephrine	↓ cAMP, cGMP	↑ Na^+ and Cl^- absorption
	cholera toxin	↑ cAMP ↑ adenylate cyclase activity	↓ HCO_3^- secretion ↑ Na^+, Cl^-, HCO_3^-, H_2O excretion
Ileum		↑ cAMP	↑ Na^+, Cl^-, secretion, NaCl absorption
Pancreas	secretin	↑ cAMP ↑ adenylate cyclase activity	↑ HCO_3^-, H_2O secretion
Colon	—	↑ cAMP ↑ adenylate cyclase activity	↑ Cl^-, H_2O secretion
Gall bladder	—	↑ cAMP	↑ Na^+ and Ca^- influx ↓ H_2O absorption
Erythrocyte	norepinephrine	↑ cAMP ↑ adenylate cyclase activity	↑ bidirectional K^+ flux ↑ net K^+ uptake

A number of different mechanisms have been proposed whereby cyclic nucleotides might alter the permeability of membranes to water and sodium[81]. Since cyclic nucleotides act ultimately by the phosphorylation of specific substrate proteins, it has been suggested that cyclic-nucleotide-dependent phosphorylation of a plasma-membrane protein alters membrane permeability. Cyclic-nucleotide-dependent protein-kinase activity has been measured in frog and toad bladder and the cyclic-nucleotide-dependent phosphorylation of a plasma membrane protein in the renal medulla has been reported[82-84], but the phosphorylation of a specified membrane-transport protein has yet to be demonstrated. A specific protein in the apical membrane of the toad urinary bladder has been observed to be dephosphorylated in response to hormone or cyclic AMP exposure, leading to the alternative hypothesis that dephosphorylation of membrane proteins may affect transport[85]. It has been suggested, however, that this protein, which has subsequently been observed in every vertebrate tissue examined, is actually a phosphorylated regulatory subunit of the protein kinase which is being coincidentally dephosphorylated upon binding of cAMP to the enzyme[86]. Whether the protein is a membrane transport protein or a regulatory subunit of the protein kinase is still not proven, and its role in the action of vasopressin on membranes is unclear. Finally, it has been proposed that cyclic nucleotides may affect transport through the regulation of microtubules and microfilaments. There is evidence to suggest that cyclic nucleotides are involved in the regulation of the assembly and disassembly of tubulin-containing microtubules and actin-containing microfilament bundles in cells. A specific cAMP-dependent protein kinase, that co-purifies with rat-brain tubulin, phosphorylates certain microtubule proteins that have been implicated as regulators of microtubule assembly[87–89]. A high molecular-weight, actin-binding protein, filamin, has also been reported to be phosphorylated by a cyclic-AMP-dependent protein kinase[90]. The antimitotic agent colchicine which disrupts microtubules, and the mold metabolite cytocholasin B which disrupts microfilaments, inhibit the effects of both vasopressin and cAMP on water permeability[91–94]. It is possible that an interaction of a cyclic-nucleotide-regulated cytoskeletal system with the membrane could be responsible for the increase in water permeability which occurs after vasopressin stimulation. However, the possibility that these observations are the result of non-specific effects of the inhibitors on the plasma membrane has not been ruled out.

Another hormone known to effect transport in the kidney is parathyroid hormone (PTH), which is produced in the parathyroid glands and functions primarily in calcium and phosphate homeostasis. In the kidney it stimulates calcium reabsorption and inhibits the reabsorption of phosphate, sodium and bicarbonate[79]. There is strong evidence that the effects of PTH are mediated by cAMP. cAMP can reproduce the effects of the hormone on phosphate, sodium and bicarbonate reabsorption in the proximal tubules[95]. PTH stimulates the adenylate cyclase of rat renal cortex, and to a lesser extent, the renal medulla, and results in an increase in the tissue concentration of cAMP[74,80]. In intestine and bone the effects of PTH are modified by the thyroid hormone, calcitonin. Although the adenylate cyclase of rat renal cortical membranes is stimulated by calcitonin, this is not true for other species examined, and a role for calcitonin in the regulation of renal phosphate, sodium and calcium has not been established[81,96].

Erythrocyte

In avian erythrocytes β-adrenergic agents affect cell volume by altering the bidirectional fluxes of primarily K^+, and to a lesser extent, Na^+ [97–99]. In the presence of norepinephrine, K^+ influx initially exceeds efflux, resulting in temporary cell swelling. β-Adrenergic stimulation of avian erythrocytes results in activation of adenylate cyclase and an increase in intracellular cAMP and the effects on K^+ flux and cell volume can be induced by exogenously-applied dibutyryl cAMP in the absence of hormonal stimulation [97–100]. Although a 240 000 molecular weight protein has been observed to be phosphorylated in a cAMP-dependent manner concurrent with changes in transport, it is not yet clear whether the phosphorylation of this protein has a causal effect on the changes observed [101,102]. Although mammalian erythrocytes also contain β-adrenergic-stimulated adenylate cyclase, cAMP-dependent protein kinase activities and cAMP-dependent phosphorylation of membrane proteins, neither catecholamines nor cAMP have been shown to have an effect on water or electrolyte transport [103–106].

Gastrointestinal tract

The small intestine normally has a net active influx of Na^+ and Cl^-, the result of a balance between a coupled uptake of sodium chloride in the brush border of the villus cells and an active secretory process for anions in crypt cells, as well as a larger net secretory efflux of HCO_3^- [81,107]. The diarrhoeagenic effects of cholera enterotoxin, secreted by the bacterium *Vibrio cholerae*, and *Escherichia coli* enterotoxins are the result of a reversal in the direction of net transport of Na^+ and Cl^- [107]. This secretion of electrolyte leads to a sustained passive efflux of water. The secretory response to cholera toxin is mediated by cAMP. The cyclic AMP content of the intestinal mucosa is increased by cholera toxin, and the time course of these changes is the same as that of alterations in ion transport [108]. Cyclic AMP and theophylline can reproduce the effects of cholera toxin *in vitro*, by inhibiting the coupled uptake process for NaCl and at the same time stimulating active anion secretion [107,109]. Although cholera toxin increases bicarbonate accumulation in the lumen of the ileum *in vivo*, neither cAMP nor cholera toxin has yet produced this effect *in vitro* [110]. Cholera toxin has been shown to activate adenylate cyclase in intestinal epithelia as well as a number of other tissue types [45] by a rather unique mechanism in which a subunit of the cholera toxin molecule penetrates through the plasma membrane, and possibly activates the enzyme intracellularly through direct covalent modification[111].

Two *E. coli* enterotoxins have been identified, one of which is immunologically crossreactive with cholera toxin, and which also activates adenylate cyclase[112,113]. The second enterotoxin does not alter cAMP levels in intestinal mucosa, but does produce rapid increases in cGMP associated with an activation of guanylate cyclase[113,114]. It also results in an inhibition of net Cl^- absorption, but does not stimulate net secretion as does cholera toxin[113]. This effect has not been demonstrated in other tissues, and may be specific for intestine[107]. It is likely, although not yet proven, that the increased levels of cGMP are related to the reversal in transport properties.

The mechanisms by which increases in cAMP and cGMP bring about alterations in transport are still being investigated. However, cholera toxin has been shown to increase the phosphorylation of proteins in intestinal membrane preparations, and both cAMP and cGMP have been shown to increase the incorporation of phosphate into brush border proteins[115,116].

The actions of a number of other agents which stimulate the active secretion of water and electrolytes in the small intestine may also be mediated by cAMP. Prostaglandins, which inhibit the intestinal absorption of Na^+ and stimulate the secretion of Cl^- and H_2O in the intestine increase the tissue levels of cAMP and stimulate adenylate cyclase activity[115,117]. Vasointestinal peptide (VIP) is an intestinal hormone which has among its diverse biological activities the inhibition of Na^+ absorption and stimulation of Na^+, Cl^- and fluid secretion from intestinal mucosa[81,118]. VIP has also been shown to increase cAMP levels and activate intestinal adenylate cyclase[119,120]. A third hormone, calcitonin, also decreases ilial Na^+ absorption and stimulates Cl^- secretion, but has not been shown to increase cAMP or cGMP levels in this tissue[121].

Besides the intestine, cAMP is believed to play a role in transport processes in other areas of the gastrointestinal tract. Cyclic AMP inhibits Na^+ and consequently, fluid absorption in the gallbladder[122,123]. In the pancreas the action of the hormone secretin, which regulates pancreatic-fluid secretion, is mediated by cAMP. Secretin-stimulated increases in fluid secretion and fluid bicarbonate composition can be mimicked by cAMP[124]. In addition, secretin stimulates pancreatic adenylate cyclase and elevates cAMP levels[125,126]. Vasoactive intestinal peptide also activates pancreatic adenylate cyclase, increasing the concentration of cAMP[127]. The effects of VIP in the pancreas are identical to those of secretin, and it is possible that they activate the same pancreatic adenylate cyclase[128].

Evidence for the role of cAMP in regulation of gastric secretions of the stomach is not clear. Although the nucleotide does stimulate acid secretion in both mammals and amphibians, the evidence as to which of the gastric hormones (gastrin, histamine, or cholinergic agents) might be mediated by cAMP is conflicting[81].

CYCLIC NUCLEOTIDES AND DISEASE: EVIDENCE FOR ABNORMAL CYCLIC NUCLEOTIDE METABOLISM IN PSEUDOHYPOPARATHYROIDISM

A transport-related disease believed to be due to a deficiency in cyclic nucleotide metabolism is pseudohypoparathyroidism (PHP). Pseudohypoparathyroidism was first described by Albright et al. in 1942 as a genetic disease closely resembling idiopathic hypoparathyroidism[129]. It is characterized by hypocalcaemia and hyperphosphataemia, but differs from idiopathic hypothyroidism in that serum Ca^{2+} and PO_4^- levels cannot be returned to normal after the administration of PTH[129]. It was later found that PTH also does not restore urinary levels of cAMP to normal as found in idiopathic hypoparathyroidism[130]. Since the action of PTH in both kidney and bone is mediated through activation of adenylate cyclase, it was hypothesized that this disorder resulted from defective PTH receptors and/or adenylate cyclase systems in these tissues. This has been supported by the fact that administration of dibutyryl cAMP to patients with PHP results in near normal serum Ca^{2+} and PO_4^- levels[131].

It is clear, however, that the pathogenesis of PHP is not simply due to a defective adenylate cyclase system. There is some evidence which directly conflicts with this concept, suggesting that PHP is not a single disorder or that it is a disorder brought about by more than one metabolic defect. It appears that some patients with PHP demonstrate a partial cAMP response to PTH; when the renal cortical adenylate cyclase from one patient with classic (type I) PHP was tested in vitro, it showed normal sensitivity to PTH[132]. Also, a syndrome known as pseudohypoparathyroidism type II has been described, in which the kidney's calcaemic and phosphaturic responses to PTH are abnormal, but in which normal increases in urinary cAMP are seen in response to PTH[133-135].

There is evidence that some of the chemical aberrations attributable to PHP are the result of abnormal vitamin D metabolism[135]. The administration of vitamin D or its metabolities has been shown to restore the normal calcaemic response to PTH[136,137]. In some patients with PHP, after serum Ca^{2+} concentrations have been normalized with vitamin D, serum PTH and PO_4 levels return to normal[138,139]. However, urinary cAMP still may not be stimulated by PTH, suggesting that at least in these cases the transport and cAMP-stimulating effects of PTH may be unrelated.

The transportation of the vitamin D metabolite $25(OH)D_3$ to the metabolically active form of the vitamin, $1,25(OH)_2D_3$ occurs in the kidney. There are some data to support the suggestion that a defect in the formation of $1,25(OH)_2D_3$ may be responsible for the diminished intestinal absorption of calcium, hypocalcaemia and secondary hypoparathyroidism seen in PHP[135]. Treatment of PHP patients with $1,25(OH)_2D_3$ can reverse these metabolic abnormalities, but does not affect the urinary cAMP response to PTH, suggesting the possibility of a non-adenylate cyclase-dependent, PTH-mediated transport[135,139]. The relationship between vitamin D metabolism and renal adenylate cyclase function is unknown, and the exact role of cyclic nucleotide metabolism in PHP is yet to be elucidated.

CONCLUSION

The elucidation of defects in cyclic nucleotide metabolism in disease depends on an understanding of the component parts of their cyclases, phosphodiesterases, and protein kinases. In addition, the substrates for the cyclic-nucleotide-dependent protein kinases need to be determined. While cyclic nucleotides are involved in transport activities in a wide variety of systems, the precise role of cAMP and cGMP have not been established, principally because their substrates for phosphorylation have not been identified. The understanding of abnormalities in second messenger systems in disease will proceed more rapidly as these normal physiological and biochemical mechanisms are uncovered.

References

1. Rall, T. W. and Sutherland, E. W. (1959). Formation of a cyclic adenine ribonucleotide by tissue particles. *J. Biol. Chem.*, **232**, 1065
2. Sutherland, E. W., Rall, T. W. and Menon, T. (1962). Adenyl cyclase I. Distribution, preparation and properties. *J. Biol. Chem.*, **237**, 1220
3. Liao, S., Lin, L. H. and Tymoczko, J. L. (1971). Adenyl cyclase of cell

nuclei isolated from rat ventral prostate. *Biochim. Biophys. Acta*, **230**, 535

4. Soifer, D. and Hechter, O. (1971). Adenyl cyclase activity in rat liver nuclei. *Biochim. Biophys. Acta*, **230**, 539

5. De Robertis, E., Arnaiz, G. R. de L., Alberici, M., Butcher, R. W. and Sutherland, E. W. (1967). Subcellular distribution of adenyl cyclase and cyclic phosphodiesterase in rat brain cortex. *Biol. Chem.*, **242**, 3487

6. Rabinowitz, M., Desalles, L., Meisler, J. and Lorand, L. (1965). Distribution of adenyl cyclase activity in rabbit skeletal muscle fractions. *Biochim. Biophys. Acta*, **97**, 29

7. Entman, M. L., Levey, G. S. and Epstein, S. E. (1969). Demonstration of adenyl cyclase activity in canine cardiac sarcoplasmic reticulum. *Biochem. Biophys. Res. Commun.*, **35**, 728

8. Rall, T. W. and Sutherland, E. W. (1962). Adenyl cyclase II. The enzymatically catalyzed formation of adenosine 3',5'-phosphate and inorganic pyrophosphate from adenosine triphosphate. *J. Biol. Chem.*, **237**, 1228

9. Rall, T. W., Sutherland, E. W. and Berthet, J. (1956). The relationship of epinephrine and glucagon to liver phosphorylase IV. Effect of epinephrine and glucagon on the reactivation of phosphorylase in liver homogenates. *J. Biol. Chem.*, **224**, 463

10. Birnbaumer, L., Pohl, S. L. and Rodbell, M. (1969). Adenyl cyclase in fat cells. I Properties and the effects of adrenocorticotropin and fluoride. *J. Biol. Chem.*, **244**, 3468

11. Drummond, G. I. and Duncan, L. (1970). Adenyl cyclase in cardiac tissue. *J. Biol. Chem.*, **245**, 976

12. Orly, J. and Schramm, M. (1976). Coupling of catecholamine receptor from one cell with adenylate cyclase from another cell by cell fusion. *Proc. Nat. Acad. Sci. USA*, **73**, 4410

13. Schramm, M., Orly, J., Eimerl, S. and Korner, M. (1977). Coupling of hormone receptors to adenylate cyclase of different cells by cell fusion. *Nature (London)*, **268**, 310

14. Limbird, L. E. and Lefkowitz, R. J. (1977). Resolution of β-adrenergic receptor binding and adenylate cyclase activity by gel exclusion chromatography. *J. Biol. Chem.*, **252**, 799

15. Haga, T., Haga, K. and Gilman, A. G. (1977). Hydrodynamic properties of the β-adrenergic receptor and adenylate cyclase from wild type and variant S49 lymphoma cells. *J. Biol. Chem.*, **252**, 5776

16. Ross, E. M. and Gilman, A. G. (1977). Reconstitution of catecholamine-sensitive adenylate cyclase activity: Interaction of solubilized components with receptor replete membranes. *Proc. Nat. Acad. Sci. USA*, **74**, 3715

17. Rodbell, M., Birnbaumer, L. and Pohl, S. I. (1970). Adenyl cyclase in fat cells. III. Stimulation by secretin and the effects of trypsin on the receptors for lipolytic hormones. *J. Biol. Chem.*, **245**, 718

18. Bird, S. J. and Maguire, M. E. (1978). The agonist-specific effect of magnesium ion on binding by β-adrenergic receptors in S49 lymphoma cells. Interaction of GTP and magnesium in adenylate cyclase activation. *J. Biol. Chem.*, **253**, 8826

19. William, L. T., Mullikin, D. and Lefkowitz, R. J. (1978). Magnesium dependence of agonist binding to adenylate cyclase-coupled hormone

receptors. *J. Biol. Chem.*, **253**, 2984

20. Rodbell, M., Krans, H. M., Pohl, S. L. and Birnbaumer, L. (1971). The glucagon-sensitive adenyl cyclase system in plasma membranes of rat liver. IV. Effects of guanyl nucleotides on binding of ^{125}I-glucagon. *J. Biol. Chem.*, **246**, 1872

21. Rodbell, M., Krans, H. M., Pohl, S. L. and Birnbaumer, L. (1971). The glucagon-sensitive adenyl cyclase system in plasma membranes of rat liver. V. An obligatory role of guanyl nucleotides in glucagon action. *J. Biol. Chem.*, **246**, 1877

22. Leray, F., Chambaut, A. and Hanoune, J. (1972). Role of GTP in epinephrine and glucagon activation. *Biochem. Biophys Res. Commun.*, **48**, 1385

23. Rodbell, M., Lin, M. C., Salomon, Y., Londes, C., Harwood, J. P., Martin, B. R., Rendell, M. and Berman, M. (1975). Role of adenine and guanine nucleotides in the activity and response of adenylate cyclase systems to hormones: Evidence for multisite transition states. *J. Cyclic Nucl. Res.*, **5**, 3.

24. Maguire, M. E., Ross, E. M. and Gilman, A. G. (1977). β-Adrenergic receptor: Ligand binding properties and the interaction with adenylate cyclase. *Adv. Cyclic Nucl. Res.*, **8**, 1

25. Pfeuffer, T. and Helmreich, E. J. M. (1975). Activation of pigeon erythrocyte membrane adenylate cyclase by guanylnucleotide analogues and separation of a nucleotide binding protein. *J. Biol. Chem.*, **250**, 867

26. Ross, E. M., Howlett, A. C., Ferguson, K. M. and Gilman, A. G. (1978). Reconstitution of hormone-sensitive adenylate cyclase activity with resolved components of the enzyme. *J. Biol. Chem.*, **253**, 6401

27. Lad, P. M., Welton, A. F. and Rodbell, M. (1977). Evidence for distinct guanine nucleotide sites in the regulation of the glucagon receptor and of adenylate cyclase activity. *J. Biol. Chem.*, **252**, 5942

28. Welton, A. F., Lad, P. M., Newby, A. C., Yamamura, H., Nicosia, S. and Rodbell, M. (1977). Solubilization and separation of the glucagon receptor and adenylate cyclase in nucleotide sensitive states. *J. Biol. Chem.*, **252**, 5947

29. Schlegel, W., Kempner, E. S. and Rodbell, M. (1979). Activation of adenylate cyclase in hepatic membranes involves interactions of the catalytic unit with multimeric complexes of regulatory proteins. *J. Biol. Chem.*, **254**, 5168

30. Sabol, S. L. and Nirenberg, M. (1979). Regulation of adenylate cyclase mediated by α-receptors. *J. Biol. Chem.*, **254**, 1913

31. Lefkowitz, R. J. and Caron, M. G. (1975). Characteristics of 5'-guanylyl imidodiphosphate-activated adenylate cyclase. *J. Biol. Chem.*, **205**, 4418

32. Cassel, D. and Selinger, Z. (1977). Mechanism of adenylate cyclase activation by cholera toxin: Inhibition of GTP hydrolysis at the regulatory site. *Proc. Nat. Acad. Sci. USA*, **74**, 3307

33. Kimura, H. and Murad, F. (1975). Subcellular localization of guanylate cyclase. *Life Sci.*, **17**, 837

34. Christman, T. D., Garbers, D. L., Parks, M. A. and Hardman, J. G. (1975). Characterization of particulate and soluble guanylate cyclases from rat lung. *J. Biol. Chem.*, **250**, 374

35. Siegel, M. I., Puca, G. A. and Cuatracasas, P. (1976). Guanylate cyclase. Existence of different forms and their regulation by nucleotides in calf uterus. *Biochim. Biophys. Acta*, **438**, 310

36. Goldberg, N. D. and Haddox, M. K. (1977). Cyclic GMP metabolism and involvement in biological regulation. *Annu. Rev. Biochem.*, **46**, 823

37. Goldberg, N. D., Graff, G., Haddox, M. K., Stephenson, J. H., Glass, D. B. and Moser, M. E. (1978). Redox modulation of splenic cell soluble guanylate cyclase activity: Activation by hydrophilic and hydrophobic oxidants represented by ascorbic and dehydroascorbic acids, fatty acid hydroperoxides, and prostaglandin endoperoxides. *Adv. Cyclic Nucl. Res.*, **9**, 101

38. Beavo, J. A., Hardman, J. G. and Sutherland, E. W. (1970). Hydrolysis of cyclic guanosine and adenosine $3',5'$-monophosphates by rat and bovine tissues. *J. Biol. Chem.*, **245**, 5649

39. Russell, T. R., Terasaki, W. L. and Appelman, M. M. (1973). Separate phosphodiesterases for the hydrolysis of adenosine $3',5'$-monophosphate and cyclic guanosine $3',5'$-monophosphate in rat liver. *J. Biol. Chem.*, **248**, 1334

40. Bergstrand, H., Lundquist, B. and Schurmann, A. (1978). Cyclic nucleotide phosphodiesterase: Partial purification and characterization of a high affinity enzyme activity from human lung tissue. *J. Biol. Chem.*, **253**, 1881

41. Cheung, W. Y. (1971). Cyclic $3',5'$-nucleotide phosphodiesterase. Evidence for and properties of a protein activator. *J. Biol. Chem.*, **246**, 2859

42. Kakiuchi, S., Yamazaki, R. and Nakajima, H. (1970). Properties of a heat-stable phosphodiesterase activating factor isolated from brain extract. Studies on cyclic $3':5'$-nucleotide phosphodiesterase II. *Proc. Jpn. Acad.*, **46**, 587

43. Teo, T. S. and Wang, J. H. (1973). Mechanism of activation of a cyclic adenosine $3':5'$-monophosphate phosphodiesterase from bovine heart by calcium ions. Identification of the protein activator as a Ca^{2+} binding protein. *J. Biol. Chem.*, **248**, 5950

44. Watterson, D. M., Harrelson, W. G., Keller, P. M., Sharief, F. and Vanaman, T. C. (1976). Structural similarities between the Ca^{2+} dependent regulatory proteins of $3',5'$-cyclic nucleotide phosphodiesterase and actomyosin ATPase. *J. Biol. Chem.*, **251**, 4501

45. Dedman, J. R., Potter, J. D. and Means, A. R. (1977). Biological crossreactivity of rat testis phosphodiesterase activator protein and rabbit skeletal muscle troponin-C. *J. Biol. Chem.*, **252**, 2437

46. Cheung, W. Y., Lynch, T. J. and Wallace, R. W. (1978). An endogenous Ca^{2+}-dependent activator protein of brain adenylate cyclase and cyclic nucleotide phosphodiesterase. *Adv. Cyclic Nucl. Res.*, **9**, 233

47. Wang, J. H. and Desai, R. (1977). Modulator binding protein. Bovine brain protein exhibiting the Ca^{2+}-dependent association with the protein activator of cyclic nucleotide phosphodiesterase. *J. Biol. Chem.*, **252**, 4175

48. Klee, C. B. and Krinks, M. H. (1978). Purification of cyclic $3',5'$-nucleotide phosphodiesterase inhibitor protein by affinity chromatography on activator protein coupled to sepharose. *Biochemistry*, **17**, 120

49. Sharma, R. K., Wirch, E. and Wang, J. H. (1978). Inhibition of Ca^{2+} acti-

vated cyclic nucleotide phosphodiesterase reaction by a heat stable inhibitor protein from bovine brain. *J. Biol. Chem.*, **253**, 3575

50. Hofmann, F., Beavo, J. A., Betchel, P. J. and Krebs, E. G. (1975). Comparison of adenosine 3',5'-monophosphate-dependent protein kinases from rabbit skeletal and bovine heart muscle. *J. Biol. Chem.*, **250**, 7795

51. Brostrom, C. O., Corbin, J. D., King, C. A. and Krebs, E. G. (1971). Interaction of the subunits of adenosine 3',5'-cyclic monophosphate-dependent protein kinase of muscle. *Proc. Nat. Acad. Sci. USA*, **68**, 2444

52. Gill, G. N. and Garren, L. S. (1970). A cyclic 3',5'-adenosine monophosphate dependent protein kinase from the adrenal cortex: comparison with a cyclic AMP binding protein. *Biochem. Biophys. Res. Commun.*, **39**, 335

53. Lee, P. D., Radloff, D., Schweppe, J. S. and Jungmann, R. A. (1976). Testicular protein kinases: Characterization of multiple forms and ontogeny. *J. Biol. Chem.*, **251**, 914

54. Costa, M., Gerner, E. and Russell, D. H. (1976). Cell cyclic specific activity of type I and type II cyclic adenosine 3',5'-monophosphate dependent protein kinases in chinese hamster ovary cells. *J. Biol. Chem.*, **251**, 3313

55. Russell, D. H. (1978). Type I cyclic AMP-dependent protein kinase as a positive effector of growth. *Adv. Cyclic Nucl. Res.*, **9**, 493

56. Rangel-Aldao, R. and Rosen, O. M. (1976). Mechanism of self-phosphorylation of adenosine 3',5'-monophosphate dependent protein kinase from bovine cardiac muscle. *J. Biol. Chem.*, **251**, 7526

57. de Jonge, H. R. and Rosen, O. M. (1977). Self-phosphorylation of cyclic guanosine 3',5'-monophosphate-dependent protein kinase from bovine lung. *J. Biol. Chem.*, **252**, 2780

58. Lincoln, T. M., Dills, W. Jr. and Corbin, J. D. (1977). Purification and subunit composition of guanosine 3',5'-monophosphate-dependent protein kinase from bovine lung. *J. Biol. Chem.*, **252**, 4269

59. Gill, G. N., Walton, G. M. and Sperry, P. J. (1977). Guanosine 3',5'-monophosphate-dependent protein kinase from bovine lung. Subunit structure and characterization of the purified enzyme. *J. Biol. Chem.*, **252**, 6443

60. Kuo, J. F., Kuo, W. N., Shoji, M., Davis, C. W., Sery, V. L. and Donnelly, T. E. Jr. (1976). Purification and general properties of guanosine 3',5'-monophosphate-dependent protein kinase from guinea-pig fetal lung. *J. Biol. Chem.*, **251**, 1759

61. Gill, G. N., Holdy, K. E., Walton, G. M. and Kanstein, C. B. (1976). Purification and characterization of 3',5'-cyclic GMP-dependent protein kinase. *Proc. Nat. Acad. Sci. USA*, **73**, 3918

62. Kuo, J. F., Shoji, M. and Kuo, W. N. (1978). Molecular and physiopathologic aspects of mammalian cyclic GMP-dependent protein kinase. *Annu. Rev. Pharmacol. Toxicol.*, **18**, 341

63. Szmigelski, A., Guidotti, A. and Costa, E. (1976). Endogenous protein kinase inhibitors. Purification, characterization and distribution in different tissues. *J. Biol. Chem.*, **252**, 3848

64. Rasmussen, H. (1970). Cell communication, calcium ion and cyclic adenosine monophosphate. *Science*, **170**, 404

65. Rasmussen, H. and Goodman, D. B. (1977). Relationships between

calcium and cyclic nucleotides in cell activation. *Physiol. Rev.*, **57**, 421

66. Handler, J. S. and Orloff, J. (1973). The mechanism of action of anti-diuretic hormone. In J. Orloff and R. W. Berliner (eds.), *Handbook of Physiology, Section 8, Renal Physiology*, (Washington: American Physiological Society)

67. Orloff, J. and Handler S. J. (1962). The similarity of effects of vasopressin, adenosine 3',5'-monophosphate (cAMP) and theophylline on the toad bladder. *J. Clin. Invest.*, **41**, 702

68. Grantham, J. J. and Burg, M. B. (1966). Effect of vasopressin and cyclic AMP on permeability of isolated collecting tubules. *Am. J. Physiol.*, **211**, 255

69. Handler, J. S., Butcher, R. W., Sutherland, E. W. and Orloff, J. (1965). The effects of vasopressin and of theophylline on the concentration of adenosine 3',5'-phosphate in the urinary bladder of the toad. *J. Biol. Chem.*, **240**, 4524

70. Brown, E., Clark, D. L., Roux, V. and Sherman, G. H. (1963). The stimulation of adenosine 3',5' monophosphate by antidiuretic factors. *J. Biol. Chem.*, **238**, 852

71. Beck, N. P., Kaneko, T., Zor, U., Field, J. B. and Davis, B. B. (1971). Effects of vasopressin and prostaglandin E_1 on the adenyl cyclase–cyclic 3',5'-adenosine monophosphate system of the renal medulla of the rat. *J. Clin. Invest.*, **50**, 2461

72. Bar, H. P., Hetcher, O., Schwartz, I. L. and Walter, R. (1970). Neurohypophysial hormone-sensitive adenyl cyclase of toad urinary bladder. *Proc. Nat. Acad. Sci. USA*, **67**, 7

73. Hynil, S. and Sharp, G. W. G. (1971). Adenyl cyclase in the toad bladder. *Biochim. Biophys. Acta*, **230**, 40

74. Chase, L. R. and Aurbach, G. D. (1968). Renal adenyl cyclase: Anatomically separate sites for parathyroid hormone and vasopressin. *Science*, **159**, 545

75. Morel, F., Chabardes, D. and Imbert, M. (1976). Functional segmentation of the rabbit distal tubule by microdetermination of hormone-dependent adenylate cyclase activity. *Kidney Int.*, **9**, 264

76. Handler, J. S., Preston, A. S. and Orloff, J. (1969). Effect of adrenal steroid hormones on the response of the toad's urinary bladder to vasopressin. *J. Clin. Invest.*, **48**, 823

77. Stoff, J. S., Handler, J. S. and Orloff, J. (1972). The affect of aldosterone on the accumulation of adenosine 3',5'-cyclic monophosphate in toad bladder epithelial cells in response to vasopressin and theophylline. *Proc. Nat. Acad. Sci. USA*, **69**, 805

78. Stoff, J. S., Handler, J. S., Preston A. S. and Orloff, J. (1973). The affect of aldosterone on cyclic nucleotide phosphodiesterase activity in toad urinary bladder. *Life Sci.*, **13**, 545

79. Goldberg, M., Agus, Z. S. and Goldfard, S. (1976). Renal handling of phosphate, calcium and magnesium. In B. M. Brenner and F. C. Rector, Jr. (eds.), *The Kidney*, pp. 344–390. (Philadelphia: Saunders)

80. Rasmussen, H. and Tenehouse, A. (1968). Cyclic adenosine monophosphate, Ca^{2+} and membranes. *Proc. Nat. Acad. Sci. USA*, **59**, 1364

81. Strewler, G. J. and Orloff, J. (1977). Role of cyclic nucleotides in the

transport of water and electrolytes. *Adv. Cyclic Nucl. Res.*, **8**, 311

82.   Jard, A. and Bastide, F. (1970). A cyclic AMP-dependent protein kinase from frog bladder epithelial cells. *Biochem. Biophys. Res. Commun.*, **39**, 559

83.   Kirchberger, M. A., Schwartz, I. L. and Walter, R. (1972). Cyclic 3',5'-AMP-dependent protein kinase activity on toad bladder epithelium. *Proc. Soc. Exp. Biol. Med.*, **140**, 657

84.   Dousa, T. P., Sands, H. and Hechter, O. (1972). Cyclic AMP-dependent reversible phosphorylation of renal medullary plasma membrane protein. *Endocrinology*, **91**, 757

85.   De Lorenzo, R. J. and Greengard, P. (1973). Activation by adenosine 3',5'-monophosphate of a membrane-bound phosphoprotein phosphatase of toad bladder. *Proc. Nat. Acad. Sci. USA*, **70**, 1831

86.   Malkinson, A. M., Kreuger, B. K., Rudolf, S. A., Casnellie, J. E., Haley, B. E. and Greengard, P. (1975). Widespread occurrence of a specific protein in vertebrate tissues and regulation by cyclic AMP of its endogenous phosphorylation and dephosphorylation. *Metabolism*, **24**, 331

87.   Sandoval, I. V. and Cuatrecasas, P. (1976). Protein kinase associated with tubulin: Affinity chromatography and properties. *Biochemistry*, **15**, 3424

88.   Sloboda, R. D., Rudolph, S. A., Rosenbaum, J. L. and Greengard, P. (1975). Cyclic AMP-dependent endogenous phosphorylation of a microtubule-associated protein. *Proc. Nat. Acad. Sci. USA*, **72**, 177

89.   Lockwood, A. H. (1978). Phosphorylation of tubulin assembly protein by cAMP-dependent protein kinase. *J. Cell Biol.*, **79**, 288a.

90.   Wallach, D., Davies, P., Bechtel, P., Willingham, M. and Pastan, I. (1978). Cyclic AMP dependent phosphorylation of the actin-binding protein filimin. *Adv. Cyclic Nucl. Res.*, **9**, 371

91.   Taylor, A., Mamelak, M., Reaven, E. and Maffly, R. (1973). Vasopressin: Possible role of microtubules and microfilaments in its action. *Science*, **181**, 347

92.   Yuasa, S., Urakabe, S., Kimura, G., Shirai, D., Takamitsu, Y., Orita, Y. and Abe, H. (1975). Effect of colchicine on the osmotic water flow across the toad urinary bladder. *Biochim. Biophys. Acta*, **413**, 277

93.   Taylor, A., Maffly, R., Wilson, L. and Reaven, E. (1975). Evidence for involvement of microtubules in the action of vasopressin. *Ann. NY Acad. Sci.*, **253**, 723

94.   Abramow, M. (1976). Effect of vasopressin on water transport in the kidney: Possible role of microtubules and microfilaments. In J. W. L. Robinson (ed.), *Intestinal Ion Transport*, pp. 173–188. (Baltimore: University Park Press)

95.   Kuntziger, J., Amill, C., Roinel, N. and Morel, F. (1974). Effects of parathyroidectomy and cyclic AMP on renal transport of phosphate calcium and magnesium. *Am. J. Physiol.*, **227**, 905

96.   Marx, S. J. and Aurbach, G. D. (1975). Renal receptors for calcitonin: Coordinate occurrence with calcitonin activated adenylate cyclase. *Endocrinology*, **97**, 448

97.   Riddick, D. H., Kregenow, F. M. and Orloff, J. (1971). The effect of norepinepherine and dibutyryl cyclic adenosine monophosphate on

cation transport in duck erythrocytes. *J. Gen. Physiol.*, **57**, 752

98. Gardner, J. D., Klaeveman, H. L., Bilezikian, J. P. and Aurbach, G. D. (1974). Stimulation of sodium transport in turkey erythrocytes by cyclic AMP. *Endocrinology*, **96**, 499

99. Kregenow, F. M., Robbie, D. E. and Orloff, J. (1976). Effect of norepinephrine and hypertonicity on K influx and cyclic AMP in duck erythrocytes. *Am. J. Physiol.*, **231**, 306

100. Bilezikian, J. P. and Aurbach, G. D. (1973). A β-adrenergic receptor of the turkey erythrocyte I. Binding of catacholamine and relationship to adenylate cyclase activity. *J. Biol. Chem.*, **248**, 5575

101. Rudolph, S. A. and Greengard, P. (1974). Regulation of protein phosphorylation and membrane permeability by β-adrenergic agents and cyclic adenosine 3′,5′-monophosphate in the avian erythrocyte. *J. Biol. Chem.*, **249**, 5684

102. Rudolph, S. A., Schafer, D. E. and Greengard, P. (1976). Effects of cholera enterotoxin on cation fluxes, cell volume and cAMP levels in the turkey erythrocyte. *Biophys. J.*, **16**, 171a.

103. Sheppard, H. and Burghardt, C. (1969). Adenyl cyclase in non-nucleated erythrocytes of several mammalian species. *Biochem. Pharmacol.*, **18**, 2576

104. Rasmussen, H., Lake, W. and Allen, J. E. (1975). The effect of catecholamines and prostaglandins upon human and rat erythrocytes. *Biochem. Biophys. Acta*, **411**, 63

105. Rubin, C. S., Erlichman, J. and Rosen, O. M. (1972). Cyclic adenosine 3′,5′-monophosphate-dependent protein kinase of human erythrocyte membranes. *J. Biol. Chem.*, **247**, 6135

106. Rubin, C. S. and Rosen, O. M. (1973). The role of cyclic AMP in the phosphorylation of proteins in human erythrocyte membranes. *Biochem. Biophys. Res. Commun.*, **50**, 421

107. Field, M. (1979). Mechanisms of action of cholera and *Escherichia coli* enterotoxins. *Am. J. Clin. Nutr.*, **32**, 189

108. Field, M., Fromm, D., Al-Awqati, Q. and Greenough, W. B. III (1972). Effect of cholera toxin on ion transport across isolated ileal mucosa. *J. Clin. Invest.*, **51**, 796

109. Field, M. (1971). Ion transport in rabbit ileal mucosa. II. Effects of cyclic 3′,5′-AMP. *Am. J. Physiol.*, **221**, 992

110. Dietz, J. and Field, M. (1973). Ion transport in rabbit ileal mucosa. IV. Bicarbonate secretion. *Am. J. Physiol.*, **225**, 858

111. Gill, D. M. (1977). Mechanism of action of cholera toxin. *Adv. Cyclic Nucl. Res.*, **8**, 85

112. Moss, J. and Richardson, S. H. (1978). Activation of adenylate cyclase by heat labile *Escherichia coli* enterotoxin. *J. Clin. Invest.*, **62**, 281

113. Field, M., Graf, L. H., Laird, W. J. and Smith, P. (1978). Heat-stable enterotoxin of *Escherichia coli*, *in vitro* effects on guanylate cyclase activity cyclic GMP concentration and ion transport in small intestine. *Proc. Nat. Acad. Sci. USA*, **75**, 2800

114. Hughes, J. M., Murad, F., Chang, B. and Guerrant, R. (1978). Role of cyclic GMP in the active heat-stable entertoxin of *Escherichia coli*. *Nature (London)*, **271**, 755

115. Lucid, S. W. and Cox, A. C. (1972). The effect of cholera toxin on the phosphorylation of protein in epithelial cells and their brush borders. *Biochem. Biophys. Res. Commun.*, **49**, 1183

116. De Jonge, H. (1976). Cyclic nucleotide dependent phosphorylation of intestinal epithelial proteins. *Nature (London)*, **262**, 590

117. Kimberg, D., Field, M., Johnson, J., Henderson, A. and Gershon, E. (1971). Stimulation of intestinal mucosal adenyl cyclase by cholera enterotoxin and prostaglandins. *J. Clin. Invest.*, **50**, 1218

118. Pierce, N. F., Carpenter, C. C. J. Jr, Elliott N. L. and Greenough, W. B. III (1971). Effects of prostaglandins, theophylline and cholera enterotoxin upon transmucosal water and electrolyte movement in canine jejunum. *Gastroenterology*, **60**, 22

119. Swartz, C. J., Kimberg, D. V., Sheerin, A. E., Field, M. and Said, S. I. (1974). Vasoactive intestinal peptide stimulation of adenyl cyclase and active electrolyte secretion in intestinal mucosa. *J. Clin. Invest.*, **54**, 536

120. Simon, B. and Kather, H. (1978). Activation of human adenylate cyclase in the upper gastrointestinal tract by vasoactive intestinal polypeptide. *Gastroenterology*, **74**, 722

121. Walling, M. W., Brasitus, T. A. and Kimberg, D. V. (1977). Effects of calcitonin and substance P on the transport of Ca, Na and Cl across rat ileum *in vitro*. *Gastroenterology*, **73**, 89

122. Mertens, R. B., Wheeler, H. O. and Mayer, S. E. (1974). Effects of cholera toxin and phosphodiesterase inhibitors on fluid transport and cyclic adenosine 3′,5′-monophosphate concentrations in rabbit gall bladder. *Gastroenterology*, **67**, 898

123. Frizzell, R. A., Dugas, M. C. and Schultz, S. G. (1975). Sodium chloride transport by rabbit gall bladder. *J. Gen. Physiol.*, **65**, 769

124. Case, R. M. and Scratcherd, T. (1972). The action of dibutyryl cyclic adenosine 3′,5′-monophosphate and methylxanthines on pancreatic exocrine secretion. *J. Physiol.*, **223**, 649

125. Rutten, W. J., de Pont, J. J. H. and Bonting, S. L. (1972). Adenylate cyclase in the rat pancreas: properties and stimulation by hormones. *Biochim. Biophys. Acta*, **370**, 573

126. Case, R. M., Johnson, M., Scratcherd, T. and Sherratt, H. S. A. (1972). Cyclic adenosine 3′,5′-monophosphate concentration in the pancreas following stimulation by secretin, cholecystokinin-pancreozymin and acetylcholine. *J. Physiol.*, **223**, 669

127. Gardner, J. D., Conlon, T. P. and Adams, T. D. (1976). Cyclic AMP in pancreatic acinar cells: Effects of gastrointestinal hormones. *Gastroenterology*, **70**, 29

128. Christophe, J. P., Conlon, T. P. and Gardner, J. D. (1976). Interaction of porcine vasoactive intestinal peptide with dispersed pancreatic acinar cells from the guinea pig: Binding of radioiodinated peptide. *J. Biol. Chem.*, **251**, 4629

129. Albright, F., Burnett, C. H., Smith, P. H. and Parson, W. (1942). Pseudoparathyroidism – an example of the 'Seabright–Bantam Syndrome'. *Endocrinology*, **30**, 922

130. Drezner, M. K., Neelon, F. A., Curtis, H. B. and Lefkowitz, H. E. (1976). Renal cyclic adenosine monophosphate: An accurate index of

parathyroid function. *Metabolism*, **25**, 1103

131. Bell, N. H., Avery, S., Sinha, T., Clark, C. M., Allen, D. O. and Johnston, C. (1972). Effects of dibutyryl adenosine 3',5'-monophosphate and parathyroid extract on calcium and phosphorus metabolism in hypoparathyroidism and pseudohypoparathyroidism. *J. Clin. Invest.*, **51**, 816

132. Marcus, R., Wilbur, J. F. and Aurbach G. D. (1971). Parathyroid hormone sensitive adenyl cyclase from the renal cortex of a patient with pseudohypoparathyroidism. *J. Clin. Endocrinol. Metab.*, **33**, 537

133. Drezner, M., Neelon, F. A. and Lebovitz, H. E. (1973). Pseudohypoparathyroidism type II: A possible defect in the reception of the cyclic AMP signal. *N. Engl. J. Med.*, **289**, 1056

134. Rodriguez, H. J., Villarreal, H. Jr, Klahr, S. and Slatopolsky, E. (1974). Pseudohypoparathyroidism type II: Restoration of normal renal responsiveness to parathyroid hormone by calcium administration. *J. Clin. Endocrinol. Metab.*, **39**, 693

135. Klahr, S. and Slatopolsky, E. (1979). Urinary phosphate and cyclic AMP in pseudohypoparathyroidism. *Adv. Exp. Med. Biol.*, **103**, 173

136. Drezner, M. K., Neelon, F. A., Haussler, M., McPherson, H. T. and Lebovitz, H. D. (1976). 1,25-Dihydroxyeholecalciferol deficiency: The probable cause of hypocalcemia and metabolic bone disease in pseudohypoparathyroidism. *J. Clin. Endocrinol. Metab.*, **42**, 621

137. Stögmann, W. and Fischer, J. A. (1975). Pseudohypoparathyroidism: Disappearance of the resistance to parathyroid extract during treatment with vitamin D. *Am. J. Med.*, **59**, 140

138. Suh, S. M., Fraser, D. and Kooh, S. W. (1970). Pseudohypoparathyroidism responsiveness to parathyroid extract induced by vitamin D therapy. *J. Clin. Endocrinol. Metab.*, **30**, 609

139. Brickman, A. S., Norman, A. W. and Coburn, J. W. (1976). Restoration of PTH-dependent phosphaturia by 1,25 (OH) 2 vitamin D_3 in pseudohypoparathyroidism I. *Kidney Int.*, **10**, 448

9

Mineralocorticoids and sodium transport

R. Fraser

INTRODUCTION

Such is the wealth of information available on the mechanisms of action of hormones at the molecular level that it is easy to forget that most, if not all, of it has been gleaned during the last 20 years. It now seems clear that although some hormones may exert direct effects on cell metabolism, most seem to influence it by one of two mechanisms: by modifying protein synthesis by an effect on the cell nucleus[1,2] or by stimulating the formation of a second messenger, a cyclic nucleotide usually cyclic adenosine monophosphate[3]. The aim of this chapter is to summarize the actions of the mineralocorticoid hormones, particularly aldosterone, on renal electrolyte metabolism, first summarizing the process of sodium transport in the distal convoluted tubule and then attempting to dissect the primary effects of aldosterone.

SODIUM TRANSPORT

In animal tissues, the extracellular sodium concentration is much higher than that inside the cell. Since the plasma membrane is semi-permeable, sodium leaks into the cell down a concentration gradient. Conversely, extracellular potassium concentration is lower than the intracellular concentration and the passive flow of these ions is in the opposite direction. Diffusion of both types of ion, although passive, obeys saturation kinetics suggesting that transport is transcellular rather than intercellular and that the number of permeable sites is finite[4]. Maintenance of differential intra- and extracellular ion concentrations is crucial to cell function and, in order to maintain them, sodium must be pumped out of, and potassium into, the cell. In many tissues these two processes are coupled and are accomplished by an energy-consuming process, the sodium pump. This is one of a variety of similar ion pumps in biological tissue[5].

The sodium pump is present in all cells and a description of its basic components, together with a summary of early literature, is available[6]. Changes in its activity in various diseases have also been reviewed[7]. As an active process, the pump must contain a mechanism for coupling metabolic energy to the process of sodium extrusion and this function has been assigned to a Na,K-dependent ATPase, universally present in cell membranes and more abundant in organs such as the kidney where the process of sodium transport is carried out most vigorously. Although a few studies have questioned the central importance of this enzyme[5], its involvement seems to have been accepted widely and there have been many studies of its properties. It is inhibited by the cardiac glycosides, ouabain and strophanthidin which it binds specifically. For a more extensive review, the reader is referred to Sachs[8].

ATP is an obligatory substrate for the sodium pump, but other high energy substrates such as arginine phosphate and phosphoenolpyruvate may be involved in the coupling of sodium and potassium translocation. It has also been suggested that energy substrate oxidation may be coupled directly to the establishment of ion gradients[8], but probably only ATP is of significance in transport across the plasma membrane. Stoichiometry indicates that three moles of sodium are exchanged for two of potassium when one mole of ATP is converted to ADP. There is no doubt that, indirectly or directly, ion transport is dependent on respiration and energy metabolism[9,10].

The possible mechanisms by which ions might be transported across the plasma membrane barrier have been summarized, superficially, by Fraser[6]. Three categories were distinguished: mobile carrier mechanisms, allosteric mechanisms and electrostatic mechanisms. Of these, the postulation of a small molecule with variable affinity for sodium and potassium which shuttled between membrane surfaces would probably be too slow to account for the rate of ion transport. The remaining two devices would rely on some as yet unidentified macromolecular membrane constituent, probably a protein or lipoprotein. In transport by allosteric change, it is suggested that, in its resting state, the molecule exposes a sodium binding site on its intracellular surface. Raising the energy level of the molecule by phosphorylation, requiring ATP and catalysed by the Na,K-dependent ATPase[11], induces a rapid change in conformation (allosteric change) during which the sodium ions are transported to the extracellular surface and a potassium binding site is exposed. Dephosphorylation reverses the process. Finally, electrostatic mechanisms rely on the fact that surfaces on which high negative electrostatic field strength exists bind sodium more readily than potassium, and vice versa. Phosphorylation alters the charge distribution and might, in this way, control the ion affinity of the membrane surface. It is possible that ion binding and transporting molecules line the channels in the plasma membrane which are thought to be important in sodium translocation[12]. In addition to Na:K exchange, Na:Na and K:K exchange have also been demonstrated and for some, as yet undiscovered, reason appear to require ADP instead of ATP[13].

Thus in most, if not all, animal cells intracellular ion concentration is kept within narrow physiological limits by a sodium pump mechanism which requires ATP and incorporates a Na,K-dependent ATPase. However, a number of specialized organs translocate sodium and potassium, not indiscriminately over the cell surface as, for example, an erythrocyte does, but in a specific direction across their epithelial lining. These organs, crucial for the control of extracellular fluid composition, include the intestine[14], probably the placenta[15], the kidney and also the urinary bladder and skin of amphibians such as the toad and frog respectively. This trans-epithelial ion transport is accomplished by a careful spatial arrangement of the constituent elements of the system described above. Entry of sodium occurs at the apical cell surface which is more permeable (i.e. contains most 'permease') and extrusion to the basolateral surface where most Na,K-dependent ATPase is to be found. Thus, in the distal convoluted tubule and early collecting duct of the nephron, sodium ions are supplied across the luminal surface and extruded across the peritubular surface, resulting in sodium reabsorption from the glomerular filtrate. In amphibian membranes, these functions are served by the mucosal and serosal surfaces, respectively[16]. Evidence of this unequal distribution of activity has been published[6,17].

A more detailed analysis of the basic mechanisms of trans-epithelial ion transport is also available[18,19]. Do mineralocorticoids affect these processes and if so how?

ACTIONS OF MINERALOCORTICOIDS

The adrenal cortex secretes a variety of biologically active steroids. They influence metabolism in two main ways – by assisting in the control of intermediary metabolism (the glucocorticoids) and by promoting sodium retention and potassium loss (the mineralocorticoids). Although all corticosteroids possess each property to some degree, one or other tends to predominate. The major mineralocorticoid is aldosterone, but 11-deoxycorticosterone, corticosterone and possibly their 18-hydroxy derivatives possess significant activity. Cortisol is the major glucocorticoïd in man. A useful synthetic mineralocorticoid is 9α-fluorocortisol ('Fludrocortisone'). Mineralocorticoid activity can be inhibited specifically by a group of steroid drugs, the spirolactones, of which the most widely used is spironolactone or 'Aldactone'. Long-term administration of mineralocorticoids to normal human subjects causes sodium retention, as evidenced by reduced urinary excretion and increased plasma concentration and weight. Blood pressure also rises. Conversely, potassium excretion rises and this is accompanied by reduced plasma levels. These effects are reversed by spironolactone[20]. Direct infusion of aldosterone into the renal artery of the dog reduces urinary Na:K ratio, but only after a well-defined delay which is not shortened by increasing the steroid dose[21-23]. Early studies of the effects of aldosterone have been reviewed by Ross[24]. Its effects are mainly, if not wholly, exerted in the distal nephron[21,22,25,26] and there have been a series of careful and ingenious attempts to discover the primary events initiated by the hormone. Although several important aspects remain unclear, a coherent picture of the sequence of hormone-dependent events is now emerging.

Since the nephron is an inconvenient and often unsatisfactory vehicle for research, early studies used the amphibian membranes, toad urinary bladder or frog skin. These tissues translocate ions in a manner similar to that of the distal convoluted tubule, but their physical nature allows them to be used in *in vitro* systems to separate two fluid compartments representing the *in vivo* serosal and mucosal compartments, the composition of which can be manipulated. Moreover, sodium transport can be followed continuously by measuring short-circuit current[27,28]. Using this preparation the following facts have been established[6]. The circulating levels of the mineralocorticoid aldosterone determine the rate of sodium transport (i.e. the short-circuit current). Tissue from toads kept in distilled water, which would tend to lose sodium and to raise their rate of aldosterone secretion[29], gave higher values than that from animals kept in saline. Adrenalectomy severely impaired the level of transport *in vitro*, but this could be prevented by prior treatment of the donor animals with aldosterone. Bladders from adrenalectomized toads could also be induced to transport sodium normally by adding aldosterone *in vitro* to the serosal fluid compartment, but the response was delayed by a period of approximately 90 min, the so-called latent period. This *in vitro* response could be blocked by spironolactone and related compounds[30]. To elicit the response, hormone and tissue need only be in contact for a short period of time, approximately 5 min. Removal of the hormone at this time did not prevent, delay or attenuate the response occurring later after the latent period has expired. The response could, however, be prevented by depleting the bladder of energy substrates before adding aldosterone. However restoring these after the latent period had elapsed elicited an immediate increase in short-circuit current, suggesting that the substrates were necessary for the expression but not the initiation of the hormone's effects.

MECHANISM OF ACTION

The occurrence of a well-defined latent period provided a strong clue that the basic mechanism of action might be similar to that described for other steroid hormones – that is, the mineralocorticoids might alter epithelial cell protein synthesis by influencing DNA transcription[31-33]. Subsequent experiments seem to have justified this assumption. Aldosterone is bound to specific receptors in the cytosol and nuclei of kidney and toad bladder prepared after incubation of the whole tissue with the steroid. It is displaced from these receptors only by hormones with mineralocorticoid activity, and the ability of these to compete with aldosterone is directly proportional to their biological potency. Attachment to the cytosol receptor is a prerequisite of nuclear binding. Specific cytosol receptors can be demonstrated in tissue previously unexposed to aldosterone, but nuclei from this tissue are incapable of binding the mineralocorticoid. If, however, aldosterone-treated cytosol is added to untreated nuclei, specific nuclear binding ensues. Binding to the cytosol receptor is inhibited by spirolactones[34,35]. From these ingenious studies it has been inferred that aldosterone is first bound to a cytosol receptor which it modifies. (Recently a group of anti-inflammatory compounds have been reported to act in a similar manner[36].) The steroid–receptor complex is then taken up by the nucleus. (It should perhaps be mentioned that lower affinity binding of aldosterone also occurs at higher hormone concentrations. These may be glucocorticoid receptors[37].) In the nucleus, the complex probably alters protein synthesis, possibly acting as a 'derepressor' of DNA transcription. Protein synthesis is necessary for the hormone's effects to occur. Actinomycin D inhibits RNA synthesis by the DNA dependent, RNA polymerase and puromycin or various amino acid analogues, which prevent protein synthesis at ribosomal level, inhibit the response to aldosterone. Other experiments have shown that mineralocorticoids increase the rate of RNA and protein synthesis in responsive tissues. Aldosterone therefore increases protein synthesis. What is the function of the aldosterone-induced protein?

Modulation of trans-epithelial ion translocation might conceivably be achieved by altering one or more of the components of the sodium pump. Sodium transport would be stimulated if the rate of supply of ions to the pump increased; that is, if permease activity increased, since sodium and potassium ions are primary substrates. On the other hand, an increase in the rate of sodium extrusion, resulting either from an increase in quantity or activity of the Na,K-dependent ATPase or, if the enzyme concentration is not rate-limiting, from an increase in energy supply in the form of ATP, would have a similar effect. These are not necessarily mutually exclusive.

If the primary and major effect of the new protein is to increase cell permeability to sodium, the size of the intracellular sodium pool should increase. Conversely, stimulation of extrusion rate should shrink the pool. Among the earliest attempts to assess changes in the size of the sodium pool were those of Crabbé[38]. Toad bladder tissue was incubated with radioactively labelled sodium in the presence or absence of aldosterone. After careful removal of excess radioactivity, tissue radioactivity was assumed to be a measure of the intracellular sodium pool and this quantity was marginally but significantly increased by the mineralocorticoid. Although there are difficulties in interpreting such data, not the least of which is whether all the radioactivity measured was intracellular, and also whether the pool labelled corresponds exactly to the sodium transport pool, this permeability effect of aldosterone seems to have been borne out by subsequent experiments. More detailed accounts of the techniques for measuring the size of the intracellular sodium pool or their difficulties are available elsewhere[39,40].

Another approach to the problem of whether mineralocorticoids alter cell permeability to sodium has been to examine the effect of the hormones on sodium transport in tissue in which permeability barriers have been lowered or destroyed by prior treatment with drugs such as amiloride or amphotericin B[38,41]. In toad bladder treated in this way, sodium transport is already augmented, mimicking the effect of aldosterone. The fact that aldosterone is unable to increase the transport rate further has been interpreted as indicating that the newly-induced protein stimulates permease activity, possibly by increasing the affinity of a sodium carrier system. Similar conclusions were reached by Leaf and McKnight[42]. The effect of aldosterone on permeability is largely undisputed, but whether it is primary or secondary to some other initial process is not certain. For example, in a recent short but important review, Edelman[33] has suggested that changes in permeability may be secondary to the improved metabolic state of the tissue, signposted by raised ATP:ADP ratio. On the other hand, intracellular sodium:potassium ratios might have a secondary effect on oxidative phosphorylation.

Changes in the activity or concentration of the Na,K-dependent ATPase in aldosterone-treated tissues has also been studied[6,43]. Cardiac glycosides specifically inhibit this enzyme and, interestingly, these compounds possess an oxygenated angular methyl group, a feature unique among corticosteroids to aldosterone. Aldosterone is also reported to bind specifically to the enzyme. Early studies of the enzyme concentration changes induced by aldosterone are inconclusive. Adrenalectomy of rats usually led to a fall in the renal concentration of the Na,K-dependent ATPase, which could sometimes[44] but not always, be corrected by aldosterone administration to the ablated animal. Sodium loading of the animals, however, could also increase enzyme activity, suggesting that the response to mineralocorticoids might not be direct, but secondary to changes in intracellular electrolyte status. Jørgensen[43] has further analysed the steroid effects into acute and chronic phases and concludes, from the finding that only the chronic phase is altered by aldosterone, that the changing enzyme activity is merely an adaptation to some unknown hormonal modulation of intracellular Na:K ratio[45]. Intracellular sodium levels can affect mitochondrial ATPase activity[46]. Edelman[33] summarizes the evidence against accepting Na,K-dependent ATPase activity and/or concentration as a primary locus of aldosterone action as follows. Little or no change in the K_m of the enzyme results from aldosterone treatment of sensitive tissues. Moreover, an effect on the enzyme concentration is only obtained with supraphysiological quantities of hormone, whereas increased hormonally-stimulated sodium transport occurs without detectable changes in enzyme activity.

The final route by which the aldosterone-induced protein might act is to increase the rate of energy supply to the process of sodium transport. The crucial importance of this energy supply, in the form of ATP, has already been mentioned. Respiratory poisons or substrate depletion of tissue prevent the expression of the effects of aldosterone which can be restored respectively by ATP or by substrates such as glucose, pyruvate, β-hydroxybutyrate, acetoacetate and oxaloacetate. Providing protein synthesis has already been induced, response to these substrates is instantaneous but can be inhibited by oxythiamine, an analogue of thiamine which is a component of the pyridine nucleotides. Again the evidence that energy metabolism is directly affected by aldosterone-induced protein has also been carefully examined by Edelman[27]. In summary, the concentrations of several enzyme components of the tricarboxylic acid cycle are increased following aldosterone treatment of target organ tissue. These enzymes include glutamate and malate dehydrogenases, glutamate–oxaloacetate transaminase and, in particular, citrate synthase. Changes in the concentration of this latter enzyme are coincident, and correlate, with alterations in sodium transport, occur in response to physiological doses of hormone and are independent of (i.e. not secondary to) changes in sodium flux. Changes in urinary Na:K ratio, a hallmark of mineralocorticoid activity, follow closely upon increases in renal tissue NADH:NAD ratio, which monitors the rate of tissue respiration. The author concludes that primary modulation of energy metabolism may be the major effect of mineralocorticoids and that the increased availability of metabolic energy may serve to increase the number of sodium channels available for ion translocation. Other hormones which affect energy metabolism, such as those from the thyroid, may also alter sodium transport[47–49]. However, it remains possible that the effects on permeability and energy metabolism are independent[50].

Thus mineralocorticoids, in common with other steroid hormones, appear to exert their influence by inducing specific changes in protein synthesis. This protein may affect energy metabolism and either in this way or independently alter permeability to sodium and also its active extrusion. However, sporadic accounts of *in vitro* effects of aldosterone on electrolyte flux in erythrocytes or erythrocyte ghosts, which of course lack nuclei, have appeared and cannot be explained by this hypothesis. In the most recent account of such studies[51] sodium flux was increased by physiological concentrations of aldosterone and inhibited by higher doses. The authors found aldosterone to bind to the Na,K-dependent ATPase and suggest that it might have a direct effect. Whether such a direct mechanism is of general importance or occurs only in the special situation of the erythrocyte is, as yet, a matter for conjecture.

References

1. King, R. J. B. and Mainwaring, W. I. P. (1974). *Steroid Cell Interactions*. (London: Butterworth)
2. O'Malley, B. W. and Means, A. R. (1974). Female steroid hormones and target cell nuclei. *Science*, **183**, 610
3. Robison, G. A., Butcher, R. W. and Sutherland, E. W. (1971). *Cyclic AMP*. (New York: Academic Press)
4. Biber, T. U. L. and Mullen, T. (1976). Saturation kinetics of sodium efflux across isolated frog skin. *Am. J. Physiol.*, **231**, 995
5. Ross, B., Leaf, A., Silva, P. and Epstein, F. H. (1974). Na,K-ATPase in sodium transport by the profused rat kidney. *Am. J. Physiol.*, **226**, 624
6. Fraser, R. (1971). The effect of steroids on the transport of electrolytes through membranes. *Biochem. Soc. Symp.*, **32**, 101
7. Patrick, J. and Hilton, P. J. (1979). Characterisation of sodium transport disorders in disease: different effects upon sodium and potassium of changes in the sodium pumps and in membrane permeability. *Clin. Sci. Molec. Med.*, **57**, 289
8. Sachs, G. (1977). Ion pumps in the renal tubule. *Am. J. Physiol.*, **233**, F359.
9. Silva, P., Torretti, J., Hayslett, J. P. and Epstein, F. H., (1976). Relation between Na,K-ATPase activity and respiratory rate in rat kidney. *Am. J. Physiol.*, **230**, 1432.
10. Nellans, H. N. and Finn, A. L. (1974). Oxygen consumption and sodium transport in the toad urinary bladder. *Am. J. Physiol.*, **227**, 670
11. Robinson, J. D. and Flaschner, M. S. (1979). The (Na+−K+) activated ATPase. Enzymatic and transport properties. *Biochim. Biophys. Acta*, **549**, 145
12. Keynes, R. D. (1979). Ion channels in the nerve cell membrane. *Sci. Am.*, **240**, 126
13. Glynn, I. M., Hoffman, J. F. and Lew, V. L. (1971). Some partial reactions of the sodium pump. *Phil. Trans. R. Soc. London*, **B262**, 91
14. Edmonds, C. J. (1972). Effect of aldosterone on mammalian intestine. *J. Steroid Biochem.*, **3**, 143
15. Weedon, A. P., Stacey, T. E., Ward, R. H. T. and Boyd, R. D. H. (1978). Bidirectional sodium fluxes across the placenta of the conscious sheep. *Am. J. Physiol.* **235**, F536
16. Erlij, D. (1971). Salt transport across isolated frog skin. *Phil. Trans. R. Soc. London*, **B262**, 153
17. Mills, J. N., Ernst, S. A. and DiBona, D. R. (1977). Localisation of Na⁺ pump sites in frog skin. *J. Cell Biol.*, **73**, 88
18. Helman, S. I. and O'Neil, R. G. (1977). Model of active transepithelial sodium and potassium transport in renal collecting tubules. *Am. J. Physiol.*, **233**, F559
19. Giebisch, G., Boulpaep, E. L. and Whittembury G. (1971). Electrolyte transport in kidney tubule cells. *Philos. Trans. R. Soc. London*, **B262**, 175
20. Nicholls, M. G., Ramsay, L. E., Boddy, K., Fraser, R., Morton, J. J. and

Robertson, J. I. S. (1979). Mineralocorticoid-induced blood pressure, electrolyte and hormone changes and reversal with spironolactone in healthy men. *Metabolism*, **28**, 584

21.   Vander, A. J., Wilde, W. S. and Malvin, R. L. (1960). Stop flow analysis of aldosterone and steroidal antagonist SC 8109 on renal tubular sodium transport kinetics. *Proc. Soc. Exp. Biol. Med.*, **103**, 525

22.   Hierholze, K. and Stolte, H. (1969). The proximal and distal tubular action of adrenal steroids on sodium reabsorption. *Nephron*, **6**, 188

23.   Barger, A. C., Berlin, R. D. and Tulenko, J. F. (1958). Infusion of aldosterone, 9 α fluorohydrocortisone and antidiuretic hormone into the renal artery of normal and adrenalectomised unanaesthetised dogs; effect on electrolyte and water excretion. *Endocrinology*, **62**, 804

24.   Ross, E. J. (1975). *Aldosterone and Aldosteronism*. (London: Lloyd Luke)

25.   Schwartz, G. J. and Black, M. B. (1978). Mineralocorticoid effects on cation transport by cortical collecting ducts *in vitro*. *Am. J. Physiol.*, **235**, F576

26.   Wiederholt, M., Behn, C., Schoormans, W. and Hansen, L. (1972). Effect of aldosterone on sodium and potassium transport in the kidney. *J. Steroid Biochem.*, **3**, 151

27.   Ussing, H. H. and Zerahn, K. (1951). Active transport of sodium as the source of electric current in the short-circuited isolated frog skin. *Acta Physiol. Scand.*, **23**, 110

28.   Ussing, H. H. (1968). The interpretation of tracer fluxes in terms of membrane structure. *Q. Rev. Biophys.*, **1**, 365

29.   Fraser, R., Brown, J. J., Lever, A. F., Mason, P. A. and Robertson, J. I. S. (1979). Control of aldosterone secretion. *Clin. Sci. Molec. Med.*, **56**, 389

30.   Porter, G. A. and Kinsey, J. (1972). The effect of a new anti-aldosterone agent SC 19886 on aldosterone-stimulated transepithelial sodium transport. *J. Steroid Biochem.*, **3**, 201

31.   Edelman, I. S. and Fimognari, G. (1968). On the biochemical mechanism of action of aldosterone. *Recent Prog. Hormone Res.*, **24**, 1

32.   Edelman, I. S. (1975). Mechanism of action of steroid hormones. *J. Steroid Biochem.*, **6**, 147

33.   Edelman, I. S. (1979). Mechanism of action of aldosterone: energetic and permeability factors. *J. Endocrinol.*, **81**, 49

34.   Funder, J. W., Feldman, D., Highland, E. and Edelman, I. S. (1974). Molecular modifications of anti-aldosterone compounds: effects on affinity of spironolactones for renal receptors. *Biochem. Pharmacol.*, **23**, 1493

35.   Sakauye, C. and Feldman, D. (1976). Agonist and antimineralocorticoid activities of spirolactones. *Am. J. Physiol.*, **231**, 93

36.   Feldman, D., Loose, D. S. and Tan, S. Y. (1978). Nonsteroidal anti-inflammatory drugs cause sodium and water retention in the rat. *Am. J. Physiol.*, **234**, F490

37.   Rousseau, G., Baxter, J. D., Funder, J. W., Edelman, I. S. and Tomkins, G. M. (1972). Glucocorticoid and mineralocorticoid receptors for aldosterone. *J. Steroid Biochem.*, **3**, 219

38.   Crabbé, J. (1978). The sodium retaining properties of sodium. In V. H. T. James, M. Serio, G. Giusti and L. Martini (eds.) *The Endocrine Function of the Human Adrenal Cortex*, p. 351. (London: Academic Press)

39. McKnight, A. D. C. and Leaf, A. (1978). The sodium transport pool. *Am. J. Physiol.*, **234**, F1
40. Civan, M. M. (1978). Intracellular activities of sodium and potassium. *Am. J. Physiol.*, **234**, F261
41. Finn, A. L. (1970). Effects of potassium and amphotericin B on ion transport in the toad bladder. *Am. J. Physiol.*, **218**, 463
42. Leaf, A. and McKnight, A. D. C. (1972). The site of aldosterone induced stimulation of sodium transport. *J. Steroid Biochem.*, **3**, 237
43. Jørgensen, P. L. (1972). The role of aldosterone in the regulation of (Na$^+$ + K$^+$) ATPase in the rat kidney. *J. Steroid Biochem.*, **3**, 181
44. Schmidt, U., Schmidt, J., Schmidt, H. and Dubach, V. C. (1975). Sodium- and potassium-activated ATPase – a possible target of aldosterone. *J. Clin. Invest.*, **55**, 655
45. Westenfelder, C., Arevalo, G. J., Baranowski, R. L., Kurtzman, N. A. and Katz, A. I. (1977). Relationship between mineralocorticoids and renal Na$^+$ K$^+$ ATPase: sodium reabsorption. *Am. J. Physiol.*, **233**, F593
46. Weiner, M. W. (1975). ATPase activity of kidney mitochondria stimulated by sodium. *Am. J. Physiol.*, **228**, 815
47. Gregg, C. M., Cohen, J. J., Black, A. J., Espeland, M. A. and Feldstein, M. C. (1978). Effects of glucose and insulin on metabolism and function of perfused rat kidney. *Am. J. Physiol.*, **235**, F52
48. Lo, C.–S. and Lo, T. N. (1979). Time course of the renal response to triodothyronine in the rat. *Am. J. Physiol.*, **236**, F9
49. Rossier, B. C., Rossier, M. and Lo, C. S. (1979). Thyroxine and sodium transport in the toad. *Am. J. Physiol.*, **236**, C117
50. Snart, R. S. (1972). The two stage nature of the aldosterone response. *J. Steroid Biochem.*, **3**, 129
51. Hamlyn, J. M. and Duffy, T. (1978). Direct stimulation of human erythrocyte membrane (Na$^+$ + K$^+$) Mg ATPase activity *in vitro* by physiological concentrations of aldosterone. *Biochem. Biophys. Res. Commun.*, **84**, 458

10

Sodium transport in cystic fibrosis
C. Garner, A. K. Khullar, V. Schwarz and N. I. M. Simpson

There can be few fields in medical science in which so much uncon-firmed, if not unconfirmable, research has been published as in that of cystic fibrosis (CF). The literature abounds with positive findings which independent investigators have been unable to repeat[1]. In these circum-stances a comprehensive and uncritical review of publications can be mis-leading and even counterproductive.

What is the evidence for abnormal sodium transport in CF and how solid is it? The definitition of the disease includes an abnormally high sodium concentration in the sweat. In contrast to a normal infant's sweat sodium concentration of about 20 mmol/l, the CF patient's may be as high as 120 mmol/l or more. This substantial difference between the normal and the pathological makes the sweat test the most useful and re-liable tool in the diagnosis of CF, compared with which other reported biochemical abnormalities are as yet inadequate.

The pancreas, even if undamaged by blockage of the duct, fails to respond to secretin[2], but no other tissue or cell has been reliably shown to evince a major defect in sodium transport. The handling of the ion by the kidney *in vivo* is normal, as also is sodium movement into and out of the red blood cells *in vitro,* although a slight abnormality has been repor-ted by some investigators. Heart, nerves and brain all function perfectly.

The thick, viscid mucus which is a dominant feature of CF has not, as yet, been shown to be connected with a sodium transport defect.

It would seem, therefore, that the faulty handling of sodium by the sweat glands is due to an abnormality of a process peculiar to these (and possibly other) glands. A generalized membrane defect would surely manifest itself in other tissues, as would interference with sodium movement by some abnormal (if somewhat elusive) protein in the blood (the 'CF factor') which has been reported by several investigators[3].

Kaiser et al.[4], in a study unconfirmed by independent investigators, found that the sweat produced by a normal gland in vivo contained more sodium than usual after perfusion with CF sweat. Mangos et al.[5] made similar observations with rat parotid gland perfused with CF fluids. These findings suggest that such fluids contain a substance which interferes with the handling of sodium by certain glands, but not by other tissues.

What exactly does handling of sodium by the sweat gland imply? The currently accepted view is that sodium ions probably diffuse into the secretory coil cell which pumps them into the lumen, followed by Cl^- and water. The precursor fluid so formed is approximately isotonic, both in the normal and in the CF gland[6], and as it passes through the coiled portion of the duct most of the Na^+ is reabsorbed into the interstitium, presumably again by diffusion into and pumping out of the cells. Reabsorption fails to be achieved to more than a limited extent in the CF gland. There must be some reabsorption, or the surface sweat would contain 140 mmol sodium/l. Since the kidney tubule regularly reabsorbs 75% or more of the sodium filtered, in the normal or CF subject, we must assume that it is not reabsorption in general which is deficient in CF, but rather a mechanism peculiar to the sweat gland (and possibly some other glands) which ensures a rapid but short-lived, intermittent sodium movement across the duct cell.

Is there such a mechanism and, if so, what could it be? It seems reasonable to suggest that it would involve an increase in permeability to sodium ions of the luminal membrane, with perhaps an enhanced capacity of the Na/K pump at the serosal membrane to transport the ions flooding into the cell. The hypothesis is based on the premise that whereas a low permeability is advantageous in conserving energy needed to maintain the cellular milieu, a high permeability may be mandatory for rapid transport.

We have been using a modified form of the standard sweat test for many years, in which we collect the sweat serially for four or five periods of 5 min following stimulation with pilocarpine, and we frequently find that the secretion rate, and with it the sodium concentration, drops over the 20–25 min sampling time[7]. The dependence of the sodium concentration of a secretion on the secretory rate is a feature of several types of gland and is presumably connected with the available contact time in the reabsorption duct. However, a review of the last 287 consecutive tests on normal individuals in our records yielded 48 in which the secretion rate either remained steady or rose throughout the collection period: of these 25 (52%) showed, nevertheless, a steady fall in sodium concentration. Two examples are given in Table 10.1. This observation is compatible with the hypothesis that the glands progressively adjust to reabsorb more salt in the course of a secretory episode. If such 'adjustment' is relatively slow, the sodium concentration would fall, as in the examples shown; if it is fast, the sodium concentration would remain steady over most of the course of 20–25 min, but might still be expected to show a fall in the first few minutes. The normal sweat test does not lend itself to a study of changes in the secretion rate or sodium concentration in the initial secretory period because individual glands come into action at different times and the secretion is collected from between 80 and 200 glands/cm^2 of skin. We therefore undertook a study of the performance of single glands *in vivo,* collecting sweat, after a 30 s stimulation with pilocarpine, under liquid paraffin into capillaries and determining the sodium by atomic absorption on an electrically-heated carbon rod. Of 22 experiments, seven showed a fall in sodium concentration despite a substantially constant or rising secretion rate over the first 4–5 min. In the remainder, the sodium concentration varied with the secretory rate. Three examples are presented in Table 10.2. These observations suggest that there may be a mechanism, which has to be switched on, for increasing the ability of the duct cells to reabsorb salt from the lumen, and thus support our hypothesis.

We have been unable to perform single-gland experiments on CF patients, but an analysis of the last 115 consecutive sweat tests on such subjects has yielded 36 in which the secretion rate was steady or rising; of these 10 (28%) showed a progressive fall in sodium concentration, albeit at the much higher level usual in CF. Two examples are shown in Table 10.3. It is thus clear that if this fall in sodium concentration betokens a slow increase in reabsorption capability, the adaptation is not altogether lacking in CF, although it may be poorly-developed or inhibited.

Turning our attention to possible mechanisms whereby the reabsorption of sodium might be enhanced, we have established that sweat contains cyclic AMP (Table 10.4). The nucleotide probably originates within the gland, an assumption which is the more likely since we have found adenylate cyclase in the tissue. The enzyme is stimulated by a number of agonists, including prostaglandins E_1 and E_2 (both at 2×10^{-4}mol/l), bradykinin (at 8×10^{-6}mol/l) and acetylcholine (at 1×10^{-5}mol/l) – Table 10.5.

TABLE 10.1 Sodium concentrations in consecutive sweat samples secreted at constant or rising rates

Control subject	Secretion rate (mg/3 cm²/5 min)	[Na] (mmol/l)
1	13.1	58
	16.0	51
	16.3	47
	16.1	45
2	14.0	22.8
	15.7	15.9
	16.4	14.7
	16.3	13.4

TABLE 10.2 Sodium concentrations in consecutive sweat samples from single glands

Expt.	Time after end of stimulation (s)	Secretion rate (nl/min)	[Na] (mmol/l)
1	55	0.72	108
	110	0.76	94
	170	0.72	88
	250	0.66	73
	300	0.66	74
2	59	0.87	91
	96	—	—
	141	1.35	75
	187	1.24	65
	239	1.30	67
3	105	4.8	103
	170	5.8	79
	255	5.2	79
	375	6.1	76
	—	6.1	69

SODIUM TRANSPORT IN CYSTIC FIBROSIS

TABLE 10.3 Sodium concentrations in consecutive sweat samples secreted at rising rates: CF subjects

CF subject	Secretion rate (mg/3 cm²/5 min)	[Na] (mmol/l)
1	21	119
	29	111
	32	106
	32	99
2	8.7	100
	11.9	99
	18.3	94
	25.5	86

TABLE 10.4 Cyclic AMP in children's sweat

	n	$cAMP$(pmol/100 mg)
Controls	(7)	0.60 ± 0.10 SEM
CF	(4)	0.66 ± 0.074 SEM

TABLE 10.5 Stimulation of adenylate cyclase

Agonist	% stimulation
PGE_1	120
PGE_2	150
Bradykinin	68
Acetylcholine	160

In view of the possibility that one of the roles of adenylate cyclase in the sweat gland might be a modification of the membrane by phosphorylation of one or more proteins, we incubated sweat gland homogenate with γ-^{32}P-ATP $\pm$ cyclic AMP and submitted the mixture to polyacrylamide gel electrophoresis. The gel was cut into 16 5 mm bands and the label was counted in each. While the ^{32}P-content of corresponding slices in ten experiments was variable, statistical analyses by the t test and by the Wilcoxon signed rank test indicated a highly significant positive deviation from the joint ($\pm$ cAMP) mean in favour of cAMP in three bands. These contain proteins of molecular weights $3\text{--}4 \times 10^4$, 1.8×10^4 and 1.0×10^4 respectively. There was an equally significant negative deviation at the top of the gel (molecular weight $> 10^6$). We tentatively conclude from this observation that the sweat gland homogenate contains proteins which are phosphorylated in the presence of cAMP, and one or more of high molecular weight which are dephosphorylated. There is no indication, at present, as to the location of these proteins within the cell or their function.

We have presented evidence that efficient reabsorption of salt in the sweat duct may be subject to a delay, which could imply that a switch-on mechanism is needed. This mechanism may involve adenylate cyclase which is present in the gland and is stimulated by a number of agonists including acetylcholine, the neurotransmitter responsible for activating the gland. Our studies of protein phosphorylation suggest that the cyclic AMP may be instrumental in phosphorylating some and dephosphorylating other cellular proteins.

The experiments we have described indicate no more than the existence of possible machinery for speeding up sodium transport. The vital link is a demonstration that the cyclic AMP system is directly involved in the movement of sodium ions. Experiments to establish whether this connection exists are now under way.

Such tests as we have done on cystic fibrosis subjects indicate, so far, no abnormality in the cyclic AMP system; but elucidation of the mechanism whereby reabsorption of sodium is controlled in the normal gland may well yield the long-sought answer.

References

1. Benke, P. J. (1976). Biochemistry of cystic fibrosis: an overview. In J. A. Mangos and R. C. Talamo (eds.). *Cystic Fibrosis: Projections into the Future*, p. 157. (New York: Stratton)
2. Hadorn, B., Johansen, P. G. and Anderson, C. M. (1968). Pancreozymin secretion test of exocrine pancreatic function in cystic fibrosis. *Canad. Med. Assoc. J.*, **98**, 377
3. Bowman, B. H. (1976). Factors related to cystic fibrosis. In J. A. Mangos and R. C. Talamo (eds.). *Cystic Fibrosis: Projections into the Future*, p. 277. (New York: Stratton)
4. Kaiser, D., Drack, E. and Rossi, E. (1971). Inhibition of net sodium transport in single sweat glands by sweat of patients with cystic fibrosis. *Pediatr. Res.*, **5**, 167

5. Mangos, J. A., McSherry, N. R. and Benke, P. J. (1967). A sodium transport inhibitory factor in the saliva of patients with cystic fibrosis. *Pediatr. Res.*, **1,** 436
6. Schulz, I. J. (1969). Micropuncture studies of the sweat formation in cystic fibrosis patients. *J. Clin. Invest.*, **48,** 1470
7. Sutcliffe, C. H., Style, P. P. and Schwarz, V. (1968). Biochemical studies of sweat secretion in cystic fibrosis. *Proc. R. Soc. Med.*, **61,** 297

11

Nephrogenic
diabetes insipidus
J. Brodehl

DEFINITION

The renal type of diabetes insipidus was recognized as a separate entity
more than 30 years ago, when it was described in the literature almost
simultaneously by two independent investigators, Forssman in Sweden[1]
and Waring and co-workers in the United States[2]. Families with this type
of defect, however, had been described many years previously[3] without
being distinguished from the central or neurohormonal diabetes insipidus. The name 'nephrogenic diabetes insipidus' was proposed by
Williams and Henry in 1947[4], and today it is used synonymously with the
terms 'vasopressin or ADH-resistant diabetes insipidus' or 'diabetes insipidus renalis'.

Nephrogenic diabetes insipidus (NDI) is characterized by a resistance
of the kidney to the antidiuretic effect of vasopressin. It can occur as a
congenital and then mostly inherited disorder, or as an acquired disturbance due to intoxication, systemic diseases or obstructive uropathy. I will
restrict myself mainly to discussion of the congenital type of nephrogenic
diabetes insipidus, since this relates to the general topic of this book and
– as in other inborn errors of transport and metabolism – allows the study
of a singular defect and its consequences for the kidney and the whole
organism. First I shall describe the clinical picture of the disease, its diagnosis, treatment and genetic transmission, and then give a short review

on the present knowledge of the cellular action of vasopressin, the function of the tubular membranes and the pathomechanism of the disease.

Congenital nephrogenic diabetes insipidus is characterized by the symptoms shown in Table 11.1. The primary defect is the unresponsiveness of the distal nephron, mainly the collecting duct, to the antidiuretic effect of vasopressin. In this way the kidney loses its ability to concentrate urine, which leads to polyuria, polydipsia, chronic dehydration, and, mainly in infants, to fever, obstipation, failure to thrive and mental retardation. Laboratory investigation reveals extracellular hyperosmolality, especially hypernatraemia, the urine remains hypotonic and has an osmolality of 50–100 mosm/kg H_2O, the osmolar U/P ratio remains constantly below 1, and cannot be reversed by exogenous application of vasopressin. The congenital type is mostly inherited and transmitted as an X-linked recessive or partially recessive trait.

TABLE 11.1   Congenital nephrogenic diabetes insipidus

Primary defect:	Unresponsiveness of distal nephron to antidiuretic effect of vasopressin
Symptoms:	Polyuria, polydipsia, dehydration (mainly in infants), fever, obstipation, failure to thrive, mental retardation
Laboratory:	Hyperosmolality, hypernatraemia, hypotonic urine, $U/P_{osm} < 1$, complete resistance to exogenous vasopressin
Heredity:	X-linked transmission

CLINICAL MANIFESTATION

The defect in congenital NDI is present from birth, and, therefore, symptoms usually appear within the first few weeks of life, depending on the kind of milk formula given to the infant. As long as the infant is fed breast milk, he usually thrives fairly well and does not develop signs of dehydration. This can be explained by the fact that human milk has a very low salt and protein content, and that its constituents are mainly assimilated by rapid cellular growth. Therefore, the osmolar load to be excreted by the infant's kidney remains in a low range (see Table 11.2). A breast-fed infant does not need to elevate his urinary osmolality above 120 mosmol/kg H_2O, which can almost be achieved even by a completely affected infant. As soon as the infant is fed with cows' milk formula, the osmolar load to the kidney is increased 2–3 fold, which increases the demand for free water by the same order. This is not provided any more by oral feeding and, therefore, dehydration appears.

TABLE 11.2 Renal osmolar load in infant feed

		Urea (mosm)	Na + K + Cl (mosm)	Total (mosm)
Human milk	1 l	48	31	79
Cows' milk	1 l	132	89	221
Strained pears	100 g	1	2	3
Strained beef + vegetables	100 g	29	28	54

From Ziegler and Fomon[5]

The main symptoms are fever, variation in weight due to hydrolability, and failure to thrive, as shown by Figure 11.1, in which the data of a 4-month-old male infant are depicted. The infant's skin is dry and mottled, he is chronically obstipated, vomits frequently, is restless and suffers occasionally from convulsions. Since enhanced thirst cannot be recognized easily in this period of life, many infants with this defect experience a series of unnecessary, and often harmful, diagnostic and therapeutic procedures, including various antibiotic treatments, X-ray examinations, spinal taps and paracentesis, until the correct diagnosis is made. It is not known how many cases have remained undiagnosed during infancy and how many have died without their disease being suspected.

Untreated, most patients fail to grow normally and develop mental retardation [6-9]. These are caused by both malnutrition and dehydration. Malnutrition is the consequence of excessive fluid intake, which provokes vomiting and anorexia. Episodes of severe dehydration and hyperelectrolytaemia can produce cerebral bleeding and organic brain damage [10-12]. Recently we have observed a moderately retarded 5-month-old infant, who had two convulsions before the diagnosis of NDI was made, and in whom the cranial computer tomography revealed a localized brain atrophy in the temporo-medio-basal area of the left hemisphere, as shown in Figure 11.2. Psychological study [13] demonstrated that three out of eight children with congenital NDI tested could be regarded as being normal in terms of psychological and personality development, while three had dull–normal or borderline levels and two had severe

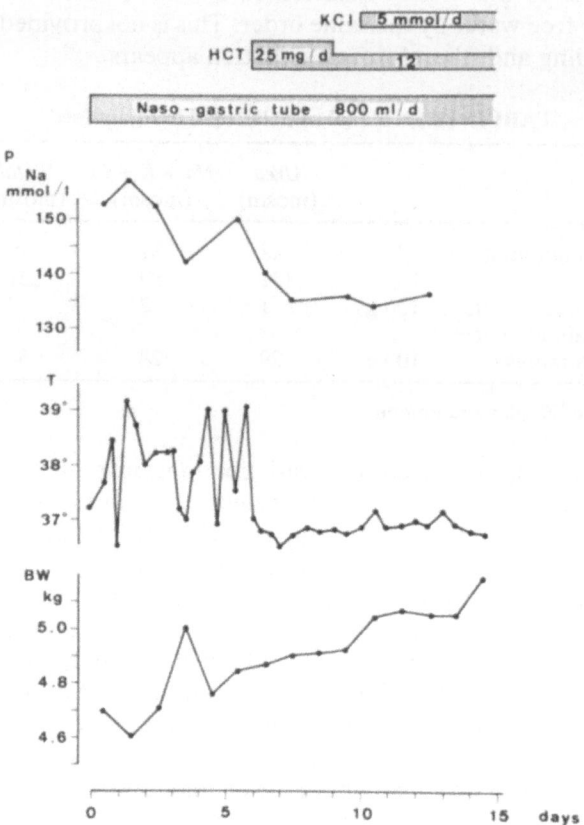

Figure 11.1 Clinical course and treatment of a 4-month-old boy with NDI. HCT – hydrochlorothiazide

mental retardation. Besides organic brain alterations the psychological development is influenced by a permanent demand for drinking and the urge for frequent voiding, which compete with playing, learning and nightly sleep. Many children with NDI, therefore, are characterized by hyperactivity, distractibility, short attention span, and restlessness. As soon as thirst becomes obvious and fluids are not withheld, the development gradually improves and many cases are reported in the literature of adults who seem to be physically and mentally quite normal, with the exception of their need to drink large amounts of water.

The urinary volume in adults with NDI is in the range of 12–20 litres

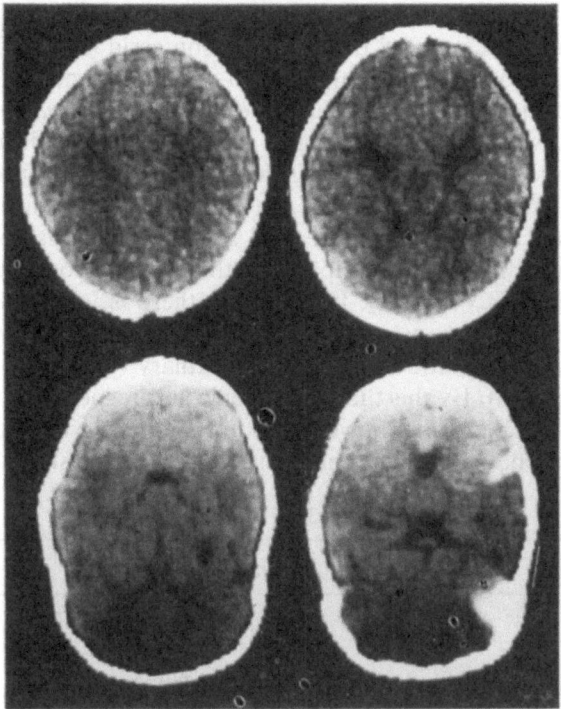

Figure 11.2 Cranial computer tomography of a 5-month-old boy with NDI (see text). By courtesy of Dr. Stoeppler, Dept. Neuroradiology, Medical School, Hannover

per day, and in infants and children proportionally lower. Theoretically, it should be in the range of 10–12% of glomerular filtration rate, since this is the percentage regulated in the kidney by vasopressin. However, in many cases the daily urinary volume is lower, because the development of chronic dehydration produces a reduction of glomerular filtration rate. A sequela of excessive water turnover is the development of hydronephrosis, hydroureter and megacystis[14-16] which do not usually need any surgical intervention, and are found in all long-lasting states of polyuria. Otherwise there are no further pathological findings.

DIAGNOSTIC PROCEDURES

The diagnosis of NDI can best be made by the vasopressin-test. This is preferred to the dehydration-test, which could be dangerous in infants and must be supervised very strictly. The vasopressin test is either performed with 1-deamino-8 D arginine-vasopressin (DDAVP), which is a synthetic analogue of natural arginine–vasopressin and is characterized by a high and prolonged antidiuretic effect and by low vasopressor activity[17,18], or with lysine–vasopressin or pitressin, as indicated in Table 11.3. In our laboratory the test is done with lysine–vasopressin which is given as a bolus in the dosage of 2 mU/kg body weight during the course of a clearance study. In Figure 11.3 a normal response, shown on the right (patient M.R.), is compared with a non-response in a case with NDI (patient C.V. – left). In the latter there is, after vasopressin, no increase in urinary osmolality, which remains in the range of 80–100 mosm/kg H_2O, and no reduction in urinary volume (V) or free water clearance (C_{H_2O}). By this the nephrogenic non-response to vasopressin is demonstrated, but this, however, is not identical with the diagnosis of NDI, as will be mentioned under differential diagnosis.

TABLE 11.3 The vasopressin test

Agent		Quantity		Reference
DDAVP	intranasal	10 μg	infants	17
		20 μg	children	17
		40 μg	adults	18
	intravenous	0.5 μg/m²	infants	17
		2 μg	children	17
		4 μg	adults	18
Lysine-vasopressin	i.v.	2 mU/kg	infants and children	(Brodehl)
		8 mU/kg/h	as infusion (for cAMP-determination)	23
Pitressin tannate oil	i.m.	0.5 U/6 kg	children	64

It is still controversial as to whether the urinary excretion of cyclic–3′,5′ adenosine monophosphate (cAMP) can be used for discrimination of vasopressin response from non-response. It is known that the tubular hydro-osmotic effect of vasopressin is initiated by activation of membrane-bound adenyl-cyclase, and it was claimed that *in vivo* the application of vasopressin is followed by an increase in the urinary excretion of cAMP in normal subjects[19-21]. This response could not be obtained in patients with NDI[22-24], which seemed to indicate that the molecular defect in NDI was indeed a lack or resistance of a receptor for vasopressin in the tubular membrane. Our own experience is limited to

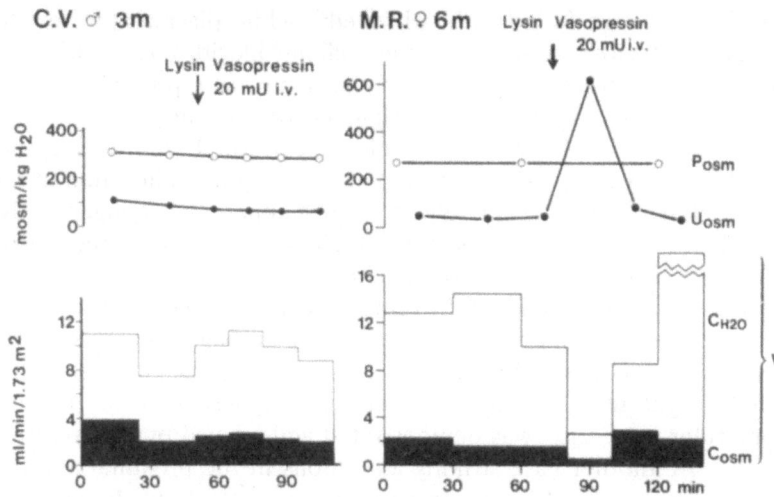

Figure 11.3 Effect of lysine–vasopressin in a normal infant (right) and in an infant with NDI (left)

two patients with NDI, in whom no significant elevation of cAMP excretion could be observed after vasopressin. However, neither the normal stimulation of cAMP excretion could consistently be seen by other investigators[25–26], nor the non-response to vasopressin registered in cases with NDI[25,27]. Therefore, one has to conclude that it is undecided whether the determination of cAMP in response to vasopressin is really meaningful for the diagnosis of NDI[28,29]. It is certain, on the other hand, that the urinary response to vasopressin is not comparable with that to parathormone, which increases urinary cAMP excretion 70–120 fold. It further seems to be important, that when attempting to measure cAMP excretion, vasopressin should not just be administered as a bolus, but as an infusion over 1–4 h.

Vasopressin measured in blood and urine by radioimmunoassay is usually elevated in NDI, and responds appropriately to the changes in fluid osmolality[30,31]. The extrarenal pituitary responsiveness to vasopressin is preserved in patients with NDI, which also is regarded as mediated by adenylate cyclase[32].

Other laboratory findings are non-specific and mainly the consequence of chronic dehydration and hyperelectrolytaemia. Glomerular filtration rate is often slightly to moderately reduced, the renal plasma flow (C_{PAH}) even more, thus elevating the filtration fraction[4,30,33,34]. In severe dehydration serum urea and creatinine could be increased.

Plasma renin was found to be elevated[35], while plasma aldosterone is reported to be low[36] or normal[37]. The sodium chloride content of sweat is increased in untreated cases[38-40] and the same was reported for saliva[38]. Uric acid was described to be significantly elevated in adults with NDI[30,33] while in children the levels were normal. It was suggested, therefore, that hyperuricaemia might be an acquired alteration of long-lasting NDI. Further renal defects are not apparent in congenital NDI and all other partial functions of the tubules are found to be undisturbed.

The macroscopic anatomy of the kidney is normal. By microdissecting the kidney, it was found that the proximal convoluted tubules are shorter in NDI cases than in normals[41,42] a disturbing finding which needs further investigation. Biopsy specimens do not show any specific tubular altera-tion by light microscopy[35,43]. In one case hypertrophy of the juxta-glomerular apparatus was demonstrated and proved by electronmicro-scopy[35]. In another case striking alterations in the proximal and distal tubules are observed by electronmicroscopy, mainly in the mitochon-dria, which contained concentric ringed structures and myelin figures suggestive of a disturbance in mitochondrial lipids[43]. The latter case had been treated with frusemide before biopsy, and therefore the signifi-cance of this finding remains unclear.

DIFFERENTIAL DIAGNOSIS

NDI has to be differentiated from many other polyuric states which are listed on Table 11.4. From the pathophysiological point of view, three types of polyuria have to be considered: a disturbance of ADH secre-tion, a disturbance of thirst manifesting as primary polydipsia, and the renal concentrating defects. The disturbance of ADH secretion[44] includes diseases with an abnormality of the osmoreceptors, in which thirst is usually also involved, and therefore hypernatraemia predomin-ates, abnormalities in ADH production and release, which can be of idiopathic or inherited origin, or be acquired due to trauma, tumour or infection, and, very rarely, an enhanced elimination of ADH in the per-iphery due to immunological processes[45]. The primary polydipsias[46] are found in central nervous lesions as in leukaemia and infections, or in cases with psychological or psychiatric disturbances. The renal concen-trating defects are either related to the osmotic gradient in the medulla, which is the prerequisite of the final concentrating procedure in the col-lecting ducts and thus include diseases such as chronic renal failure, nephronophthisis, amyloid nephropathy, sickle cell disease and others, or alternatively, the renal concentrating defect may be due to the changes in water permeability in the distal tubules, which is regulated by vasopressin. In this group NDI is just one entity, the others are acquired as hypokalaemic or hypercalcaemic nephropathies or intoxications[47]. The classification of the renal concentration defects is somewhat arbitrary, since in many systemic diseases or diffuse renal diseases both mechanisms for urinary concentrations are involved. The diagnosis of these defects requires a series of investigations, including clearance studies, vasopressin-response in osmotic mannitol diureses[48,49], other tubular function studies, endocrinological and immunological studies and the renal biopsy. A correct diagnosis should be attempted in each case, since the therapeutic approach could be very specific for different types of polyuric states.

TABLE 11.4   **Differential diagnosis of polyuric states**

1. *Disturbance of ADH secretion*
   1.1.   Abnormality of osmoreceptors
   1.2.   Abnormality of ADH production and release
            (idiopathic, inherited, acquired DI)
   1.3.   Enhanced peripheral ADH elimination

2. *Disturbance of thirst*
   2.1.   Central-nervous lesions
            (infections, leukaemia, trauma)
   2.2.   Psychogenic (compulsive) polydipsia

3. *Renal concentrating defects*
   3.1.   Failure of medullary osmolar gradient
        3.1.1.   Chronic renal failure
        3.1.2.   Nephronophthisis
        3.1.3.   Amyloid nephropathy
        3.1.4.   Osmotic diuresis
        3.1.5.   Postobstructive uropathy
        3.1.6.   Sickle cell disease
        3.1.7.   Complex tubulopathy   (Fanconi-S.)
   3.2.   Failure in vasopressin induced hydro-osmotic
        response
        3.2.1.   Congenital NDI
        3.2.2.   Hypokalaemic nephropathy
        3.2.3.   Hypercalcaemic nephropathy
        3.2.4.   Intoxications with lithium
              demethylchlortetracycline,
              methoxyflurane

TREATMENT

The aim of any treatment of NDI is to prevent dehydration and hyper-electrolytaemia and, at the same time, to reduce the daily fluid intake to amounts which are tolerable for the patients and do not interfere with their daily activities and nightly sleep. Fluids have to be offered freely as soon as thirst regulates the need. In infants, a naso gastric tube allows a continuous drip of solute-free fluid, especially at night. A diet low in salt and protein keeps the obligatory fluid loss low and is therefore recommended. Since vasopressin and its analogues are totally ineffective in NDI, this is also true for those agents which either stimulate ADH release, such as clofibrate[50], or enhance hormone activity, such as chlorpropamide and carbamazepine[51,52] which are used in central diabetes insipidus. The administration of cAMP has no effect on urinary concentrating ability[53,54]. Thus saluretic agents introduced into the treatment of NDI almost 20 years ago[55,56] still remain the drugs of choice. Hydrochlorothiazide is usually used[57-61] although other saldiuretics, seem to be equally effective, such as ethacrynic acid[37,62] and frusemide[63,64].

The acute effect of hydrochlorothiazide is striking as shown in Figure 11.1: the fever subsides immediately, weight is gained and hypernatraemia is quickly normalized. If the saluretic treatment is combined with a diet low in sodium and protein, the reduction of daily urinary volume amounts up to 1/3 of the original value. However, if dietary restrictions are not kept, the antidiuretic effect diminishes or disappears completely.

Balance studies show that the paradoxical antidiuretic effect of saluretics in HDI is mainly produced by sodium depletion. In Figure 11.4 the water balance of a 5-month-old infant with NDI is shown over a period of 40 days. The balance data are depicted in the usual way: water intake is represented by the upper line from which the stool water and urine are subtracted. The open part of the column represents retention. In the period without hydrochlorothiazide great weight changes can be noticed. The average water retention, shown on the left-hand column above the graph, is low. Stool water is also minimal, which reflects the obstipation of the patient. Under treatment with hydrochlorothiazide and additional supplementation with potassium chloride, the average water retention increased markedly, and the stool water doubled, while the urinary volume reduced by 20%. Thus, the water economy improved strikingly, which was reflected in the well being of the infant. The changes in the water balance are produced by the changes in sodium metabolism, as shown in Figure 11.5. Hydrochlorothiazide first provokes a heavy natriuresis, which leads to sodium depletion, and reduced extracellular sodium concentrations, which are not shown on this graph. During the second period of treatment, the renal sodium excretion was markedly reduced, from an average of 2.22 without treatment to 1.58 mmol/day under hydrochlorothiazide. In this way the need for obligatory free water in the distal tubules was also reduced, and therefore the total urinary volume decreased.

It was first postulated by Brown and co-workers[65] that the antidiuresis after saluretics might be mediated by renin and angiotensin: Sodium depletion stimulates renin production, which produces increased amounts of angiotensin, and this in turn stimulates sodium reabsorption in the proximal tubules. In this way the sodium and water delivery to the distal tubules is diminished and antidiuresis might appear without the presence or effectiveness of vasopressin. This hypothesis is supported by findings of greatly increased plasma renin levels in saluretic-treated patients with diabetes insipidus[65] and NDI[35] (Brodehl, unpublished). Furthermore, angiotensin can indeed produce a marked antidiuresis in nephrogenic diabetes insipidus[66–68] as shown in Figure 11.6. where the effect of angiotensin infusion in a 4-year-old girl with complete NDI is depicted: there is a marked decrease of free-water clearance and urinary volume, which obviously is produced by a increased sodium reabsorption since sodium clearance is more reduced than glomerular filtration rate. The urinary osmolality is only slightly increased and does not reach isotonicity. Thus the effects of renin and angiotensin are indeed very similar to those produced by saluretic agents and therefore might mediate the antidiuresis under saluretic treatment.

Recent reports about successful treatment of NDI with prostaglandin inhibitors have appeared in the literature[69,70]. It was found in two patients with NDI, that the excretion of prostaglandin E was elevated, which could be reduced by indomethacin and ibuprofen, respectively and was followed by a slight reduction in urinary volume[69]. The addition of a saluretic agent enhanced this effect. Monn[70] reported an infant with NDI, in whom treatment with aspirin successfully reduced the urinary volume. We, therefore, gave aspirin to a 5-month-old infant with NDI, as is shown in Figure 11.7. The results, however, were disappointing and there was no significant improvement in water economy as compared with the period before aspirin administration. Prostaglandin excretion (PGE and $PGF_{2\alpha}$) was not high in this case. Therefore treatment with aspirin was discontinued. On theoretical and experimental grounds, however, a trial with a more potent inhibitor of prostaglandin synthetase, i.e. indomethacin, seems to be justified, since prostaglandins were shown to antagonize the effects of angiotensin[71].

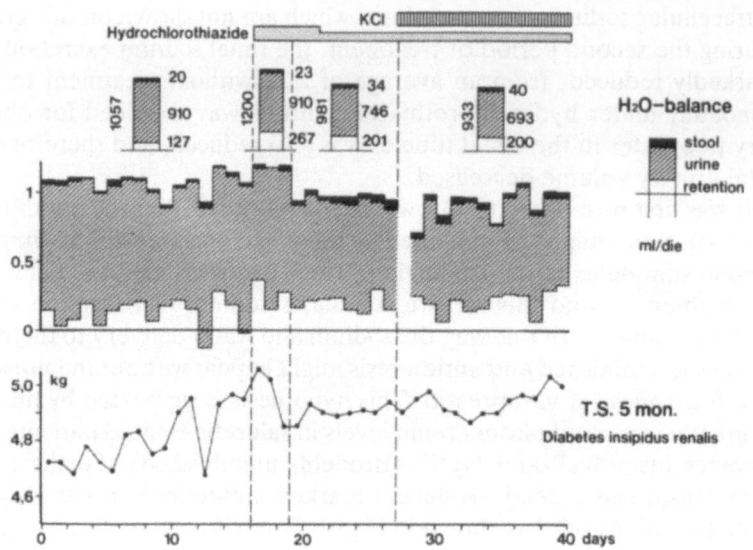

Figure 11.4   The effect of hydrochlorothiazide on water balance in a 5-month-old boy with NDI

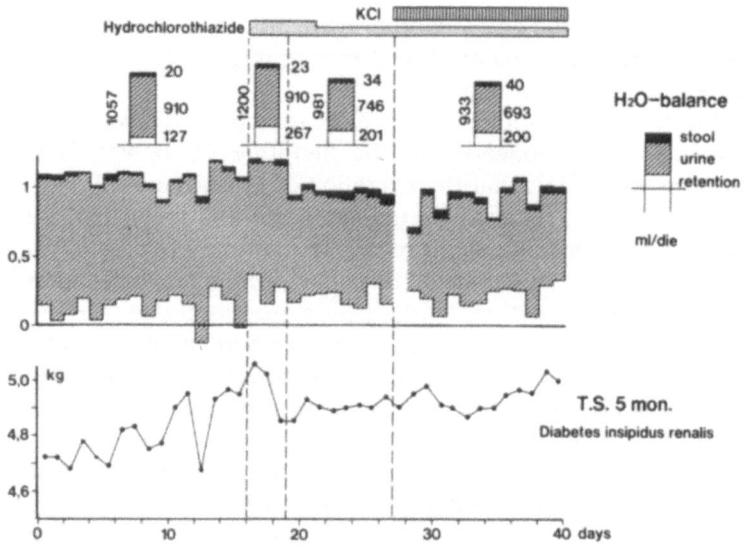

Figure 11.5   The effect of hydrochlorothiazide on sodium balance in a 5-month-old boy with NDI (same balance study as in Figure 11.4)

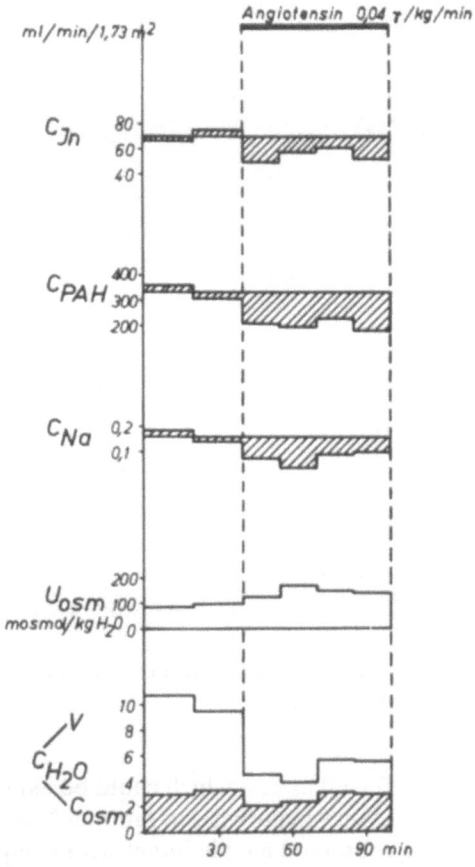

Figure 11.6 Effect of angiotensin II-infusion on kidney function in a 4-year-old girl with complete NDI. From Brodehl and Gellissen[67]

HEREDITY

The hereditary pattern observed by Forssman[1,72] and Williams and Henry[4] in their first descriptions of NDI showed clearly that only males exhibited complete unresponsiveness to vasopressin, and that a male-to-male transmission did not occur. This indicated that familial NDI was transmitted as a sex-linked recessive trait. Incomplete forms of the disease, however, could occur in female sibs, female 'carriers' and

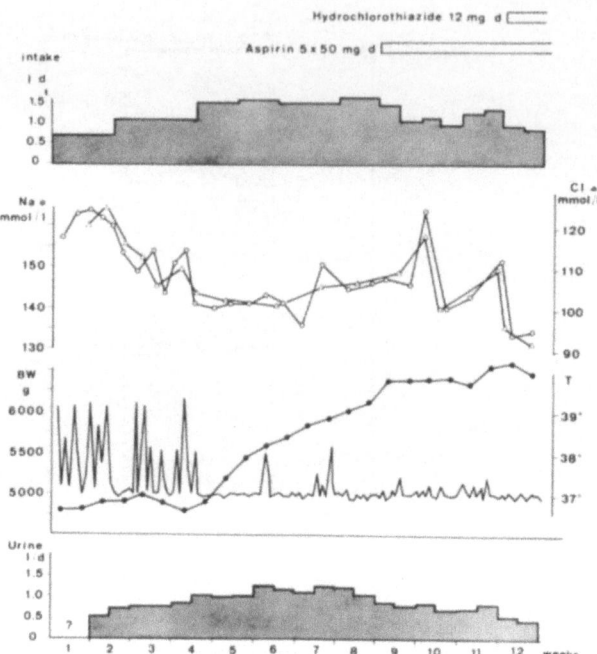

Figure 11.7 Effect of aspirin on the clinical course of a 5-month-old boy with NDI (propositus in Figure 11.8)

female relatives of affected males, which could be explained by a partial recessive gene or by Lyon's hypothesis of random X chromosome inactivation[73]. We recently observed a male infant with complete NDI, whose pedigree revealed the characteristic type of inheritance of familial NDI (Figure 11.8). Males of the trait showed the complete vasopressin resistance, while females suffered from a partial defect, manifested by polydipsia and polyuria. So far, we have only measured the concentration of the urine of the mother of the propositus which was 280 mosm/kg H_2O.

Females certainly can exhibit the complete form of NDI. This was first reported by Dancis and co-workers[74] and later by others[61,75]. This finding and the report of a large Mormon pedigree by Cannon[76] raised doubts about whether X-linked inheritance is the only type of transmission in NDI. Cannon observed apparent male-to-male transmissions on six occasions and postulated an autosomal dominant inheritance with incomplete penetrance in the females. This was also favoured by Robinson and Kaplan[77]. A critical re-evaluation, however, of old and newly

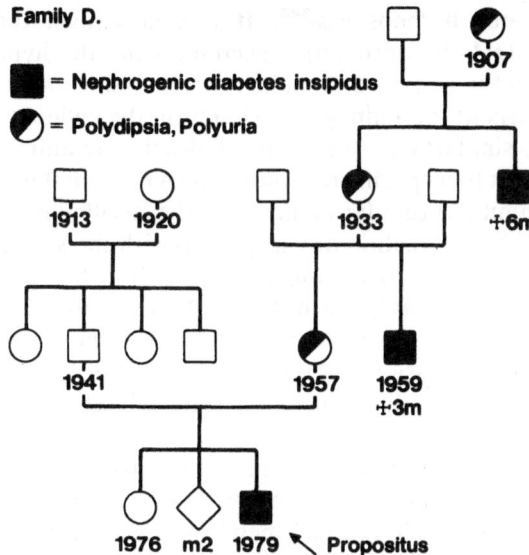

Figure 11.8 Pedigree of family D with NDI

described pedigrees led Bode and Crawford[7] to suggest that the original proposal of X-linked inheritance is probably correct and might even fit for Cannon's pedigree, since all six cases of male-to-male transmission occurred in early generations, in which one was forced to rely on historical data for the diagnosis as well as for the exclusion of consanguinity.

Attempts to identify heterozygotes of NDI have been made by estimation of urinary concentrating ability[78] and by cAMP excretion after vasopressin[29]. The great majority of carriers indeed manifest a partial concentrating defect[7], although discrimination is not perfect and both methods might fail in the individual case[29,79].

The incidence of NDI is not known. Families with NDI have been described from all parts of the world[7,25,80-82]. The rate of new mutations is unknown. Bode and Crawford[7] postulated that it may be extremely low, and suggested that almost all families with NDI in North America could be traced to the Ulster Scots who arrived in Nova Scotia aboard the ship *Hopewell* in 1761.

PATHOGENESIS OF NDI

Before the pathogenesis of NDI is discussed a few words are necessary to describe the present state of knowledge about the physiological regulation of water homeostasis[83-85]. It is well known that antidiuretic hormone (ADH=vasopressin) is secreted from the hypothalamus and pituitary gland in response to an increase in extracellular osmolality. In its effector organ, the kidney, ADH acts on the collecting ducts and on functionally similar late segments of distal convoluted tubules. The hormone binds to a specific receptor, which is located in the peritubular (i.e. contraluminal) tubular membrane (the socalled basolateral plasma membrane)[86,87]. Interaction of vasopressin with the specific receptor stimulates the enzymatic formation of cyclic AMP, which serves as an intracellular mediator of vasopressin. Cyclic AMP, in turn, elicits, directly or indirectly, an increase in water permeability of the luminal membrane. In this way the diffusion of free water from the luminal site into the hypertonic medullary interstitium is achieved, which leads to the final concentration of the urine.

On a molecular basis many steps are involved in the effect of vasopressin increasing water permeability. The vasopressin-sensitive receptor in the basolateral plasma membrane is closely associated with adenylate cyclase, an enzyme that catalyses the formation of cyclic AMP from adenosine triphosphate (ATP). The vasopressin receptor is probably located on the outer surface of the plasma membrane, while adenylate cyclase faces the inside of the cell. The intracellular concentration of cAMP is determined not only by its rate of formation, but also by its rate of breakdown, which is catalysed by cAMP-phosphodiesterase. cAMP formed in response to vasopressin administration leads to increased water permeability. This may be mediated through activation of one or more protein kinases, which catalyse the transfer of γ-phosphorus from ATP onto the serine or threonine in side chains of polypeptides. Hypothetically, water permeability would be associated with a specific membrane protein, which serves as substrate for a cyclic-AMP-dependent protein kinase. Phosphorylation of this protein would cause a change in the structure of the membrane, which in turn would increase the water permeability. The membrane can be returned to its original resting, relatively water-impermeable state by enzymatic removal of phosphate from protein through the action of protein phosphatase.

The role of microtubules, which are linear unbranched structures polymerized from a soluble protein called tubulin, and of microfilaments, which are fibrous linear structures composed of proteins with biochemical properties similar to those of muscle actin, in the water transport across the cell is still uncertain[88]. There is enough experimental evidence which suggests that the integrity of those structures is required for the cellular action of vasopressin since chemicals that disrupt microtubules and microfilaments such as colchicine and vinblastin, block the hydro-osmotic effect of vasopressin[89].

The vasopressin sensitive adenylate cyclase is not only found in the collecting ducts of the medulla[90], but also in high concentration in the ascending limb of Henle's loop[91]. The physiological significance of this finding remains controversial. It was postulated by Atherton and co-workers[92] that vasopressin may have at least two sites of action in the kidney, one in the collecting ducts on water permeability, and the other in the thick portion of the ascending limb of Henle's loop on sodium-chloride reabsorption. Experimental data on this aspect are at variance. In this connection it is worthwhile mentioning that in patients with NDI, in whom the hydro-osmotic action of vasopressin is absent, vasopressin can exert an effect on electrolyte excretion, as was shown by ourselves many years ago[34]. The acute administration of lysin vasopressin in a patient with NDI produced an immediate increase in free-water clearance (C_{H_2O}), and a delayed increase in the clearance of sodium (C_{Na}), as shown in Figure 11.9. These findings were hypothetically interpreted as an indication that vasopressin might stimulate sodium reabsorption in tubular segments prior to the distal diluting tubule, probably in the ascending limb of Henle's loop, and by this could increase the sodium concentration in the medullary interstitium.

The investigation of the molecular pathogenesis of various types of diabetes insipidus was greatly facilitated by the discovery of animal models. In rats there is a strain with hypothalamic diabetes insipidus, the Brattleboro rat[93]. In mice there are three different strains, one with oligosyndactyly and a medullary gradient type of diabetes insipidus[94,95], a second strain with a unique kidney lesion and progressive polyuria[96], and a third strain with vasopressin-resistant diabetes insipidus, that very closely resembles human congenital NDI[83]. In the last model almost all biochemical steps involved in the effect of vasopressin, could be measured[83]. It was found that the affinity of adenylate cyclase for vasopressin was normal in the affected mice. The stimulation of adenylate cyclase by saturating concentrations of vasopressin was however markedly reduced from control values. The activities of phosphodiesterase and protein kinase and their content in microtubules were normal. It was therefore concluded that impaired stimulation of renal medullary adenylate cyclase by vasopressin might be the sole or a contributing cause of the vasopressin-resistant concentrating defect in the mice[83].

It is still open whether the human NDI is caused by the same molecular defect as that recognized in the mouse NDI model. The experimental data accumulated in the mouse and the clinical findings in man are

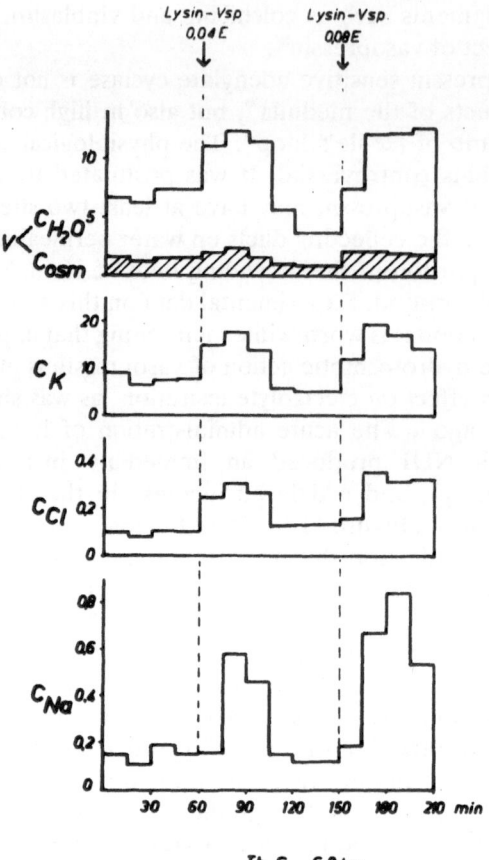

Figure 11.9   Effect of lysine vasopressin on water and electrolyte excretion in a 16-month-old boy with NDI. From Brodehl *et al.*[34]

indeed very similar, with the exception of the mode of hereditary transmission. However, the final proof for the same molecular defect is still missing, since it has not been possible to measure adenylate cyclase activity and its stimulation with vasopressin in human kidney specimens of NDI patients, and the urinary excretion of cAMP does not, unfortunately, consistently reflect the activity of adenylate cyclase in the collecting ducts, as mentioned above. There are many steps from vasopressin-receptor binding on basolateral plasma membrane to the hydro-osmotic effect of vasopressin on the luminal membrane, and, as in many other diseases, the same pathophysiological effects could be produced by more than one disturbance at various levels of a biochemical chain. Therefore, what today is called the entity 'congenital nephrogenic diabetes insipidus', could turn out to be more than one molecular defect tomorrow. It is hoped that further investigations on the pathomechanism of NDI will result in an even better understanding of the disease and provide a more effective treatment for the affected patients.

References

1. Forssman, H. (1945). On hereditary diabetes insipidus with special regard to a sex linked form. *Acta Med. Scand. Suppl.* **159**
2. Waring, A. J., Kajdi, L. and Tappan, V. (1945). Congenital defects of water metabolism. *Am. Dis. Child.*, **69**, 323
3. McIlraith, C. H. (1892) Notes on some cases of diabetes insipidus with marked family and hereditary tendencies. *Lancet,* **II**, 767
4. Williams, R. H. and Henry, C. (1947). Nephrogenic diabetes insipidus: transmitted by females and appearing during infancy in males. *Ann. Int. Med.*, **27**, 84
5. Ziegler, E. E. and Fomon, S. J. (1971). Fluid intake, renal solute load, and water balance in infancy. *J. Pediatr.*, **78**, 561
6. Forssman, H. (1955). Is hereditary diabetes insipidus of nephrogenic type associated with mental deficiency? *Acta Psychiatr. Neurol. Scand.*, **30**, 577
7. Bode, H. H., and Crawford, J. D. (1969). Nephrogenic diabetes insipidus in North America – the Hopewell hypothesis. *N. Engl. J. Med.*, **280**, 750
8. Hillman, D. A., Neyzi, O., Porter, P., Cushman, A. and Talbot, N. B. (1958). Renal (vasopressin-resistant) diabetes insipidus. Definition of the effects of a homeostatic limitation in capacity to conserve water on the physical, intellectual and emotional development of a child. *Pediatrics*, **21**, 430
9. Kirman, B. H., Black, S. A., Wilkinson, R. H. and Evans, P. R. (1956). Familial pitressin-resistant diabetes insipidus with mental defect. *Arch. Dis. Child.*, **31**, 59
10. MacAulay, D. and Watson, M. (1967). Hypernatremia in infants as a cause of brain damage. *Arch. Dis. Child.*, **42**, 485
11. Morris-Jones, P. H., Houston, I. B. and Evans, R. C. (1967). Prognosis of the neurological complications of acute hypernatremia. *Lancet*, **II**, 1385
12. Habel, A. H. and Simpson, H. (1976). Osmolar relation between cerebro-spinal fluid and serum in hyperosmolar hypernatraemic dehydration. *Arch. Dis. Child.*, **51**, 660
13. Ruess, A. L. and Rosenthal, I. M. (1963). Intelligence in nephrogenic diabetes insipidus. *Am. J. Dis. Child.*, **105**, 358
14. Manson, A. D., Yalowitz, P. A., Randall, R. V. and Greene, L. F. (1970). Dilatation of the urinary tract associated with pituitary and nephrogenic diabetes insipidus. *J. Urol.*, **103**, 327
15. Ten Bensel, R. W. and Peters, E. R. (1970). Progressive hydronephrosis,

hydroureter and dilatation of the bladder in siblings with congenital nephrogenic diabetes insipidus. *J. Pediatr.*, **77**, 439

16. Wiggelinkhuizen, J., Retief, P. J. M., Wolff, B., Fisher, R. M. and Cremin, B. J. (1973). Nephrogenic diabetes insipidus and obstructive uropathy. *Am. J. Dis. Child.*, **126**, 398

17. Aronson, A. S. and Svenningsen, N. W. (1974). DDAVP test for the estimation of renal concentrating capacity in infants and children. *Arch. Dis. Child.*, **49**, 654

18. Radó, J. P. (1978) 1-desamino-8-D-arginine vasopressin (DDAVP) concentration test. *Am. J. Med. Sci.*, **275**, 43

19. Taylor, A. L., Davis, B. B., Pawlson, L. G., Josimovich, J B. and Mintz, D. H. (1970). Factors influencing urinary excretion of 3′,5′ adenosine monophosphate in humans. *J. Clin. Endocrinol. Metab.*, **30**, 316

20. Pawlson, L. G., Taylor, A., Mintz, D. H., Field, J. B. and Davis, B. B. (1970). Effect of vasopressin on renal cyclic AMP generation in potassium deficiency and patients with sickle hemoglobin. *Metabolism*, **19**, 694

21. Joppich, R., Kollmann, D., Ingrisch, U. and Weber, P. (1977). Urinary cyclic AMP and renal concentrating capacity in infants. *Eur. J. Pediatr.*, **124**, 113

22. Fichman, M. P. and Brooker, G. (1972). Deficient renal cyclic adenosine 3′,5′-monophosphate production in nephrogenic diabetes insipidus. *J. Clin. Endocrinol. Metab.*, **35**, 35.

23. Bell, N. H., Clark, C. M., Avery, S., Sinha, T., Trygstad, C. W. and Allen, D. O. (1974). Demonstration of a defect in the formation of adenosine 3′,5′-monophosphate in vasopressin-resistant diabetes insipidus. *Pediatr. Res.*, **8**, 223

24. McConnell, R. F., Lorentz, W. B., Berger, M., Smith, E. H., Carvajal, H. F. and Travis, L. B. (1977). The mechanism of urinary concentration in nephrogenic diabetes insipidus. *Pediatr. Res.*, **11**, 33

25. Takahashi, K., Kamimura, M., Shinko, T. and Tsuji, S. (1966). Effects of vasopressin and water-load of urinary adenosine-3′,5′ cyclic monophosphate. *Lancet*, **II**, 967

26. Broadus, A. E., Hardman, J. G., Kaminsky, N. I., Ball, J. H., Sutherland, E. W. and Liddle, G. W. (1971). Extracellular cyclic nucleotides. *Ann. N.Y. Acad. Sci.*, **85**, 50

27. Monn, E., Osnes, J. B. and Øye, I. (1976). Basal and hormone-induced urinary cyclic AMP in children with renal disorders. *Acta Paediatr. Scand.*, **65**, 739

28. Broadus, A. E., Mahaffey, J. E., Bartter, F. C. and Neer, R. M. (1977). Nephrogenic cyclic adenosine monophosphate as a parathyroid function test. *J. Clin. Invest.*, **60**, 771

29. Uttley, W. S., Atkinson, B., Adams, A. and Shirling, D. (1975). Cyclic adenosine monophosphate excretion in urine of patients and carriers of congenital nephrogenic diabetes insipidus. Abstract, *9th Meet. Eur. Soc. Paediatr. Nephrol. Cambridge*

30. Gorden, P., Robertson, G. L. and Seegmiller, J. E. (1971). Hyperuricemia, a concomitant of congenital vasopressin-resistant diabetes insipidus in the adult. *N. Engl. J. Med.*, **284**, 1057

31. Robertson, G. L., Shelton, R. L. and Athar, S. (1976). The osmoregula-

tion of vasopressin. *Kidney Int.*, **10**, 25
32. Sober, A. J. and Gorden, P. (1972) Pituitary responsiveness to aqueous vasopressin in patients with congenital vasopressin-resistant diabetes insipidus. *J. Clin. Endocrinol. Metab.*, **35**, 924
33. Cutler, R. E., Kleeman, C. R., Maxwell, M. H. and Dowling, J. T. (1962). Physiologic studies in nephrogenic diabetes insipidus. *J. Clin. Endocrinol. Metab.*, **22**, 827
34. Brodehl, J., Gellissen, K. and Hagge, W. (1965). Die Wirkung des Vasopressins beim Diabetes insipidus renalis. *Klin. Wochenschr.*, **43**, 72
35. Dembowski, J., Gekle, D., Thoenes, W. and Wernze, H. (1973). Hyperreninämie und Hypertrophie des juxtaglomerulären Apparates bei familiärem Diabetes insipidus renalis. *Klin. Wochenschr.*, **51**, 1159
36. Godard, C., Mégevand, A., deSousa, R. C. and Muller, A. F. (1968). Etude du metabolisme de l'aldostérone dans un cas de diabète insipide néphrogénique congenital. *Pediatr. Res.*, **2**, 22
37. Brown, D. M., Reynolds, J. W., Michael, A. F. and Ulstrom, R. A. (1966). The use and mode of action of ethacrynic acid in nephrogenic diabetes insipidus. *Pediatrics*, **37**, 447
38. Gautier, E. and Prader, A. (1956). Un cas de diabète insipide néphrogène chez un nourisson avec absence initiale de soif ("diabète insipide occulte"). *Helv. Paediatr. Acta*, **11**, 45
39. Lobeck, C. C., Barta, R. A. and Mangos, J. A. (1963). Study of sweat in pitressin resistant diabetes insipidus. *J. Pediatr.*, **62**, 868
40. Plöchl, E. and Stur, O. (1965). Schweissuntersuchungen bei Diabetes insipidus während der Behandlung mit Saluretika. *Helv. Paediatr. Acta*, **20**, 331
41. Darmady, E. M., Offer, J., Prince, J. and Stranack, F. (1964). The proximal convoluted tubule in the renal handling of water. *Lancet*, **II**, 1254
42. Fettermann, G. H., Fabrizio, N. S. and Strudnicki, F. M. (1966). The study by microdissection of structural tubular defects in certain examples of the hereditary nephropathies. *Proc. Third Int. Congr. Nephrology, Washington*, Vol. 2, 235
43. Abelson, H. (1968). Nephrogenic diabetes insipidus. A study of the fine structure of the kidney in a seven month old male. *Pediatr. Res.*, **2**, 271
44. Maffly, R. H. (1977). Diabetes insipidus. In T. E. Andreoli, J. J. Grantham and F. C. Rector (eds.), *Disturbances in Body Fluid Osmolality*, p. 285. (Bethesda: American Physiological Society)
45. Bisset, G. W., Black, A., Hilton, P. J., Jones, N. F. and Montgomery, M. (1976). Polyuria associated with an antibody to vasopressin. *Clin. Sci. Molec. Med.*, **50**, 277
46. Barlow, E. D. and de Wardener, H. E. (1959). Compulsive water drinking. *Q. J. Med.*, **28**, 235
47. Singer, I. and Forrest, J. N. (1976). Drug-induced states of nephrogenic diabetes insipidus. *Kidney Int.*, **10**, 82
48. Oetliker. H., Simon, J. and Tietze, H. U. (1974). Diagnostic value of mannitol-induced diuresis in children. *Acta Paediatr. Scand.*, **62**, 113
49. Simon, J., Zamora, I., Martinez-Sanchez, F. and Bartolome, V. (1978). Mannitol osmolar clearance in diabetes insipidus of children. *Acta Paediatr. Scand.*, **67**, 433

50. Moses, A. M., Numann, P. and Miller, M. (1973). Mechanism of chlorpropamide induced antidiuresis in man: evidence for release of ADH and enhancement of peripheral action. *Metabolism*, **22**, 59

51. Radó, J. P., Szende, L., Borbély, L. and Takó, J. (1970). Clinical value and mode of action of chlorpropamide in diabetes insipidus. *Am. J. Med.*, **260**, 359

52. Meinders, A. E., Cejka, V. and Robertson, G. L. (1974). The antidiuretic action of carbamazepine (Tegretol) in man. *Clin. Sci. Molec. Med.*, **47**, 289

53. Jones, N. F., Barraclough, M. A., Barnes, N. and Cottom, D. G. (1972). Nephrogenic diabetes insipidus. Effects of $3',5'$ cyclic-adenosine monophosphate. *Arch. Dis. Child.*, **47**, 794

54. Proesmans, W., Eggermont, E., Vanderschueren-Lodeweyckx, M., Tiddens, H. and Eeckels, R. (1975). The effect of exogenous $3', 5'$-adenosine-monophosphate on urinary output in children with vasopressin-resistant diabetes insipidus. *Pediatr. Res.*, **9**, 509

55. Crawford, J. D., Kennedy, G. C. and Hill, L. E. (1960). Clinical results of treatment of diabetes insipidus with drugs of the chlorothiazide series. *N. Engl. J. Med.*, **262**, 737

56. Reerink, H. (1961). A new treatment of renal diabetes insipidus. In *Symposium on Water and Electrolyte Metabolism, Amsterdam*, p. 121 (Amsterdam: Elsevier)

57. Calesnick, B. and Brenner, S. A. (1961). An observation of hydrochlorothiazide in diabetes insipidus. *J. Am. Med. Assoc.*, **176**, 1088

58. Goodman, A. D. and Carter, R. D. (1962). A study on the mechanism of the anti-diuretic action of chlorothiazide in diabetes insipidus. *Metabolism*, **11**, 1033

59. Earley, L. E. and Orloff, J. (1962). The mechanism of antidiuresis associated with the administration of hydrochlorothiazide to patients with vasopressin resistant diabetes insipidus. *J. Clin. Invest.*, **41**, 1988

60. Schotland, M. G., Grumbach, M. M. and Strauss, J. (1963). The effects of chlorothiazide in nephrogenic diabetes insipidus. *Pediatrics*, **31**, 741

61. Brodehl, J. and Braun, L. (1964). Familiaerer nephrogener Diabetes insipidus mit voller Ausprägung bei einem weiblichen Säugling. *Klin. Wochenschr.*, **42**, 563

62. Ramos, G., Rivera, A., Peña, J. C. and Dies, F. (1967). Mechanism of the antidiuretic effect of saluretic drugs. *Clin. Pharmacol. Ther.*, **8**, 557

63. Reimold, E. W. (1967). Angiotensin and Saluretika beim Diabetes insipidus renalis im frühen Säuglingsalter. *Z. Kinder.*, **101**, 6

64. Von Brenndorf, A. I. and Hagge, W. (1973). Die Furosemidbehandlung des Diabetes insipidus renalis bei eineiigen Zwillingen. *Monatsschr. Kinder.*, **121**, 494

65. Brown, J. J., Chinn, R. H., Lever, A. F. and Robertson, J. I. S. (1969). Renin and angiotensin as a mechanism of diuretic-induced antidiuresis in diabetes insipidus. *Lancet*, **1**, 237

66. Gautier, E. (1964). Neonatal hyperosmolarity, an instance of unresponsiveness to antidiuretic hormone. In *Nutricia symposium. The Adaption of the Newborn Infant to Extrauterine Life*. (Leiden: Stenfert Kroese)

67. Brodehl, J. and Gellissen, K. (1966). Die antidiuretische Wirkung des Angiotensins beim Diabetes insipidus. *Klin. Wochenschr.*, **44**, 101

68. Orr, F. R. and Filipich, R. L. (1967). Studies with angiotensin in nephrogenic diabetes insipidus. *Canad. Med. Assoc. J.*, **97**, 841
69. Fichman, M., Zipser, R., Kaye, Z., Lee, A. and Zia, P. (1978). Antidiuresis with suppression of elevated urinary prostaglandin E (PGE) by ibuprofen in nephrogenic diabetes insipidus (NDI) and 1-desamino-8-D arginine vasopressin (DDAVP) in primary diabetes insipidus. Abstract, *7th Int. Congr. Nephrology, Montreal* Q2
70. Monn, E. (1979) Effect of prostaglandin synthetase inhibitors on urine volume in nephrogenic diabetes insipidus. *Thirteenth Meet. Eur. Soc. Paediatr. Nephrol.* Capri, Italy
71. Aiken, J. W. and Vane, J. R. (1973). Intrarenal prostaglandin release attenuates the renal vasoconstrictor activity of angiotensin. *J. Pharmacol. Exp. Ther.*, **184**, 678
72. Forssman, H. (1975) The recognition of nephrogenic diabetes insipidus. *Acta. Med. Scand.*, **197**, 1
73. Lyon, M. F. (1962). Sex chromatin and gene action in mammalian X chromosome. *Am. J. Genet.*, **14**, 135
74. Dancis, J., Birmingham, J. R. and Leslie, S. H. (1948). Congenital diabetes insipidus resistant to treatment with pitressin. *Am. J. Dis.*, **75**, 316
75. Schreiner, R. L., Skafish, P. R., Anand, S. K. and Northway, J. D. (1978). Congenital nephrogenic diabetes insipidus in a baby girl. *Arch. Dis. Child.*, **53**, 906
76. Cannon, J. F. (1955) Diabetes insipidus: clinical and experimental studies with considerations of genetic relationship. *Arch. Int. Med.*, **96**, 215
77. Robinson, M. G. and Kaplan, S. A. (1960) Inheritance of vasopressin-resistant ("nephrogenic") diabetes insipidus. *Am. J. Dis. Child.*, **99**, 164
78. Carter, C. and Simpkiss, M. (1956). The 'carrier state' in nephrogenic diabetes insipidus. *Lancet*, **II**, 1069
79. Uttley, W. S. and Thistlethwaite, D. (1972). Failure to detect the carrier in congenital nephrogenic diabetes insipidus. *Arch. Dis. Child.*, **47**, 251
80. Nakano, K. K. (1969). Familial nephrogenic diabetes insipidus. *Hawaii Med. J.*, **28**, 205
81. Feigin, R. D., Fimoin, D. L. and Kaufman, R. L. (1970). Nephrogenic diabetes insipidus in a Negro kindred. *Am. J. Dis, Child.*, **120**, 64
82. Schultz, P. and Lines, D. R. (1975). Nephrogenic diabetes insipidus in an Australian aboriginal kindred. *Humangenetik*, **26**, 79
83. Dousa, T. P. and Valtin, H. (1974). Cellular action of antidiuretic hormone in mice with inherited vasopressin–resistant urinary concentrating defects. *J. Clin. Invest.*, **54**, 753
84. Berliner, R. W. (1976). The concentrating mechanism in the renal medulla. *Kidney Int.*, **9**, 214
85. Robertson, G. L., Athar, S. and Shelton, R. L. (1977). Osmotic control of vasopressin function. In T. E. Andreoli, J. J. Grantham, and F. C. Rector (eds.), *Disturbances in Body Fluid Osmolality*, p. 125. (Bethesda: American Physiological Society).
86. Grantham, J. J. and Burg, M. B. (1966). Effect of vasopressin and cyclic AMP on permeability of isolated collecting tubules. *Am. J. Physiol.*, **211**, 255
87. Schwartz, I. L., Shlatz, L. J., Kinne-Saffran, E. and Kinne, R. (1974).

Target cell polarity and membrane phosphorylation in relation to the mechanism of action of antidiuretic hormone. *Proc. Natl. Acad. Sci. USA,* **71,** 2595

88.   Taylor, A. (1977). Role of microtubules and microfilaments in the action of vasopressin. In T. E. Andreoli, J. J. Grantham, and F. C. Rector (eds.). *Disturbances in Body Fluid Osmolality,* p. 97 (Bethesda: American Physiological Society)

89.   Dousa, T. P. and Barnes, L. D. (1974). Effect of colchicine and vinblastine on the cellular action of vasopressin in mammalian kidney. *J. Clin. Invest.,* **54,** 252

90.   Chase, L. R. and Aurbach, G. D. (1968). Renal adenyl cyclase: anatomically separate sites for parathyroid hormone and vasopressin. *Science,* **159,** 545

91.   Imbert-Teboul, M., Chabardés, D., Montégut, M., Clique, A. and Morel, F. (1978). Vasopressin-dependent adenylate cyclase activities in the rat medulla: evidence for two separate sites of action. *Endocrinology,* **102,** 1254

92.   Atherton, J. C., Green, R. and Thomas, S. (1970). Influence of lysin-vasopressin dosage on the time course of changes in renal tissue and urinary composition in the conscious rat. *J. Physiol.,* **213,** 291

93.   Valtin, H. and Schroeder, H. A. (1964). Familial hypothalamic diabetes insipidus in rats (Brattleboro strain). *Am. J. Physiol.,* **206,** 425

94.   Falconer, D. S., Latsyzewski, M. and Isaacson, J. H. (1964). Diabetes insipidus associated with oligosyndactyly in the mouse. *Genet. Res.,* **5,** 473

95.   Naik, D. V. and Valtin, H. (1969). Hereditary vasopressin-resistant urinary concentrating defects in mice. *Am. J. Physiol.,* **217,** 1183

96.   Virgo, N. S. and Miller, J. R. (1974). Hereditary vasopressin-resistant diabetes insipidus in SWV mice. *Canad. J. Physiol. Pharmacol.,* **52,** 995

12

Mendelian hypophosphataemias as probes of phosphate and sulphate transport by mammalian kidney

(X-linked hypophosphataemia and autosomal hypophosphataemia in man and the *Hyp* mutation in mouse)

H. S. Tenenhouse, D. E. C. Cole and C. R. Scriver

In earlier work pertaining to the renal transport of amino acids in man and other mammals[1-5], we used the Mendelian errors of membrane transport[6,7] to delineate the specificity of carrier-dependent amino-acid transport systems in renal epithelium. Almost a decade later it is satisfying to see how closely the description of the Na^+/amino-acid cotransport systems by formal biochemical and physiological analyses[8] approximates the genetic view of the tubular reabsorptive systems. Encouraged by our success with genetic probes in one area, we have chosen to use the inborn errors of transport again, this time to learn something about renal reabsorption of phosphate and sulphate in man.

At the Heidelberg meeting of SSIEM in 1975, we discussed X-linked hypophosphataemia and its relationship to other Mendelian forms of rickets[9] Since then, we have identified a new autosomal form of hypophosphataemia[10]. We have also been able to study a hypophosphataemic mouse homologue of the X-linked condition[11]. In the following discussion we will use evidence from the X-linked and autosomal conditions in man, together with findings in the hypophosphataemic mouse and elsewhere, to develop an hypothesis about phosphate reabsorption in mammalian kidney. We will also use the same genetic probes to offer some preliminary observations on sulphate reabsorption.

EVOLUTIONARY OUTLOOK ON
CELLULAR TRANSPORT OF PHOSPHATE

Phosphate is a water-soluble anion. In solution its effective ion radius is greater than that depicted in Figure 12.1. Since the distribution ratio of phosphate (inside:outside) in the intact living cell can deviate from the permeability expected of its oil:water partition coefficient, one is led to consider mediated permeation of this anion in some biological systems. The evidence that membrane transport serves phosphate entry into cells reaches far back in the evolution of biological systems. Eukaryotes would have utilized phosphate transport to sustain aerobic metabolism as long ago as 1.5 billion years and prokaryotes might have utilized membrane phosphate carriers in forms evolving as far back as 3 billion years[12]. Moreover, we are aware that phosphate has an important place in the geological history of the Earth[13]. Since the appearance of the anion at significant concentrations in primitive oceans and the emergence of aerobic prokaryotes and eukaryotes are apparently concordant in time, one can presume that phosphate was a key bioelement in the early evolution of Earth's biosphere. Development and refinement of aerobic metabolism, as we know it[14], could prosper only if organisms could collect phosphate efficiently. Thus, membrane transport of the anion, as a general process, is apparently an old attribute of cells.

Evolution undertook a major experiment with vertebrates that began about 400 million years ago. As the rigid skeleton of higher vertebrates evolved, it acquired large amounts of phosphate in hydroxyapatite. At the same time, maintenance of phosphate homeostasis in the vertebrate became coupled to complex mechanisms of hormonal regulation that also encompassed calcium (see Figure 12.2 and later section on homeostatic adaptation to phosphorus deprivation). Mammals, including man,

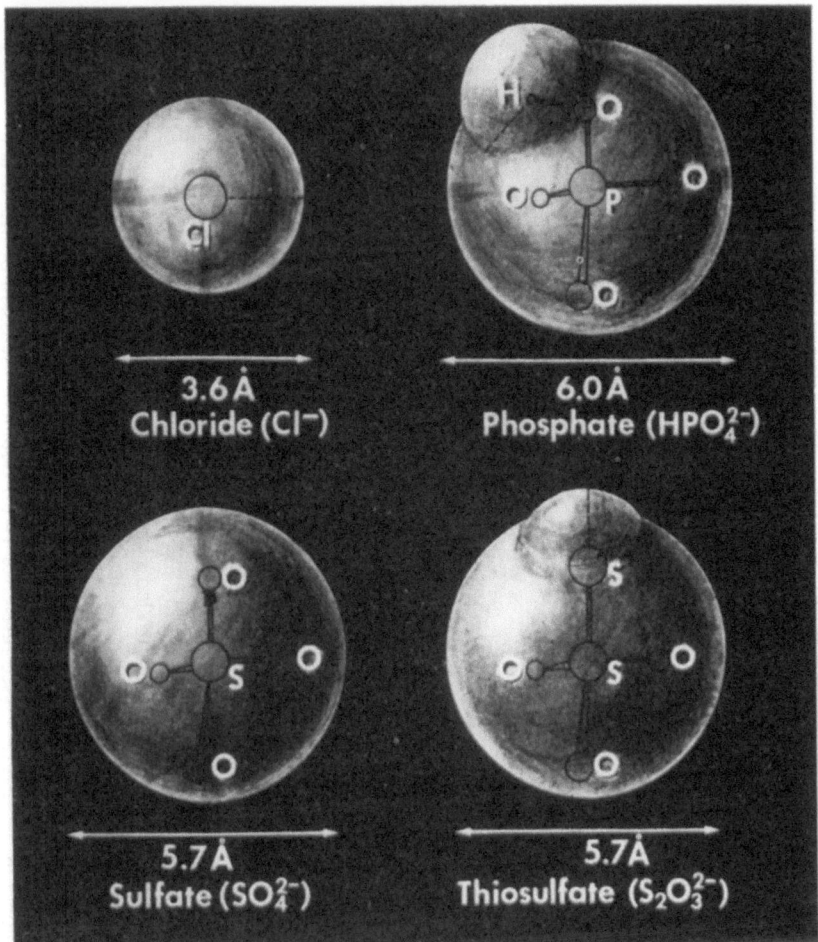

Figure 12.1 Physical dimensions of some anions; dimensions are larger when ions are hydrated in solution; membrane transport proteins strip off water of hydration when positioning solute at active site

are now dependent on their diet for intake of phosphate, and to a great extent on the kidney for maintenance of phosphate homeostasis (Table 12.1)[15,16]. Oscillations in fractional renal excretion of phosphate quickly modulate the extracellular phosphate concentration and vice versa. Accordingly, it is not surprising that disorders which comprise phosphate reabsorption are accompanied by attrition of the extracellular pool

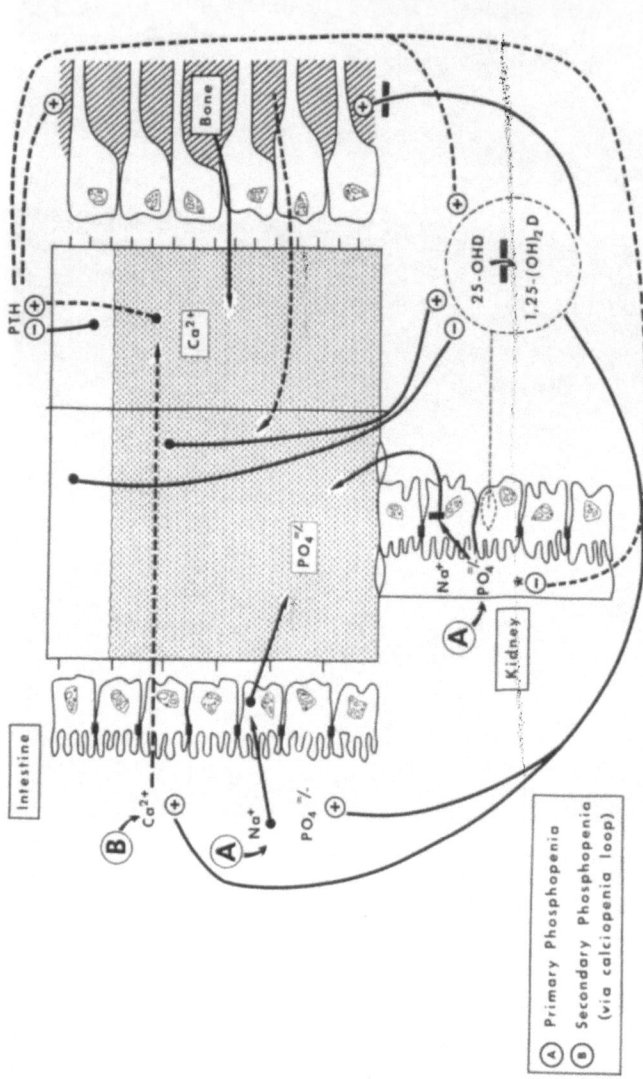

Figure 12.2 Diagram of some controlling and controlled signals in the feedback loops and cascades of plasma (extracellular) phosphate and calcium homeostasis. (See also Figure 12.9 for a further description of phosphate homeostasis.) Origins of Mendelian phosphopaenia (originating in defective renal reabsorption) and of Mendelian calcipaenia leading to secondary phosphopaenia (in defective 1,25-(OH)$_2$D$_3$ biosynthesis (type-I vitamin D-dependency) or action on target tissues (type-II vitamin D-dependency)[21], are shown in the diagram: (see reference 17 for detailed discussion of Mendelian phosphopaenic and calciopaenic rickets)

(reflected by hypophosphataemia) and of the bone pool (reflected by rickets and osteomalacia). Because net phosphate balance is influenced not only by its renal reabsorption and intestinal absorption, but also by vitamin D and parathyroid hormone, we have proposed the terms 'calcipaenia' and 'phosphopaenia'[12,17] for clinical use, to draw attention to the primary mechanisms of hypophosphataemia (Figure 12.2), recognizing, of course, that hypophosphataemia is obligatory in both the calcipaenic and phosphopaenic states, for the pathogenesis of rickets and osteomalacia[17,18]. X-linked hypophosphataemia (XLH) and autosomal hypophosphataemic bone disease (HBD) are Mendelian phosphopaenic disorders.

TABLE 12.1 Components of phosphate* homeostasis in average human adult

1.	*Daily intake (net absorption from intestine)*		1000 mg
2.	*Distribution in body pools*		
	Extracellular	400 mg	
	Intracellular	900 mg	
	Bone	40 000 mg	
3.	*Renal handling (mg/day)*		
	Filtered†	6500	
	Reabsorbed	5500	
	Excreted	1000	1000 mg
		Net balance:	0

* Expressed as phosphorus
† Assuming a Donnan equilibrium across membranes of 1.09 and that approximately 20% of phosphorus is bound to plasma proteins, then filtered fraction is about $0.95 \times GFR \times [P]$ plasma[16]. Fractional excretion of phosphate anion ($FE_{PO_4} = 1 -$ Reabsorbed PO_4) is 0.153 in this example. If phosphorus balance is zero (net intestinal absorption = renal loss) and is not altered in the short term, it follows that any concomitant change in FE_{Pi} must alter the extracellular pool and do so rapidly

GENETIC PROBES AND PHOSPHATE TRANSPORT IN MAN AND MOUSE

Human diseases

XLH is the most frequently encountered form of 'familial vitamin D-resistant rickets'[5]. X-linked dominant inheritance of hypophosphataemia in this disease was first reported by Winters and colleagues in 1958[19] and more than 20 years after Albright and co-workers[20] published their original clinical report* Now, after 40 years of controversy regarding the precise nature of the disease[22], one can capitalize on the X-linkage to resolve some important aspects of the debate, with the assistance of an X-linked mouse model. The autosomal form of hypophosphataemia (HBD) emerged as a clinical entity[10] only when the characteristics of XLH had been sufficiently defined to permit recognition of the analogue (Table 12.2). The splitting of a clinical phenotype (in this case hypophosphataemia) into more than one form is now a conventional exercise in Mendelian genetics[23] that recognizes genetic heterogeneity[24] and, in this case, serves to delineate more than one gene product controlling phosphate homeostasis in man.

HBD is autosomal dominant, with a key pedigree[10] showing male-to-male transmission of the hypophosphataemia phenotype. Rickets, a severe complication of XLH, is rarely encountered during the period of bone growth in HBD despite a comparable degree of hypophosphataemia in the two conditions. While osteomalacia affects endosteal trabecular bone in both conditions during childhood, the HBD adult with hypophosphataemia can have completely normal bone mineralization (C. R. Scriver et al, unpublished observations), something that does not occur in the affected adult hemizygote with XLH. Renal handling of phosphate is also different in the two conditions, in at least two ways[10]: first, tubular reabsorption (TR_{Pi}) is greater in HBD than in XLH at similar levels of hypophosphataemia, yet both have a similar reduction of maximal tubular reabsorption capacity (Tm_{Pi}); secondly, the residual process of phosphate reabsorption in the mutant phenotype is quite resistant to the inhibitory effect of parathyroid hormone in XLH, yet it is still responsive in HBD. We perceive these phenotypic differences in bone mineralization and renal conservation of phosphate in HBD and XLH as insights into the way the bone phosphate pool is maintained and the nephron conserves phosphate under normal conditions (Figure 12.3).

Physiological studies have already provided evidence for more than one mode of phosphate transport in kidney. Whereas parathyroid hormone interacts with the nephron to inhibit net phosphate reabsorption at both proximal and distal sites[16,25], in the proximal portion of the nephron there are at least two modes of phosphate transport[26]: one of high capacity but quite insensitive to parathyroid hormone; the other of

---

* Albright and colleagues (1937) proposed that vitamin D-resistant rickets was the result of target-organ resistance to vitamin D. Their hypothesis appears not to be correct for XLH. However, the disease they anticipated has been discovered – at last; it is Type-II (autosomal recessive) vitamin D dependency[21].

TABLE 12.2 Salient phenotypic features in human HBD and XLH and in the murine counterpart of XLH (*Hyp*)

Feature	HBD	XLH*	Hyp*
1. *Inheritance*	Autosomal dominant	X-linked dominant	X-linked dominant
2. *Serum composition*			
Phosphorus	low	low	low
PTH	normal	normal†	normal
1,25-$(OH)_2D$	normal	normal‡	—
AP	normal or slightly elevated	elevated	elevated
3. *Renal handling of phosphorus*			
FE_{Pi}	normal	elevated	elevated
Tm_{Pi}	reduced	reduced	reduced
PTH effect on FE_{Pi}	brisk increase	blunted or absent increase	(see ref. 32)
Urine cAMP	increased excretion	increased excretion	—
4. *Somatotype*			
Body length	normal (> 3rd centile) (leg bowing)	shortened (< 3rd centile) (lower segment particularly)	shortened (particularly hind limbs and tail)
Bone lesion	osteomalacia (rickets rare)	rickets and osteomalacia	rickets and osteomalacia

Abbbreviations: HBD, human hypophosphataemic bone disease[10]; XLH, human X-linked hypophosphataemia[9,22]; *Hyp*, murine hypophosphataemia on C57Bl/6J background[11]; PTH, parathyroid hormone; 1,25-$(OH)_2D$, 1,25-dihydroxyvitamin D; AP, alkaline phosphatase; FE_{pi}, fractional excretion of phosphorus; Tm_{Pi}, maximal tubular reabsorption of phosphorus; cAMP, cyclic adenosine-3′,5′-phosphate

* XLH and *Hyp* are presumed to be homologues for the gene product affected by mutation. However, the mutations (DNA sequences) are not necessarily homologous

† Some XLH patients, under some conditions, have modest elevation of serum immunoreactive (C-terminal) PTH

‡ Some XLH patients – particularly those on treatment with phosphate and vitamin D – have serum 1,25-$(OH)_2D$ levels below the normal range[29a]

lesser capacity but more responsive to inhibition by hormone. It does not follow that these two modes of phosphate transport, so clearly segregated in the proximal convoluted segment and pars recta respectively in the rabbit nephron[26], must be segregated thus in other species. The ultimate relevance of this physiological observation lies in the unveiling of different forms of phosphate transport in the proximal nephron. We propose that an X-linked gene may control the proximal tubular transport process more sensitive to parathyroid hormone, while the autosomal gene may control the less-sensitive process in this region of the nephron. The hormone-sensitive system of distal tubule may be yet another independent mode of phosphate transport. We suggest further that the X-linked gene may also control phosphate transport in the bone compartment (Figure 12.3), and we can assume the phosphate transport in the plasma membrane of erythrocyte is not like renal membrane carriers since phosphate permeation of erythrocytes not only has different characteristics from phosphate transport in kidney[29] but it is also unaffected by the XLH and HBD mutations[27].

The *Hyp* mouse

The *Hyp* mutation in mouse is helping us to understand how the X-linked gene in man contributes to phosphate homeostasis. *Hyp* stands for hypophosphataemia[11] and the *Hyp* gene is located at a distal locus on the X-chromosome. Accordingly, the *Hyp* phenotype (on the C57Bl/6J background) observes the characteristics of any X-linked phenotype, that is, affected males are mutant hemizygotes and affected females are heterozygotes which as a group show milder expression of the mutant allele than their male counterparts. In addition to the hypophosphataemia, the *Hyp* mouse shares dwarfism, rickets, and elevated renal fractional excretion of phosphate with XLH (Table 12.2[11, 28, 29]). *Hyp* mice and XLH patients thus appear to be counterparts; the important question is: are they analogues or homologues? If *Hyp* is a homologue, it is then a powerful probe of the primary mechanism of hypophosphataemia in XLH, and of the appropriate treatment in XLH, and it can also reveal, in ways impossible to achieve in human subjects, the cellular mechanisms of renal phosphate transport under control of the X-linked gene. Fortunately, we can be quite confident that the X-linked phosphate transport processes displayed in man with XLH and the *Hyp* mouse are homologous, because of the exceptional conservation of the X-chromosome that has characterized mammalian evolution[30]. Genes on the X-chromosome in different species code for gene products with identical function in the mammal. Therefore, the *Hyp* mouse can be expected to reveal the abnormal gene product in human XLH.

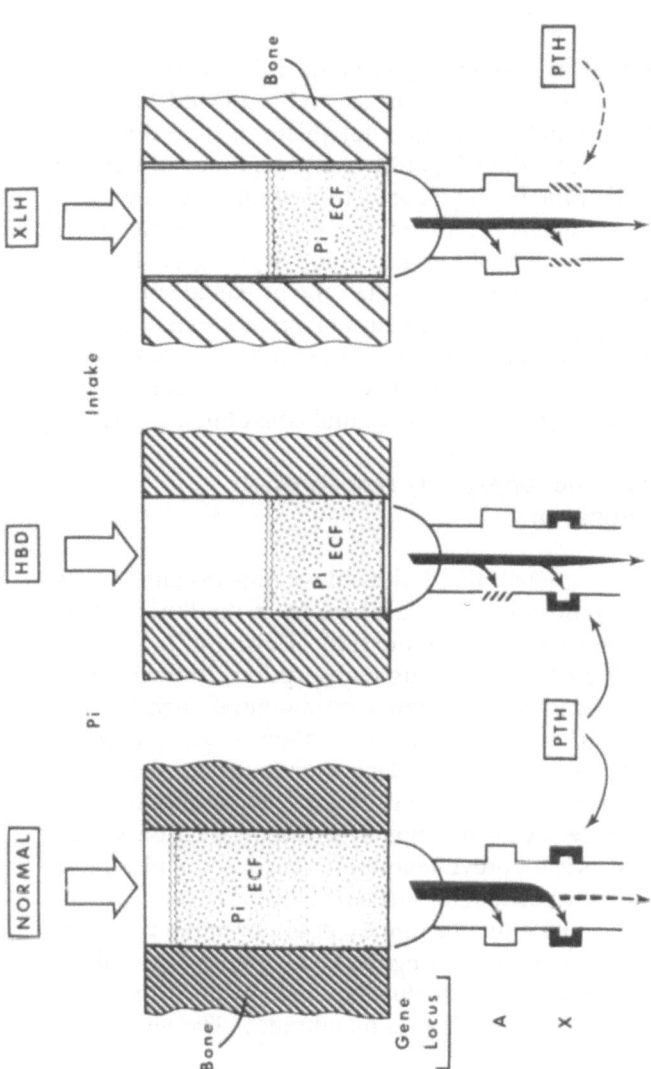

Figure 12.3 Hypothesis for principal phenotypic findings in hemizygotes with X-linked hypophosphataemic rickets (XLH) and patients with autosomal dominant hypophosphataemic bone disease (HBD). Both conditions have comparable hypophosphataemia (central compartment) when dietary intake of phosphorus is similar. Bone mineralization (lateral compartment) is severely compromised in XLH (rickets and osteomalacia) and less so in HBD (osteomalacia only). Renal loss of phosphate (arrow for outflow at bottom) is increased in both conditions but defect in reabsorption (lateral arrows) involves different tubular transport systems: X is responsive to parathyroid hormone and the product of an X-linked gene; A is unresponsive to hormone and the product of an autosomal gene. The presumed order of A and X system in series along nephron may be relevant. An X-linked phosphate transport system in bone compartment is one explanation for severe defect in bone mineralization in XLH

STUDIES OF PHOSPHATE TRANSPORT
IN THE *HYP* MOUSE

Renal handling of phosphate *in vivo*

Whole kidney fractional excretion of phosphate is increased in *Hyp* males *(Hyp/*Y) (Figure 12.4)[29, 31, 33] and in severely affected heterozygotes *(Hyp/*+)[33]*. Parathyroidectomy does not ablate the defect in renal reabsorption of phosphate[32] although parathyroid hormone does modify the degree of phosphaturia in *Hyp* mice. Micropuncture studies[31, 32] reveal reduced fractional and absolute reabsorption of phosphate in the proximal portion of superficial nephrons accessible to puncture. Involvement of the nephron at a site more distal than the proximal convoluted segment, perhaps pars recta, or involvement to a greater extent in deep nephrons is also apparent because the whole-kidney rate of delivery of phosphate to bladder urine in *Hyp* mice exceeds that accounted for simply by failure of reabsorption in the proximal convoluted segment.

The normal process of net phosphate reabsorption
in the mammalian nephron

It will be helpful to the argument that follows if we now examine briefly what determines *net* reabsorption of phosphate from the lumen of the nephron (this discussion is developed more fully elsewhere[34]).

Renal epithelial cells control phosphate reabsorption. Epithelial cells are asymmetric, possessing luminal and contraluminal surfaces that differ in morphology and are characterized by their respective brush-border and basal–lateral membranes. Tight junctions at the apical (luminal) pole join adjacent epithelial cells to form a continuous brush-border membrane surface facing the lumen. In topological terms, the luminal surface of the brush-border membrane encounters phosphate that is *outside* the body; the peritubular surface of the basal–lateral membrane is exposed to phosphate in a secondary pool *inside* the body; the primary internal pool encountered during the transcellular flux of phosphate is the intracellular space of epithelium bounded by the cytoplasmic surfaces of brush-border and basal–lateral membranes. The net flux re-

---

* Heterozygous (Hyp/+) offspring from Hyp/+ × +/Y matings are identified by selecting dwarfed rachitic females; the phenotype is confirmed by demonstrating hypophosphatae-mia[11]. Mildly affected females cannot be recognized consistently by this protocol. Studies of the heterozygous phenotype will be enhanced when it is possible to breed *Hyp/*Y mice to +/X dams and obtain obligate heterozygotes.

Infusion Protocol

Diet Protocol
with Phosphate

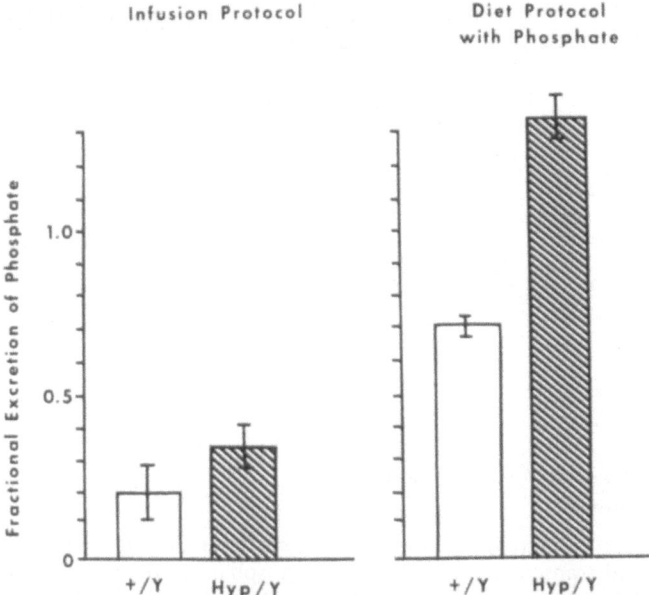

Figure 12.4   Fractional excretion of phosphate (FE_{pi}) in the *Hyp* mouse monitored by inulin clearance (infusion protocol)[29] and under conditions of dietary
phosphorus loading monitored by creatinine clearance. FE_{Pi} is significantly elevated ($p < 0.01$) in *Hyp* mouse and exceeds unity ('negative' reabsorption) in the
loaded state ($p < 0.001$) – as it can in XLH, the homologous human phenotype[56].
Data in right panel provided by F. H. Glorieux

sulting in complete internalization of anion during reabsorption encounters two membranes in series. There are four components in the
transmembrane series of fluxes (Figure 12.5): influx and efflux at the
brush-border membrane and a corresponding pair of fluxes at the basal–
lateral membrane.

Putting aside the role that diffusion plays in the reabsorption of the
divalent and monovalent species of phosphate anion under physiological
conditions[34], let us consider just the mediated component that is
apparently involved in net reabsorption of this anion. Only the net flux at
the brush-border membrane need be considered initially to explain net
reabsorption from the lumen. The relationship is simple: influx must
exceed efflux (backflux). What then prevents intracellular phosphate
from achieving the effective intracellular concentration (activity) at
which backflux equals influx at the cytoplasmic surface of the brush-
border membrane? Two possibilities come to mind: the first is *metabolic
runout*, where phosphate is converted to a different chemical form and

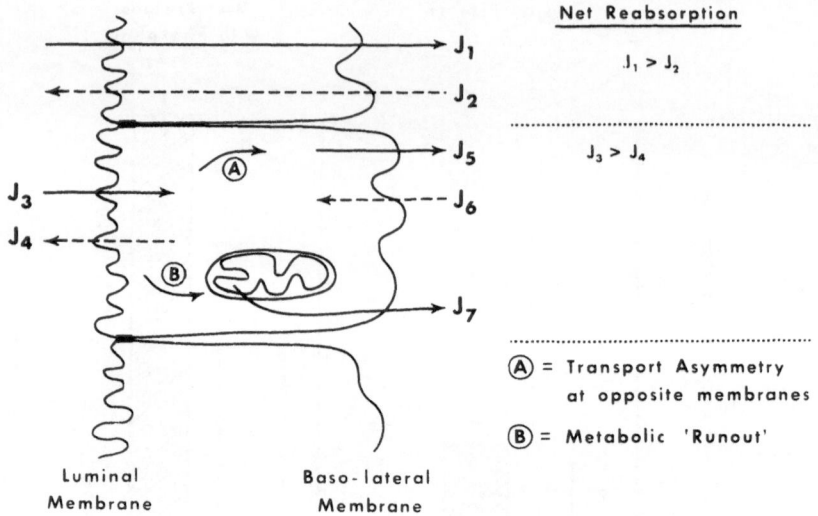

Figure 12.5 Diagram of fluxes (J_1-J_6) that occur during reabsorption cellular uptake and transcellular movement of phosphate in renal epithelium. Net reabsorption occurs when $J_1 > J_2$ or $J_3 > J_4$. 'Runouts' involving differential permeability Ⓐ at membranes (brush-border and basal–lateral) or metabolic conversion Ⓑ, keep cellular phosphate at cytoplasmic surface of luminal membrane below effective concentration (activity) that would allow $J_4 = J_3$. J_7 is flux of chemically modified solute participating in metabolic runout

moves in that form to gain access to the peritubular space; the second is *transport runout,* where phosphate leaves the cell at the basal–lateral membrane under conditions of permeability that differ from those pertaining to the brush-border membrane. Both mechanisms appear to be important for phosphate: incorporation of phosphate into organic pools is large in kidney[23]; a difference in transport properties at apical and basal poles of renal epithelium has been clearly demonstrated in purified brush-border and basal–lateral membranes of mammalian kidney[35].

In vitro studies in *Hyp* kidney

Slices The *Hyp* mouse maintains renal-cortex phosphorus content in the normal range[29,33] despite an intrinsic defect in net reabsorption of anion (Figure 12.6). How this is accomplished is not yet known but it is probably achieved by an unimpaired system of phosphate uptake in the

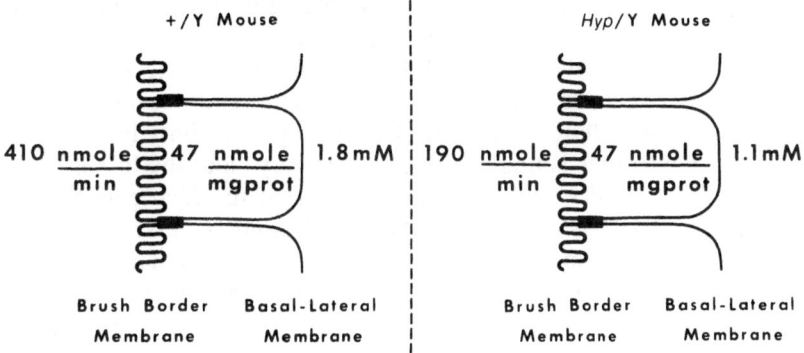

Figure 12.6 Relationships between phosphorus concentrations in urine, cells and peritubular fluid (plasma) in normal (+/Y) and mutant (*Hyp*/Y) male *Hyp* mice (data from reference 29). Note that cellular [P] is apparently unchanged in *Hyp* phenotype

basal–lateral membrane of epithelial cells[29]. Whether the phosphate content of renal cells is kept at the same level in all parts of the cell, or in all segments of *Hyp* nephron, is also unknown; perhaps epithelial cells of distal convoluted segments have higher phosphate levels while proximal segments are partially depleted.

Slices of *Hyp* renal cortex take up phosphate normally, distribute it to inorganic and organic pools in normal fashion, and allow anion to efflux at the same rate as normal slices[29]. Since basal–lateral membranes are apparently exposed predominantly in renal cortex slices, and solute in the incubating medium has reduced access to the lumen and brush-border membrane[36,37] these results indicate that intracellular metabolic runout and permeability runout at the basal–lateral membrane are not perturbed in *Hyp* kidney. A defect in phosphate transport at the brush-border membrane is implied.

Brush-border membrane vesicles Isolated brush-border membranes can be prepared and used for the study of phosphate transport[33,35,38]. Phosphate enters renal brush-border membrane vesicles by an electroneutral process on a saturable, Na^+-dependent, arsenate-inhibited component and also by a diffusional component[35]. The characteristics of sodium phosphate-cotransport are similar in mouse and rat renal brush-border membranes[38]. Transport of phosphate in isolated basal–lateral membrane vesicles is mainly Na^+-independent[35]. The apparent K_m value for phosphate transport in the brush-border preparation is of the order of 50–80 μM at pH 7.4 in the presence of Na$^+$. Phosphate is not bound or incorporated significantly by renal membranes.

The specific activity of brush-border enzymes is the same in renal membrane vesicles isolated from normal and mutant mice[33,38]. However, about half of the phosphate transport activity in renal brush-border membranes is missing in *Hyp*/Y kidney[33] and the loss is comparable in *Hyp*/+ mice with severe expression of the *Hyp* gene[38]. Loss of transport activity is confined to the Na$^+$-dependent, arsenate-inhibited component and is specific for phosphate (Figure 12.7). The apparent K_m for phosphate transport is not altered significantly in the *Hyp* brush-border membrane (Figure 12.8).

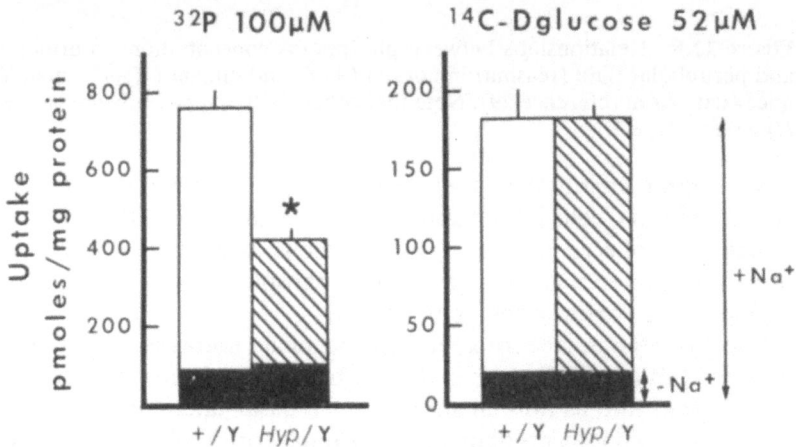

Figure 12.7 Simultaneous net uptakes of inorganic phosphate and D-glucose by renal brush-border membrane vesicles at 60 s, pH 7.4. Total uptakes in NaCl ($+$Na$^+$) and diffusional uptake in CKl ($-$Na$^+$) are shown. Difference (*) in Na$^+$/PO$_4$-contransport between normal ($+$/Y) and mutant (*Hyp*/Y) membranes is significant ($p < 0.001$). Simultaneous Na$^+$/D-glucose-cotransport is not different in the two strains. Phosphate and D-glucose do not inhibit cotransports of each other at concentrations designated (methods described in reference 29)

Evers *et al.*[39] have observed 30% loss of *in vitro* phosphate transport activity in rat renal brush border membranes exposed to parathyroid hormone *in vivo*. The loss of transport activity is confined to the Na$^+$-dependent uptake system, is selective for phosphate, is specific for parathyroid hormone, and is a membrane effect. The quantitative loss of phosphate transport *in vitro* approximates that found by micropuncture of the proximal tubule in the rat following *in vivo* exposure of the

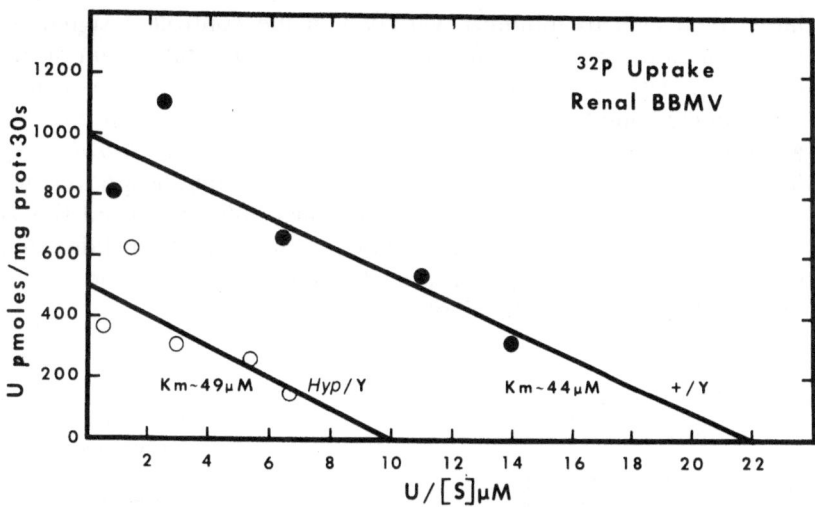

Figure 12.8 Concentration-dependent Na^+/PO_4-cotransport at 30s by renal brush-border membrane vesicles prepared from $+/Y$ and Hyp/Y mice; Na^+ concentration was kept constant; phosphate concentration was varied. The apparent K_m for phosphate is unchanged but V_{max} is about half normal in Hyp/Y membranes

nephron to an equivalent dose of parathyroid hormone. The inhibition observed *in vitro* is not accompanied by a change in the apparent K_m for phosphate uptake by brush-border membrane vesicles[39]. The findings in rat membranes prepared from kidney exposed to parathyroid hormone *in vitro* and in *Hyp* membranes are striking in their similarity: they suggest that the transport process specified by the X-linked gene and the process inhibited by parathyroid hormone may be one and the same.

HOMEOSTATIC ADAPTATION TO PHOSPHORUS DEPRIVATION

Phosphate homeostasis involves controlled and controlling systems (Figure 12.9). Intracellular phosphate is a *controlled system*. The *controlling system*, emitting controlling signals, presumably involves parathyroid hormone acting on bone and kidney and $1,25-(OH)_2D_3$ acting on bone and gut. Oscillations in the cellular phosphate pool lead to oscillations in controlled signals sent to the controlling system; the latter then acts to minimize variation in the controlled signal, thus achieving homeostasis. In the intact organism the total system of 'feedback loops' and 'cascade effects' involved in the process of homeostasis is exceedingly complex (Figure 12.2). Accordingly, it is often difficult to analyse the mechanism of homeostasis in response to a *disturbing signal* introduced from outside the system. Environmental phosphorus deprivation is a disturbing signal in the mammal. We have used the *Hyp* mouse to examine how one particular component acts to sustain homeostasis in the controlled system: renal brush-border membrane transport of phosphate proves to be adaptive.

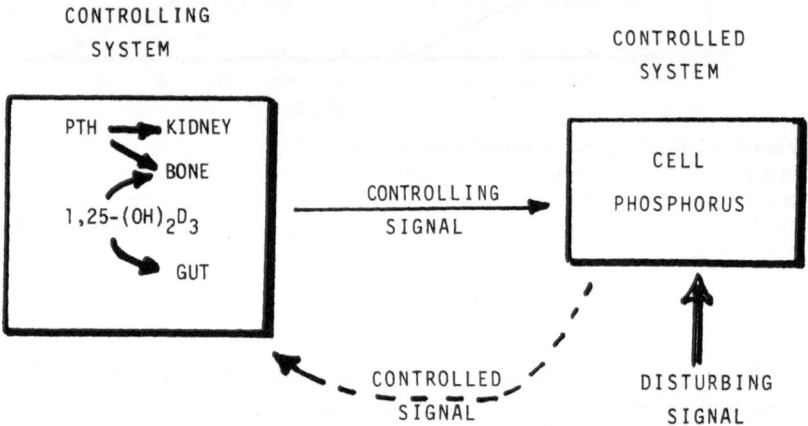

Figure 12.9 Components and signals in system exhibiting metabolic homeostasis of cellular phosphate. The effect of phosphorus deprivation (a disturbing **signal**) on homeostasis was studied (see Figure 12.2). From Neer[15].

Human subjects modify renal excretion of anion when the dietary supply of phosphate is diminished: urinary output of phosphate falls abruptly[40] and the venous plasma renal threshold (Tm_p/GFR) rises[41]. The renal adaptation to phosphorus deprivation has been studied extensively in other mammals. Fractional reabsorption of filtered phosphate rises in the intact rat, and also in the thyroparathyroidectomized rat and dog[42–47]. The response is not dependent on the integrity of parathyroid or thyroid glands, the status of vitamin D nutrition, plasma calcium, extracellular volume, or urinary pH. Moreover, the adapted kidney becomes relatively resistant to the normal inhibitory effect of parathyroid hormone on phosphate reabsorption[45]. The adaptive response appears within a few days in man[40] and rat[42], but in the dog a much longer time, weeks rather than days, is required[47]. *In situ* micropuncture studies show that fractional reabsorption of phosphate is increased in proximal segments of the nephron in the adapted kidney[42]. The response reflects duration of the disturbing signal more than the level of plasma phosphorus. This finding is important because it suggests that plasma phosphorus *per se* is not the controlled signal that initiates the adaptive response.

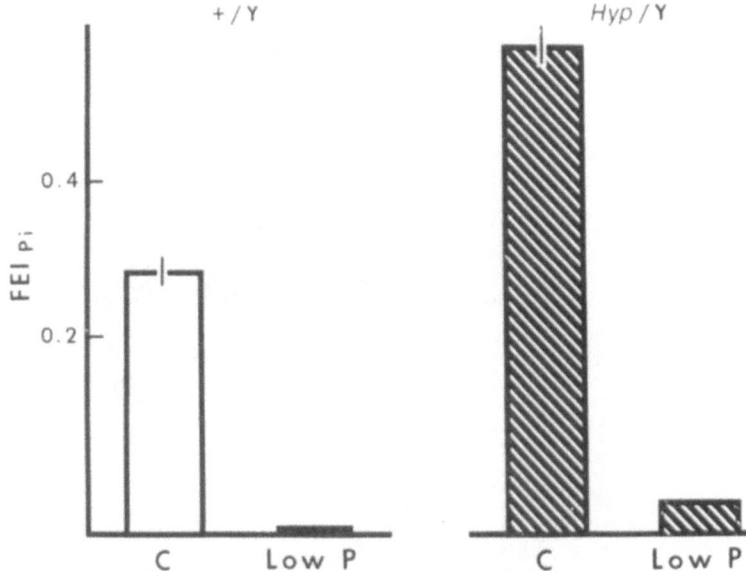

Figure 12.10 *In vivo* renal adaptation after 2 weeks on low-phosphorus diet (low-P) (0.03% P, w/w); control diet (C) contained 0.6% P, w/w. Normal (+/Y) and mutant hemizygous (*Hyp*/Y) mice both adapt to low-P diet by reducing fractional phosphate excretion index (FEI$_{Pi}$ and C$_{Pi}$/C$_{Cr}$) significantly ($p < 0.001$); *Hyp*/Y mice retain abnormally high FEI$_{Pi}$ compared to +/Y mice (see Figure 12.4) even in adapted state, implying that adaptation does not only involve tubular transport system under control of X-linked gene (data from reference 49)

The *Hyp* mouse also adapts to phosphorus deprivation[33,49]. Urinary phosphate excretion is suppressed dramatically (Figure 12.10). Yet, even in the adapted state, fractional excretion of phosphate is still greater in the *Hyp* animal than in the adapted normal littermate. These findings indicate two points of interest: first, the *Hyp* mouse, under normal dietary conditions, has not adapted to the 'intrinsic' signal of chronic hypophosphataemia, and one recalls here that the renal tissue phosphorus content is not diminished in the *Hyp* animal (Figure 12.6); secondly, renal adaptation can occur in the mutant animal which lacks an X-linked component of phosphate reabsorption in the nephron.

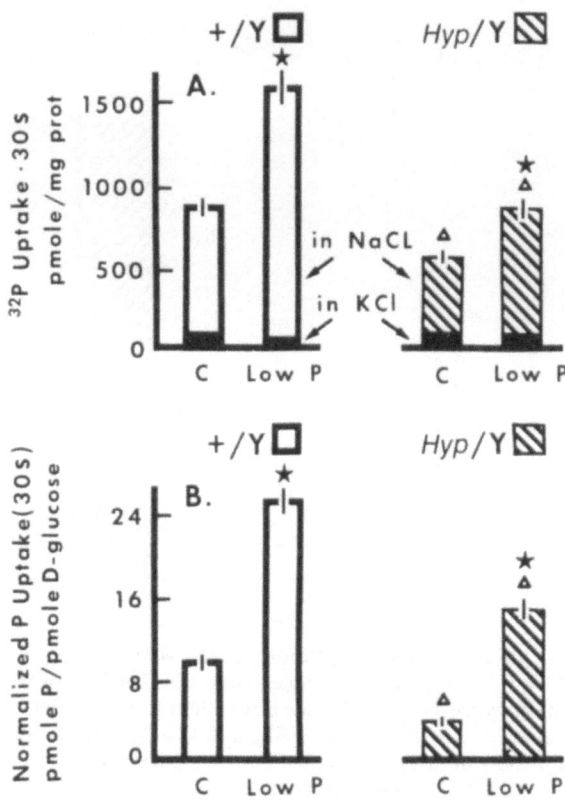

Figure 12.11 Na^+-dependent transport of phosphate (upper graphs) and of phosphate normalized to simultaneous D-glucose transport (lower graphs) by renal brush-border membrane vesicles prepared from mice fed on control and low-phosphorus diets (see Figure 12.10 for details of diets and data on *in vivo* adaptation). Na^+/PO_4 cotransport is significantly decreased in mutant (*Hyp*/Y) membranes ($\triangle$, $p < 0.01$) vs normal (+/Y) membranes in both control and adapted states. Adapted (low-P) membranes transport phosphate at increased rates (*, $p < 0.01$) vs control membranes in both +/Y and *Hyp*/Y mice. Data indicate also that Na^+/D-glucose cotransport is decreased in the adapted state. (Data from reference 49)

Renal brush-border membrane vesicles in adapted mice transport phosphate on the Na^+-dependent system at about twice the rate of membranes prepared from non-adapated mice (Figure 12.11). The effect is specific for phosphate, and *Hyp* and normal mice are comparable in their adaptive response. Mice are also similar to rats[50]: both adapt to the disturbing signal with a selectively enhanced capacity for brush-border membrane Na^+/PO_4^- cotransport. Parathyroid hormone is not essential for the membrane adaptation in the rat and the adapted membrane is resistant to inhibition of phosphate transport by parathyroid hormone[50]. While the transport V_{max} is increased, the apparent K_m is unchanged in the adapted membranes in both mouse and rat[33, 49, 50] (Figure 12.12). The renal content of phosphorus in the adapted mouse is of particular interest: 2 weeks after phosphorus deprivation has begun, renal phosphorus is no different from normal in adapted *Hyp* and control mice[33]. Another finding, still unexplained, is decreased transport of D-glucose by renal brush-border membrane vesicles during phosphorus deprivation[33, 50].

We[33, 49] and others[50] view these findings as strong evidence that a specific Na^+/PO_4^- cotransport mechanism in the renal brush-border membrane acts independently of the parathyroid-hormone-controlling signal, is responsive to the disturbing signal of phosphorus deprivation, and is not designated by the X-linked gene. The adaptive value of such a system is obvious, but how adaptation is achieved at the molecular level, and by what specific controlling cellular signal, is a fascinating problem for further study.

RELATIONSHIP BETWEEN ALKALINE PHOSPHATASE AND PHOSPHATE TRANSPORT IN RENAL BRUSH-BORDER MEMBRANES IN *HYP* AND NORMAL MICE

It has been proposed[51, 52] that alkaline phosphatase in kidney might be involved in phosphate reabsorption. We have investigated this hypothesis with isolated brush-border membrane vesicles prepared from normal and *Hyp* mice. The *Hyp* mutation and chronic phosphorus deprivation, both strong modifiers of phosphate transport activity in the mouse renal brush-border membrane preparation, have no corresponding effect on membrane alkaline phosphatase activity (Figure 12.13). Moreover, levamisol (2×10^{-5} mol/l) and ethylene diamine tetra-acetic acid (EDTA; 10^{-3} mol/l), both potent inhibitors of renal alkaline phos-

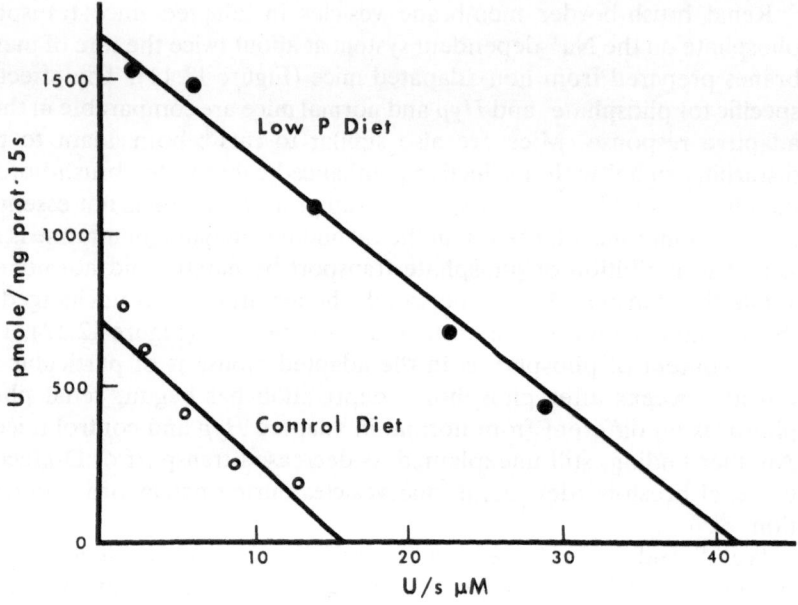

Figure 12.12 Concentration-dependent uptake of phosphate on the Na^+-dependent system in renal brush-border membrane vesicles prepared from normal ($+/Y$) mice fed on control and low-P diets. Renal adaptation to P deprivation is accompanied by increased activity (V_{max}) of Na^+/PO_4 cotransport but no change in apparent K_m; Hyp/Y mice show the same mode of adaptation

phatase activity in renal brush-border membranes *in vitro*, have no effect on phosphate transport by membrane vesicles (Figure 12.13). We conclude that alkaline phosphatase does not play a direct role in phosphate transport across the brush-border membrane of the mouse nephron. Studies in the phosphorus deprived rat[50] yield similar evidence: the large increase in phosphate transport in the adapted rat kidney is accompanied by only small ($< 20\%$) increases in alkaline phosphatase activity.

UNRESOLVED PROBLEMS IN X-LINKED HYPOPHOSPHATAEMIA

Intestinal phosphate transport

There is controversy whether intestinal transport of phosphate is normal or impaired in the human disorder (cited in detail elsewhere[22]). *Hyp*

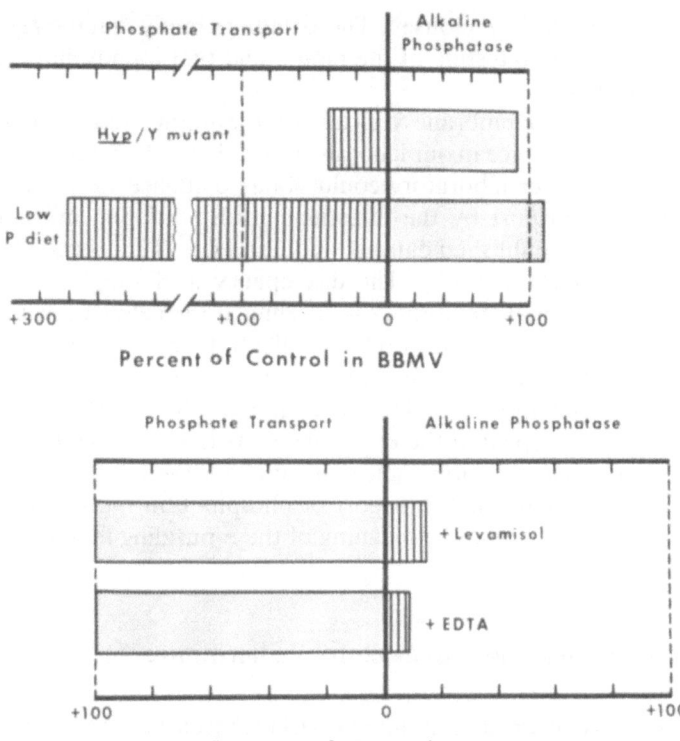

Figure 12.13   Relationship between alkaline phosphatase activity, measured at pH 10, and Na^+/PO_4 cotransport activity in isolated renal brush-border membranes under various conditions. Data show effect of experimental procedures expressed as percent of control; hatched bars indicate a significant ($p < 0.01$) effect

mice have been used to investigate expression of the X-linked gene in the intestine[53,54]. Everted jejunal sacs from vitamin D-fed *Hyp*/Y mice transport phosphate at about 40% of the normal rate, as measured by the transmural phosphate distribution ratio. Calcium transport in everted duodenal sacs is similar in *Hyp* and normal mice. *In vivo* administration of 1,25-$(OH)_2D_3$ stimulates intestinal calcium transport in both *Hyp* and normal animals, but has an effect on intestinal phosphate transport only in the normal animal[53]. Phosphorus deprivation does not stimulate intestinal phosphate transport in either the normal or *Hyp* animal[54]. Vitamin D deprivation diminishes intestinal phosphate transport in the normal mouse, but has no additional effect on the blunted transport of phosphate in the *Hyp* mouse[54]. These findings imply that the *Hyp* gene is expressed in the intestine of the mouse and that a phosphate transport process is involved.

Brush-border membrane vesicles from jejunum were prepared from *Hyp*/Y and +/Y mice in our laboratory and also by Sacktor's group using our mice. Neither laboratory could obtain evidence for impairment of phosphate transport by the intestinal brush-border membrane in the *Hyp* mouse (unpublished data: D. K. Fast, H. S. Tenenhouse and C. R. Scriver; B. Sacktor *et al.*). The discrepancy in findings obtained with renal and intestinal membranes is puzzling, if the cellular location of the phosphate-transport gene product is likely to be similar in renal and intestinal epithelia, and if one accepts the prior evidence for a defect in transmural transport of phosphate in the *Hyp* mouse intestine[53,54]. Therefore, we repeated the experiments with everted jejunal sacs prepared from *Hyp* and normal mice: in our hands there is no significant difference in the intestinal transport of phosphate in mutant and normal mice. We are pursuing the meaning of these puzzling findings.

Renal responsiveness to calciotropic hormones

Phosphate reabsorption in human XLH is insensitive to elevated levels of circulating parathyroid hormone[55] or to infused parathyroid hormone[56]. However, urinary cyclic AMP excretion rises briskly after parathyroid hormone infusion in XLH[9,56]. On the other hand, calcium infusion enhances net reabsorption of phosphate[57] and restores the renal phosphaturic response to parathyroid hormone[58]. It is the view of Short *et al.*[58] that these findings indicate both a requirement for normal circulating levels of parathyroid hormone for expression of the mutation in the XLH kidney, and a hyper-responsiveness of the mutant kidney to normal amounts of hormone. The failure of parathyroidectomy to restore the normal capacity for phosphate reabsorption both in human patients[9] and in the *Hyp* mouse[32] is considered as evidence against this hypothesis. Nonetheless, renal responsiveness to parathyroid hormone in the X-linked disease continues to be of interest.

Two laboratories have now studied the *in vitro* renal responsiveness of *Hyp* mouse to the calciotropic agents, synthetic (1–34 fragment) parathyroid hormone and salmon calcitonin. Both found reduced responsiveness to parathyroid hormone and increased responsiveness to calcitonin in *Hyp* kidney. Brunette *et al.*[59] used a microassay of adenylcyclase activity to measure responsiveness in specific segments of isolated single nephrons. They found a blunted response to parathyroid hormone at graded doses (0.01–10 units/ml) in the proximal convoluted tubule of *Hyp* mice; pars recta and distal convoluted segments were normally responsive to the hormone. Distal convoluted tubule segments were markedly hyper-responsive to calcitonin. Sacktor and colleagues (unpublished data) used renal cortex homogenates enriched in tubular basal–lateral membranes in their experiments. They found that stimulation of adenylcyclase activity by parathyroid hormone in graded doses (1–60 units/ml) was blunted in *Hyp* kidney (Figure 12.14). They also

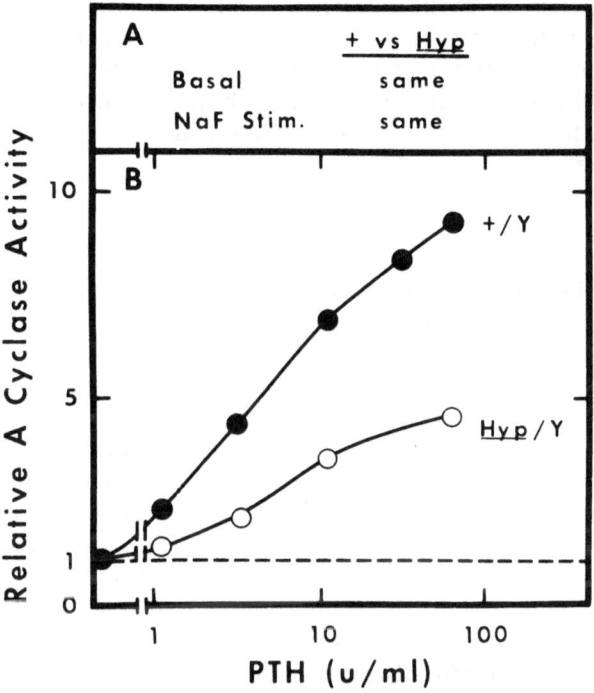

Figure 12.14 Relative adenyl cyclase activity (experimental: control (no PTH added)) in basal–lateral membrane-enriched renal cortex homogenates prepared from mutant hemizygous (*Hyp*/Y) and normal male (+/Y) mice. Dose–response data (lower portion) shown for synthetic parathyroid hormone (1–34 fragment) (PTH) added *in vitro*. Upper portion indicates that adenylcyclase activity in basal state and after NaF stimulation are not different in *Hyp*/Y and +/Y mice, in contrast to blunted response to PTH in *Hyp*/Y phenotype. (Unpublished data, Sacktor, B., Tenenhouse, H. S. and Scriver, C. R.).

found that the adenylcyclase response was enhanced in the presence of calcitonin (0.3 and 3 μg/ml) in the *Hyp* mouse. Intracellular coupling events and protein kinase activity were both normal in *Hyp* kidney. These findings, which corroborate those of Brunette *et al.*, imply that cellular responsiveness to calciotropic hormones is modified, apparently in the way the hormonal signal is perceived at the membrane level in the *Hyp* nephron. Since the basic defect in the *Hyp* nephron seems to be one of proximal tubular reabsorption of phosphate, with an increased load of the anion delivered to the distal tubule *in vivo*, one wonders whether an imbalance of phosphate distribution in the nephron has something to do with the altered responsiveness to calciotropic hormones. These findings may offer an explanation for a puzzling observation made in earlier studies[29]. Urinary cyclic AMP excretion is elevated in *Hyp* mice (41 nmol/mg creatinine in *Hyp* vs 32 nmol/mg creatinine in normal mice fed normal diets, $p < 0.05$). Hyper-responsiveness of the distal tubule to calcitonin, which circulates at normal levels in *Hyp* mice[59], may be the explanation for augmented urinary excretion of cyclic AMP in the mutant phenotype.

RENAL HANDLING OF SULPHATE IN HYPOPHOSPHATAEMIC STATES

Inorganic sulphate (Figure 12.1) is utilized by the body for numerous purposes, some of which are of special importance to cartilage and bone. The extracellular concentration of sulphate is determined to a considerable extent by the kidney, the ion being filtered by the glomerulus and reabsorbed by the tubule[60,61], reabsorption is limited by a maximal rate of tubular transport (Tm_{SO_4})[62]. The normal Tm_{SO_4} value in human subjects is said to show considerable inter- and intra-individual variation, but this finding may reflect technical problems in the early analysis of sulphate as much as physiological phenomena. There is some evidence for renal adaptation in sulphate excretion to low protein intake; this observation stems from studies in the dog (cited in reference 61). Modern studies with renal brush-border membrane vesicles prepared from rat kidney cortex[62] show that sulphate is transported by an electroneutral Na^+/SO_4^{2-}-cotransport process that has many of the characteristics of phosphate transport in this membrane. Phosphate anion does not appear to interact with the sulphate transport system in the renal brush-border membrane[62].

Because we are interested in the renal handling of sulphate anion in hypophosphataemic states, and because the measurement of serum sulphate is cumbersome by conventional methods, we developed a simple microassay for accurate analysis of the anion both in urine and in small volumes (100 μl) of deproteinized serum[63]. The method utilizes selective precipitation of ^{133}Ba; phosphate anion does not interfere with the assay. Serum sulphate levels in healthy adult and child subjects (0.29 ± 0.03 mM, mean and SD) are lower than values reported in earlier studies[61]. Some preliminary studies suggest that young infants have about two-fold higher serum sulphate levels than older subjects; patients with diminished glomerular filtration have three- to five-fold elevated serum sulphate levels. Renal clearance of sulphate is not responsive to parathyroid hormone in man in our experience (Cole, D. E. C. and Scriver, C. R., unpublished observations).

We have examined serum sulphate levels in our patients with the X-linked forms of hypophosphataemia and we have determined net tubular reabsorption of the anion under fasting conditions in these subjects. Serum sulphate is not diminished in the hypophosphataemic patients (Table 12.3) and their renal reabsorption of sulphate is not different from normal (Figure 12.15). These findings suggest that the major process of sulphate reabsorption in the human nephron is independent of the systems serving phosphate reabsorption.

TABLE 12.3   Fasting serum inorganic sulphate (mM) in
normal subjects and patients with Mendelian
hypophosphataemias

Subjects	n	Inorganic serum sulphate (mM) (mean ± SD)
Normal adults	14	0.29 ± 0.03
X-linked hypophosphataemia		
Mutant hemizygotes	5	0.29 ± 0.06
Obligate heterozygotes	8	0.32 ± 0.09
Non X-linked		
hypophosphataemia (HBD)	4	0.27 ± 0.06

Serum sulphate was measured by a microassay[63], using selective precipitation of inorganic sulphate with ^{133}Ba

We have also made some preliminary studies of sulphate excretion by the *Hyp* mouse. Urinary sulphate is increased in the mutant animal (Table 12.4). However, plasma sulphate is also raised in the *Hyp* mouse; accordingly, the excretion index is not different from normal (Table

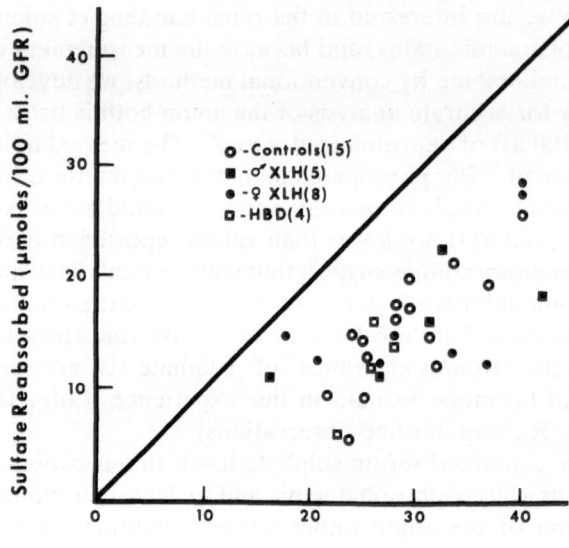

Filtered Sulfate(μmoles/100 ml. GFR)

Figure 12.15   Renal reabsorption of sulphate related to filtered load in normal age-equivalent controls and patients with X-linked hypophosphataemia (XLH) (mutant hemizygotes and heterozygotes) and with autosomal hypophosphataemic bone disease (HBD). The Mendelian hypophosphataemias XLH and HBD do not compromise sulphate reabsorption

TABLE 12.4   Inorganic sulphate in serum and urine of *Hyp* mice

Genotype	Phenotype	Serum, inorganic sulphate (mM) (mean ± SD)	Urine inorganic sulphate (mM) (nmol/g creatinine)	Excretion index excretion/serum conc.
+/Y	Normal male	0.91 ± 0.03 (n = 13)	49.2 ± 3.9 (n = 11)	56.2 ± 4.2 (11)
Hyp/Y	Hypophos phataemic male	1.21 ± 0.04* (n = 12)	69.8 ± 3.7† n = 9	58.5 ± 4.2 (n = 9)

* $p > 0.001$ by Student's t test (*Hyp*/Y) vs +/Y
† > 0.005 by Student's t test (*Hyp*/Y) vs +/Y
Sulphate in serum and urine measured by microassay[36]. Mice were studied fasting after normal overnight feeding; urines were untimed collections, obtained simultaneously with blood samples

12.4). We propose that these findings reflect a known difference in glomerular filtration rate in *Hyp* mice. GFR is reduced by about 25% in the mutant strain[32,39] and reduced filtration of sulphate could be sufficient to raise the serum level in the *Hyp* mouse. Since whole kidney excretion of sulphate is elevated under these conditions, we assume that tubular reabsorption takes place at or near the Tm in the normal mouse. Under these conditions, sulphate may also enter urine directly from tubular cells when the endogenous concentration is elevated. It is not yet apparent to us why the sulphate concentration of normal murine serum is three- to four-fold higher than in man, but the finding is analogous to the inter-species difference in serum phosphate levels.

CONCLUSION

The Mendelian hypophosphataemias of man (XLH and HBD), one X-linked, the other autosomal, provide convincing evidence for more than one mechanism of phosphate reabsorption in the nephron. A murine homologue (*Hyp*) for the X-linked disease offers a valuable opportunity to study phosphate transport by isolated renal brush-border membranes when reabsorption *in vivo* is modified by mutation. The *in vitro* evidence indicates that the mutant process controlling net reabsorption of phosphate *in vivo* is located in the brush-border membrane. We recognize, of course, that brush-border membrane events are not the sole determinants of net transcellular reabsorption; they are simply the most important.

Parathyroid hormone acts to modulate a component of brush-border membrane Na^+/PO_4^- cotransport and reduce phosphate transport. Studies in the *Hyp* phenotype, and in mice under conditions of phosphorus deprivation, suggest that this brush-border membrane component may be controlled by an X-linked gene. Another Na^+/PO_4^- cotransport component, in the same membrane, is rather unresponsive to parathyroid hormone but responds to the signal of phosphorus deprivation; this component appears to be designated by an autosomal gene. Thus, the nephron is provided with membrane components that contribute to homeostasis in the controlled system by responding in opposite ways to the opposing signals of phosphate excess and phosphate deficiency. Neither the X-linked nor autosomal component seems to serve renal reabsorption of sulphate, which is also mediated by a Na^+-dependent mechanism in the brush-border membrane. The possibility of additional systems for phosphate transfer in the brush-border membrane of tubular cells, beyond the two proposed, is, of course, not excluded. A precise description of the total process must await isolation and chacterization of membrane components *in vitro*.

There is now sufficient evidence to say that the phosphate carrier (or carriers) in the basal–lateral membranes of renal epithelium differ(s) from those in the brush-border membrane. We know also that the mode of phosphate transport in the erythrocyte membrane is quite different from that of the renal brush-border membrane. Thus, we have further evidence for the diversity of gene products serving whole body cellular phosphate homeostasis in the mammal. We suspect, but have no proof, that mineralization of bone might also be served by mediated phosphate transport processes in that tissue; the peculiar discrepancy in the intensity of bone pathology in XLH and HBD, when serum phosphate is similarly compromised in the two conditions, suggests that X-linked and autosomal genes may have independent expression in bone.

We see the Mendelian disorders of phosphate transport as useful probes that will help to delineate how cellular membranes regulate phosphate and sulphate homeostasis in man and other mammals. It requires no great insight to predict that this interesting area of research has just begun.

Acknowledgements

Our research is supported by the Medical Research Council of Canada and the Quebec Network of Genetic Medicine. Dr Cole is an MRC Fellow. We are grateful to Bertram Sacktor for his interest and for permission to use Figure 12.14 from our joint study.

References

1. Scriver, C. R. (1962). Hereditary aminoaciduria. In A. Bearn and A. G. Steinberg (eds). *Progress in Medical Genetics,* Vol. 2, p. 83. (New York: Grune and Stratton)
2. Scriver, C. R. (1969). The human biochemical genetics of amino acid transport. *Pediatrics,* **44,** 348
3. Scriver, C. R. and Hechtman, P. (1970). Human genetics of membrane transport with emphasis on amino acids. *Adv. Hum. Genet.,* **1,** 211
4. Scriver, C. R. and Bergeron, M. (1974). Amino acid transport in kidney. The use of mutation to dissect membrane and trans-epithelial transport. In W. L. Nyhan (ed.). *Heritable Disorders of Amino Acid Metabolism,* p. 515. (New York: Wiley)
5. Scriver, C. R., Chesney, R. W. and McInnes, R. R. (1976). Genetic aspects of renal tubular transport: diversity and topology of carriers. *Kidney Int.,* **9,** 149

6. Scriver, C. R. (1977). Hereditary and acquired aminoacidopathies, Entry 75. In P. L. Altman and D. D. Katz (eds). *Human Health and Disease*, p. 97. (Bethesda, Md: FASB)

7. Scriver, C. R. (1981). Inborn errors of membrane transport: mechanisms and implications for treatment. In C. Bartsocas (ed.). *Management of Genetic Disorders*. (New York: Liss). (In press)

8. Ullrich, K. J. (1979). Sugar, amino acid and Na^+ cotransport in the proximal tubule. *Annu. Rev. Physiol.*, **41**, 181

9. Scriver, C. R., Glorieux, F. H., Reade, T. M. and Tenenhouse, H. S. (1976). X-linked hypophosphatemia and autosomal recessive vitamin D dependency: Models for the resolution of Vitamin D refractory rickets. In H. Bickel and J. Stern (eds). *Inborn Errors of Calcium and Bone Metabolism*, p. 150. (Baltimore: Univ. Park Press)

10. Scriver, C. R., MacDonald, W., Reade, T., Glorieux, F. H. and Nogrady, B. (1977). Hypophosphatemic nonrachitic bone disease: an entity distinct from X-linked hypophosphatemia in the renal defect, bone involvement, and inheritance. *Am. J. Med. Genet.*, **1**, 101

11. Eicher, E. M., Southard, J. L., Scriver, C. R. and Glorieux, F. H. (1976). Hypophosphatemia: mouse model for human familial hypophosphatemic (vitamin D-resistant) rickets. *Proc. Natl. Acad. Sci. USA*, **73**, 4667

12. Scriver, C. R. (1979). The William Allan Memorial Award Address: On phosphate transport and genetic screening. "Understanding backward – living forward" in human genetics. *Am. J Hum. Genet.*, **31**, 243

13. Griffith, E. J., Ponnamperuma, C. and Gabel, N. (1977). Phosphorus, a key to life on the primitive earth. *Origins Life*, **8**, 71

14. Schwartz, R. M. and Dayhoff, M. O. (1978). Origins of prokaryotes, eukaryotes, mitochondria and chloroplasts. *Science*, **199**, 395

15. Neer, R. (1979). Calcium and inorganic phosphate homeostasis. In L. J. DeGroot, G. F. Cahill, L. Martini, D. H. Nelson, W. D. Odek, S. T. Potts Jr., E. Steinberger and A. I. Winegrad (eds.). *Endocrinology*, p. 669. (New York: Grune and Stratton)

16. Goldberg, M., Agus, Z. S. and Goldfarb, S. (1975). Renal handling of phosphate, calcium and magnesium. In B. H. Brenner and F. C. Rector Jr. (eds.). *The Kidney*, Vol. 1, p. 344. (Philadelphia: Saunders)

17. Fraser, D. and Scriver, C. R. (1976). Familial forms of vitamin D-resistant rickets revisited. X-linked hyophosphatemia and autosomal recessive vitamin D dependency. *Am. J. Clin. Nutr.*, **29**, 1315

18. Bronner, F. (1976). Vitamin D deficiency and rickets. *Am. J. Clin. Nutr.*, **29**, 1307

19. Winters, R. W., Graham, J. B., Williams, T. F., McFalls, V. W. and Burnett, C. H. (1958). A genetic study of familial hypophosphatemia and vitamin D resistant rickets with a review of the literature. *Medicine*, **37**, 97

20. Albright, F., Butler, A. M. and Bloomberg, E. (1937). Rickets resistant to vitamin D therapy. *Am. Dis. Child.*, **54**, 529

21. Brooks, M. H., Bell, N. H., Lowe, L., Stern, P. H., Orfei, E., Queener, S. F., Hamstra, A. J. and DeLuca, H. F. (1978). Vitamin-D-dependent rickets type II. Resistance of target organs to 1,25-dihydroxyvitamin D. *N. Engl. J. Med.*, **298**, 996

22. Rasmussen, H. and Anast, C. (1978). Familial hypophosphatemic

(Vitamin D-resistant) rickets and vitamin D-dependent rickets. In J. B. Stanbury, J. B. Wyngaarden and D. S. Fredrickson, (eds.). *The Metabolic Basis of Inherited Disease*, 4th Edn, p. 1537. (New York: McGraw-Hill)

23. McKusick, V. A. (1978). Mendelian inheritance in man. *Catalogs of Autosomal Dominant, Autosomal Recessive and X-Linked Phenotypes*. 5th Edn. (Baltimore: Johns Hopkins Univ. Press)

24. Childs, B. and Der Kaloustian, V. M. (1968). Genetic heterogeneity. *N. Engl. J. Med.*, **279**, 1205 and 1267

25. Morel, F., Charbardès, D., Imbert, M., Montegut, M. and Clique, A. (1976). Functional segmentation of the rabbit distal tubule by microdetermination of hormone-dependent adenylate cyclase activity. *Kidney Int.*, **9**, 264

26. Dennis, V. W., Bello-Reuss, E. and Robinson, R. R. (1977). Response of phosphate transport to parathyroid hormone in segments of rabbit nephron. *Am. J. Physiol.*, **233**, F29

27. Tenenhouse, H. S. and Scriver, C. R. (1975). Orthophosphate transport in the erythrocyte of normal subjects and of patients with X-linked hypophosphatemia. *J. Clin. Invest.*, **55**, 644

28. Meyer, R. A. Jr., Jowsey, J. and Meyer, M. H. (1979). Osteomalacia and altered magnesium metabolism in the X-linked hypophosphatemic mouse. *Calcified Tissue Int.*, **27**, 19

29. Tenenhouse, H. S., Scriver, C. R., McInnes, R. R. and Glorieux, F. H. (1978). Renal handling of phosphate in vivo and in vitro by the X-linked hypophosphatemic male mouse: evidence for a defect in the brush border membrane. *Kidney Int.*, **14**, 236

29a. Scriver, C. R., Deade, T. M., DeLuca, H. F. and Hamstra, A. J. (1978). Serum 1,25-dihydroxyvitamin D levels in normal subjects and in patients with hereditary rickets or bone disease. *N. Engl. J. Med.*, **299**, 976

30. Ohno, S. (1967). *Sex Chromosomes and Sex Linked Genes*, p. 46. (New York: Springer)

31. Giasson, S. D., Brunette, M. G., Danan, G., Vigneault, N. and Carriere, S. (1977). Micropuncture study of renal phosphorus transport in hypophosphatemic vitamin D resistant rickets mice. *Pflugers Arch.*, **371**, 33

32. Cowgill, L. D., Goldfarb, S., Goldberg, M., Slatopolsky, E. and Agus, Z. S. (1979). Demonstration of an intrinsic renal tubular defect in mice with familial hypophosphatemic rickets. *J. Clin. Invest.*, **63**, 1203

33. Tenenhouse, H. S. and Scriver, C. R. (1979a). Renal adaptation to phosphate deprivation in the *Hyp* mouse with X-linked hypophosphatemia. *Canad. J. Biochem.*, **57**, 938

34. Scriver, C. R., Stacey, T. E., Tenenhouse, H. S. and MacDonald, W. A. (1977a). Transepithelial transport of phosphate anion in kidney. Potential mechanisms for hypophosphatemia. *Adv. Exp. Med. Biol.*, **81**, 55

35. Hoffman, N., Thees, M. and Kinne, R. (1976). Phosphate transport by isolated renal brush border vesicles. *Pflugers Arch.*, **362**, 147

36. Wedeen, R. P. and Weiner, B. (1973). The distribution of p-aminohippuric acid in rat kidney slices. I. Tubular localization. *Kidney Int.*, **3**, 205

37. Arthus, M. F., Bergeron M. and Scriver, C. R. (1980). Restriction of transport between medium and liminal membrane of nephron during incubation of renal cortex slices. *Clin. Res.*, **28**, 695A

38. Tenenhouse, H. S. and Scriver, C. R. (1978). The defect in transcellular transport of phosphate in the nephron is located in brush-border membranes in X-linked hypophosphatemia (*Hyp* mouse model). *Canad. J. Biochem.*, **56**, 640

39. Evers, C. A., Murer, H. and Kinne, R. (1978). Effect of parathyrin on the transport properties of isolated renal brush-border vesicles. *Biochem. J.*, **172**, 49

40. Lotz, M., Zisman, E. and Bartter, F. C. (1968). Evidence for a phosphorus-depletion syndrome in man. *N. Eng. J. Med.*, **278**, 409

41. Bijvoet, O. L. M. (1969). Relation of plasma phosphate concentration to renal tubular reabsorption of phosphate. *Clin. Sci.*, **37**, 23

42. Trohler, U., Bonjour, J.-P. and Fleisch, H. (1976). Inorganic phosphate homeostasis. Renal adaptation to the dietary intake in intact and thyro-parathyroidectomized rats. *J. Clin. Invest.*, **57**, 264

43. Trohler, U., Bonjour, J.-P. and Fleisch, H. (1976). Renal tubular adaptation to dietary phosphorus. *Nature (London)*, **261**, 145

44. Steele, T. H. and DeLuca, H. F. (1976). Influence of dietary phosphorus on renal phosphate reabsorption in the parathyroidectomized rat. *J. Clin. Invest.*, **57**, 867

45. Steele, T. H., Underwood, J. L., Stromberg, B. A. and Larmore, C. A. (1976). Renal resistance to parathyroid hormone during phosphorus deprivation. *J. Clin. Invest.*, **58**, 1461

46. Mulhlbauer, R. C., Bonjour, J.-P. and Fleisch, H. (1977). Tubular localization of adaptation to dietary phosphate in rats. *Am. J. Physiol.*, **233**, F342

47. Wen, S.-F., Boynar, J. W. Jr. and Stoll, R. W. (1978). Effect of phosphate deprivation on renal phosphate transport in the dog. *Am. J. Physiol.*, **234**, F199

48. Goldfarb, S., Westby, G. R., Goldberg, M. and Agus, Z. A. (1977). Renal tubular effects of chronic phosphate D depletion. *J. Clin. Invest.*, **59**, 770

49. Tenenhouse, H. S. and Scriver, C. R. (1981) Renal brush-border membrane adaptation to phosphorus deprivation in the *Hyp*/Y mouse. *Nature (London)*. (In press)

50. Stoll, R., Kinne, R. and Murer, H. (1979). Effect of dietary phosphate intake on phosphate transport by isolated rat renal brush-border vesicles. *Biochem. J.*, **180**, 465

51. Melani, F., Ramponi, G., Farnararo, M., Cocucci, E. and Guerritorre, A. (1967). Regulation by phosphate of alkaline phosphatase in rat kidney. *Biochim. Biophys. Acta*, **138**, 411

52. Kempson, S. A., Kim, J. K., Northrup, J. E., Hui, Y., Knox, F. G. and Dousa, T. P. (1977). Enzyme changes in the renal cortex induced by low phosphate diet. *Kidney Int.*, **12**, 563

53. O'Doherty, P. J. A., DeLuca, H. F. and Eicher, E. M. (1976). Intestinal calcium and phosphate transport in genetic hypophosphatemic mice. *Biochem. Biophys. Res. Commun.*, **71**, 617

54. O'Doherty, P. J. A., DeLuca, H. F. and Eicher, E. M. (1977). Lack of effect of vitamin D and its metabolites on intestinal phosphate transport in familial hypophosphatemia of mice. *Endocrinology*, **101**, 1325

55. Arnaud, C., Glorieux, F. and Scriver, C. R. (1971). Serum parathyroid

hormone in X-linked hypophosphatemia. *Science*, **173**, 845

56. Glorieux, F. and Scriver, C. R. (1972). Loss of a parathyroid hormone-sensitive component of phosphate transport in X-linked hypophosphatemia. *Science*, **175**, 997

57. Glorieux, F. H. and Scriver, C. R. (1973). Transport metabolism and clinical use of inorganic phosphate in X-linked hypophosphatemia. In B. Frame, A. M. Parfitt and H. Duncan (eds.). *The Clinical Aspects of Metabolic Bone Disease*, ICS 270, p. 421. (Amsterdam: Excerpta Medica)

58. Short, E., Morris, R. C. Jr., Sebastian, A. and Spencer, M. (1976). Exaggerated phosphaturic response to circulating parathyroid hormone in patients with familial X-linked hypophosphatemic rickets. *J. Clin. Invest.*, **58**, 152

59. Brunette, M. G., Chabardes, D., Imbert-Teboul, M., Clique, A., Montegut, M. and Morel, F. (1979). Hormone-sensitive adenylate cyclase along the nephron of genetically hypophosphatemic mice. *Kidney Int.*, **15**, 357

60. Smith, H. W. (1951) Sulfate clearance. In *Kidney: Structure and Function in Health and Disease*, p. 121. (New York: Oxford Univ. Press)

61. Becker, E. L., Heinemann, H. O., Igarashi, K., Hodler, J. E. and Gershberg, H. (1960). Renal mechanisms for the excretion of inorganic sulfate in man. *J. Clin. Invest.*, **39**, 1909

62. Lucke, H., Strange, G. and Murer, H. (1979). Sulfate-ion/sodium-ion cotransport by brush-border membrane vesicles isolated from rat kidney cortex. *Biochem. J.*, **182**, 223

63. Cole, D. E. C., Mohyuddin, F. and Scriver, C. R. (1979). A microassay for analysis of serum sulfate. *Anal. Biochem.*, **100**, 339

13

Renal transport of cystine by isolated renal tubules and brush-border membrane vesicles

J. W. Foreman, P. D. McNamara and S. Segal

INTRODUCTION

Human cystinuria, an inherited disease characterized by increased excretion of cystine and the dibasic amino acids, lysine, ornithine, and arginine, has focused attention on the nature of the renal tubule reabsorption of these amino acids. In 1951, Dent and Rose[1] proposed that cystine and the dibasic amino acids were handled by a common system in the kidney that was defective in human cystinuria. This hypothesis was strengthened by the fact that lysine infusion in both man[2,3] and dog[4] increased the excretion of cystine and the other dibasic amino acids. A common system for the accumulation of dibasic amino acids in renal tubule cells has been demonstrated using cortical slices from both human[5] and rat kidney[6]. Further support for a common system came from microperfusion studies in rat proximal tubules, demonstrating arginine inhibition of cystine uptake from the tubule lumen[7].

On the other hand, evidence for cystine uptake separate from the dibasic amino acids has been demonstrated. Cystine uptake by renal cortical slices from both humans[5] and rats[6] was not inhibited by the dibasic amino acids. Further, dibasic amino-acid uptake by cortical slices from cystinuric patients was defective, but cystine uptake was not[5]. Additional support for the separate nature of renal transport processes came from descriptions of patients with cystinuria without dibasic aminoaciduria[8] and patients with hyperdibasic aminoaciduria without cystinuria[9,10]. In canine cystinuria, some dogs have only an increase in cystine excretion without significant dibasic amino acid excretion[11].

Because of these ambiguities, we examined the nature of cystine and dibasic amino-acid transport using the isolated renal tubule and isolated brush-border membrane vesicles from the rat. The isolated tubule offered advantages over the cortical slice in that concerns about substrate penetration, tissue thickness and oxygenation, which could obscure the interaction of cystine and dibasic amino acids, were minimized. The isolated brush-border membrane vesicle preparation allowed the examination of the interaction of cystine and dibasic amino acids at the membrane locus of transport, without complications of cellular metabolism.

ISOLATED RENAL TUBULES

Isolated renal tubules were prepared using a modification[12,13] of the method described by Burg and Orloff[14]. Renal cortex from adult male Sprague–Dawley rats was finely minced and then digested in 0.375% collagenase for 45 min. The tubules were then washed free of collagenase and filtered through surgical gauze, such that only cortical tubular fragments remained, as shown in Figure 13.1. The uptake studies were performed in Krebs–Ringer bicarbonate buffer containing 5% fetal calf serum and 10 mmol/l sodium acetate in special flasks, which allowed continuous bubbling of O_2:CO_2 (95:5) through the incubation mixture. The results are expressed as a distribution ratio of radioactivity [ratio of cpm/ml of intracellular fluid to the cpm/ml of the medium].

Figure 13.2 demonstrates the progressive uptake of 0.025 mmol/l [^{35}S] cystine until a steady state, where influx of the tracer equalled efflux, was reached after 60 min of incubation with a distribution ratio of 38.58 ± 0.76. With 0.5 mmol/l [^{35}S]cystine as the substrate, the distribution ratio of radioactivity at each time point was lower than that observed with 0.025 mmol/l cystine, suggesting that the uptake of cystine by isolated renal tubules was saturable and carrier-mediated.

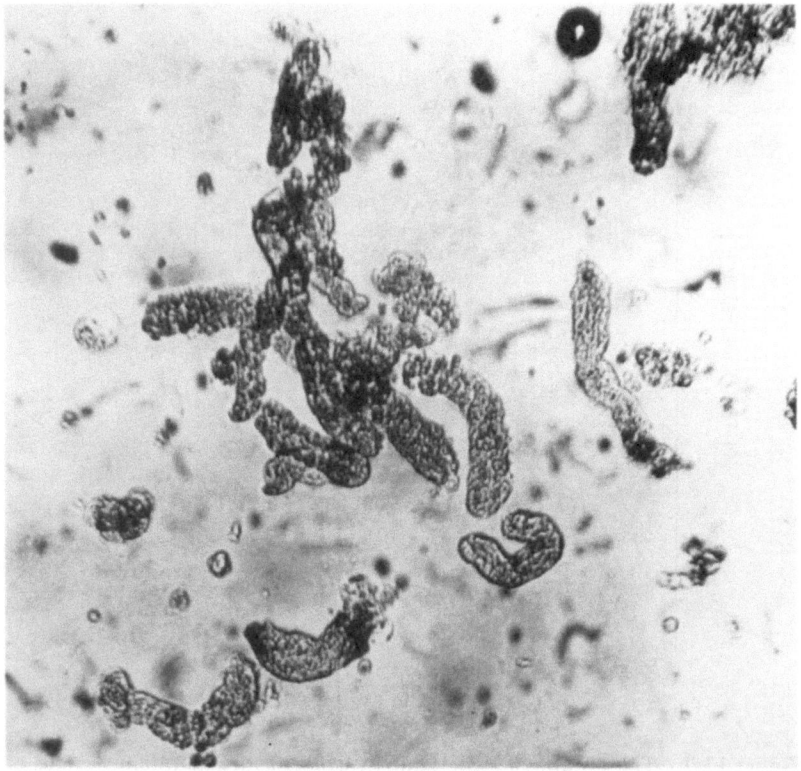

Figure 13.1 Microscopic appearance of isolated rat renal cortical tubule fragments. The tubule fragments were wet mounted in Krebs–Ringer bicarbonate buffer and stained with methylene blue (0.5%). Magnification 177×

The intracellular pool of radioactivity was analysed by thin-layer chromatography using N-ethylmaleimide to form stable adducts with cysteine and reduced glutathione. With 0.025 mmol/l [^{35}S]cystine as the substrate, over 90% of the intracellular ^{35}S was associated with the reduced form, cysteine. The remainder of the label was associated with cystine and reduced glutathione. With 0.5 mmol/l [^{35}S]cystine as the substrate, 45–50% of the intracellular ^{35}S was associated with cystine, while cysteine accounted for about 37–45% and reduced glutathione 11–14% of the label. Thus, a significant fraction of the [^{35}S]cystine taken up by the renal tubule cell was reduced to cysteine with lesser amounts incorporated into glutathione, findings similar to previous data obtained in

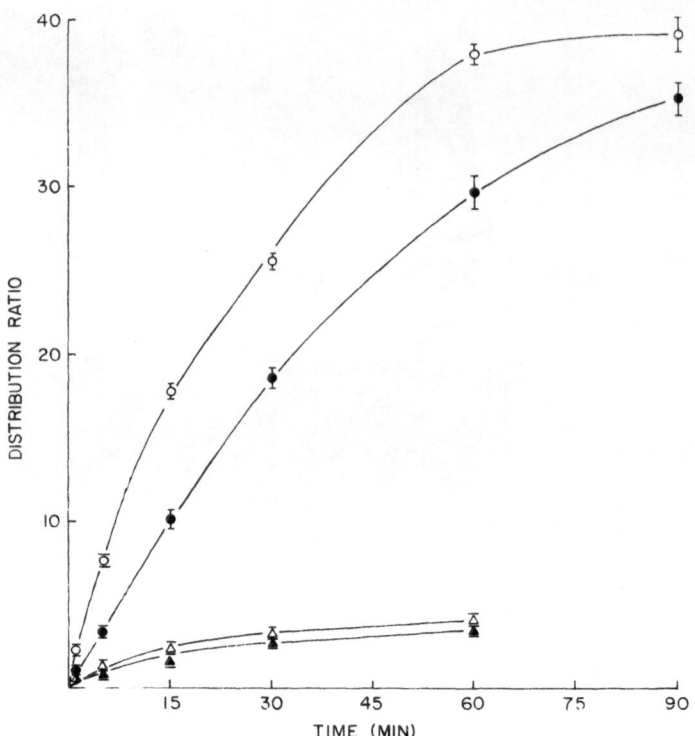

Figure 13.2   The uptake of [^{35}S]cystine by isolated cortical tubules versus time. Distribution ratio represents the ratio of cpm/ml intracellular fluid to cpm/ml of medium. Open circles represent the distribution ratios of 0.025 mmol/l [^{35}S] cystine and closed circles represent 0.025 mmol/l [^{35}S]cystine plus 3 mmol/l lysine. Open triangles represent the distribution ratios of 0.5 mmol/l [^{35}S]cystine and closed triangles represent 0.5 mmol/l [^{35}S]cystine plus 3 mmol/l lysine. From Foreman J. W. Hwang, S. M. and Segal, S. (1980). *Metabolism*, **29**, 53–61. Copyright 1980 Grune & Stratton, Inc.

renal cortical slices[15,16]. The distribution ratios of radioactivity do not, therefore, represent true concentration gradients.

   To study the effect of dibasic amino acids on the uptake of cystine, the uptake of 0.025 mmol/l and 0.5 mmol/l cystine was examined in the presence of 3 mmol/l lysine. As can be seen in Figure 13.2, lysine significantly inhibited the uptake 0.025 mmol/l cystine throughout the 90 min ($p<0.001$). However, the percentage of inhibition progressively declined from 51% after 1 min of incubation to 20% after 90 min, as the timed uptake curves of 0.025 mmol/l cystine in the presence and absence of 3 mmol/l lysine approached one another. With 0.5 mmol/l cystine as the substrate, there was only a slight reduction of cystine uptake by 3 mmol/l lysine. Similar results were obtained when the other dibasic amino acids, ornithine and arginine, were substituted for lysine.

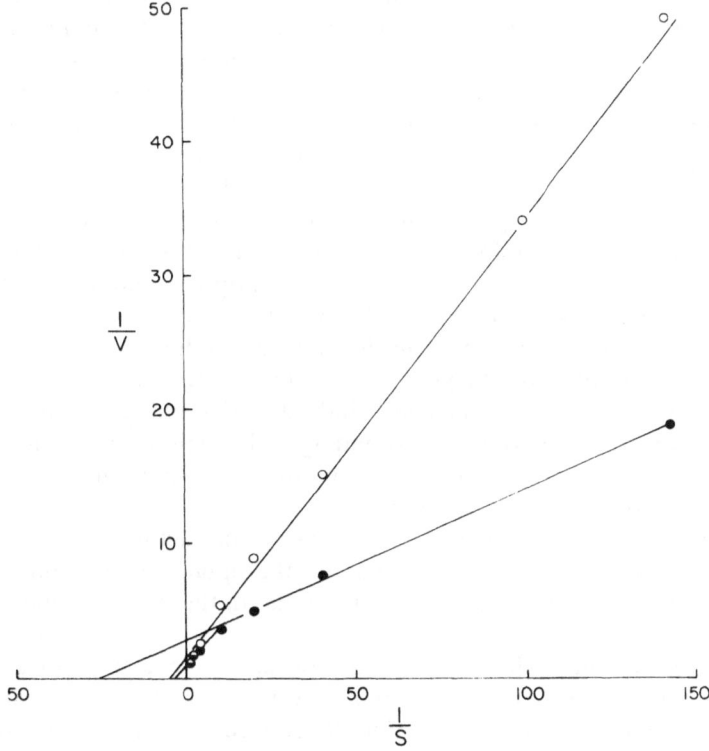

Figure 13.3 Lineweaver–Burk plot of the concentration dependence of cystine uptake after 5 min of incubation in the presence (○) and absence (●) of 3 mmol/l lysine. V represents the velocity of uptake (mmol/l intracellular fluid per 5 min) and S represents the substrate concentration (mmol/l). From Foreman, J. W., Hwang, S. M. and Segal, S. (1980). *Metabolism*, **29**, 53–61. Copyright 1980 by Grune & Stratton, Inc.

To examine more closely the nature of this inhibition of cystine uptake by lysine, the concentration dependence of cystine uptake was studied over the concentration range from 0.007 to 0.7 mmol/l cystine in the presence and absence of 3 mmol/l lysine. As shown in Figure 13.3 a Lineweaver–Burk plot of the concentration dependence revealed a two-limbed curve that is consistent with multiple transport systems for cystine uptake. The observed kinetic parameters from this plot were K_{m1} of 0.036 mmol/l, V_{max1} of 0.136 mmol/l intracellular fluid per 5 min and K_{m2} of 0.325 mmol/l, V_{max2} of 1.140 mmol/l intracellular fluid per 5 min. Using regression analysis of these data, the calculated kinetic parameters were K_{m1} of 0.012 mmol/l, V_{max1} of 0.096 mmol/l intracellular fluid per 5 min and K_{m2} of 0.55 mmol/l, V_{max2} of 1.280 mmol/l intracellular fluid per 5 min. In Figure 13.4, the percentage of total uptake via the low and high K_m systems vs. the media concentration of cystine is plotted. At a substrate concentration of 0.03 mmol/l, the uptake of cystine was equally divided between the two transport systems. With increasing concentrations, the percentage of the total uptake via the high K_m system assumed greater importance and vice-versa for the low K_m system. At the physiological concentration of cystine (0.06 mmol/l), both systems were important since 60% of total uptake entered via the high K_m system and 40% via the low K_m system.

When similar concentration dependence studies were performed in the presence of 3 mmol/l lysine (Figure 13.3), a Lineweaver-Burk plot of these data gave only a single line, indicating that only one component of transport was observed, corresponding to the high K_m system for cystine uptake. This suggested that the inhibition of cystine uptake by lysine occurred on the low K_m system.

Further support for cystine and lysine interacting with a common system came from studies examining the uptake of 0.01 mmol/l [14C] lysine by isolated rat renal-cortical tubules in the presence and absence of
1 mmol/l cystine. The distribution ratio after 5 min of incubation with 0.01 mmol/l lysine was 7.64 ± 0.08, but fell to 6.19 ± 0.17 ($p<0.01$) in the presence of 1 mmol/l cystine. Therefore, not only could the inhibition of cystine uptake by lysine be demonstrated, but the inhibition of lysine uptake by cystine could also be shown, strongly suggesting a common transport system.

ISOLATED RENAL BRUSH-BORDER MEMBRANE VESICLES

With the advent of the ability to isolate brush-border membranes from the proximal tubule and prepare vesicles from these membranes, the interaction of cystine and dibasic amino acids could be examined at the membrane locus of transport in the absence of cellular metabolism.

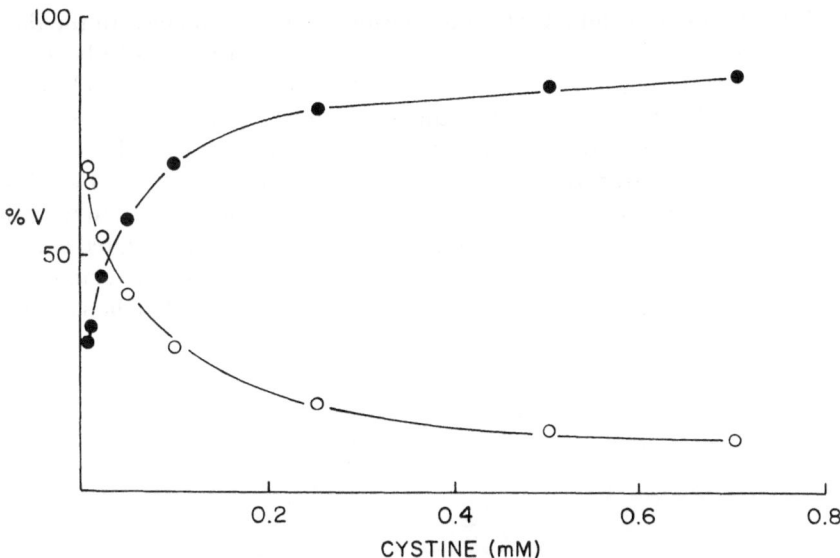

Figure 13.4   The percentage of total velocity ($\%V$) mediated via the high ($\bullet$) and low ($\circ$) K_m systems for cystine uptake versus the substrate concentration. From Foreman, J. W., Hwang, S. M. and Segal, S. (1980). *Metabolism*, **29**, 53–61. Copyright 1980 by Grune & Stratton, Inc.

These brush-border membrane vesicles were prepared by homogenization, Mg^{2+} precipitation and differential centrifugation of renal cortex from male Sprague–Dawley rats, according to the method described by Booth and Kenny[17]. An electron micrograph of a 'wet preparation' of these membrane vesicles which have been negatively stained with 4% phosphotungstic acid, pH 7.0, is shown in Figure 13.5 where the characteristic microvillar shape of the membranes can be seen. The membrane preparation showed an alkaline phosphatase enrichment of 12-fold compared to the starting material, supporting the contention that these vesicles are derived from the brush-border membrane. The uptake of [^{14}C]cystine into these vesicles was measured in the presence of a 100 mmol/l sodium gradient directed into the vesicle according to previously described methods[18]. Figure 13.6 shows a Lineweaver-Burk plot of the concentration dependence of the initial rate (0.5 min) of vesicle uptake of cystine from 0.018 to 0.89 mmol/l. The data revealed a two-limbed curve similar to that obtained with isolated cortical tubules. The observed transport parameters were K_{m1} of 0.031 mmol/l, V_{max1} of 0.322 nmol/mg protein per 0.5 min, and K_{m2} of 0.481 mmol/l, V_{max2} of

1.80 nmol/mg protein per 0.5 min. Using regression analysis of the data, the calculated kinetic parameters of transport were found to be K_{m1} of 0.033 mmol/l, V_{max1} of 0.205 nmol/mg protein per 0.5 min, and K_{m2} of 0.93 mmol/l, V_{max2} of 1.98 nmol/mg protein per 0.5 min. In the presence of 1 mmol/l lysine, the kinetic parameters were altered such that only one component of transport could be discerned, corresponding to the high K_m system (Figure 13.6). It thus appeared that lysine interacted with the low K_m system, again similar to the results obtained with isolated cortical tubules. However, no reduction of cystine to cysteine was detected when membrane vesicles were incubated for up to 30 min with labelled cystine.

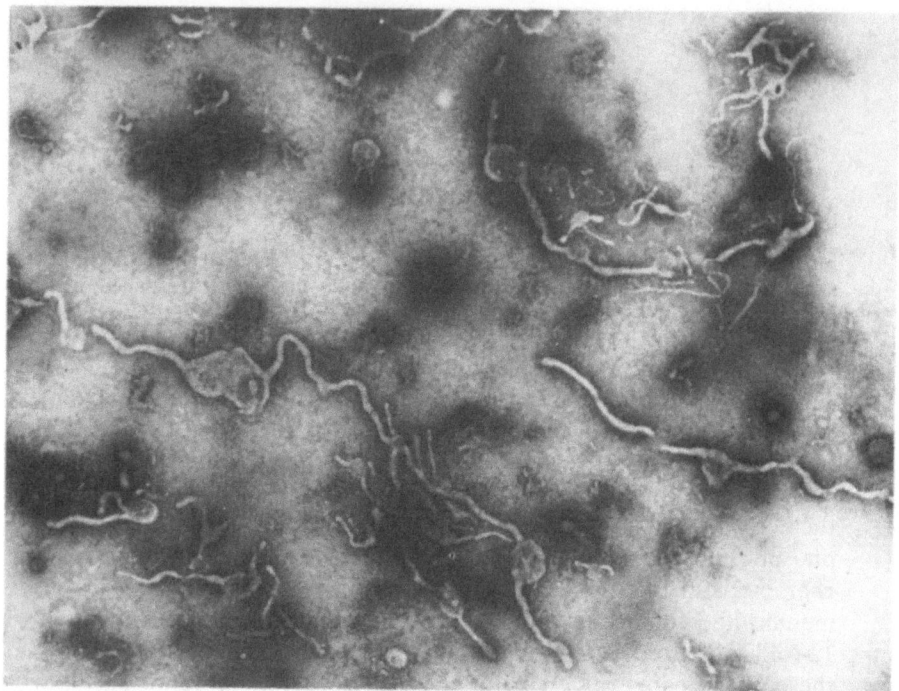

Figure 13.5 Electron micrograph of a 'wet preparation' of isolated renal brush-border membrane vesicles. These vesicles were negatively stained with 4% phosphotungstic acid (pH 7.0). Magnification 21 000 ×

The effect of several amino acids on the initial rate (0.5 min) of vesicle uptake of cystine in the presence of an inward sodium gradient was also examined (Table 13.1). At 0.027 mmol/l cystine, only dibasic amino acids at 1 mmol/l concentration caused a 55% inhibition. When the concentration of the competitor dibasics, arginine and lysine, was raised to 3 mmol/l, the inhibition of cystine uptake was increased to 67%. This 67% inhibition of 0.027 mmol/l cystine uptake by 3 mmol/l lysine and arginine correlated with the cessation of that amount of entry expected from the low K_m component (62%) of total transport. It can also be seen in Table 13.1 that a 25% reduction of vesicle uptake of 0.27 mmol/l cystine occurred in the presence of 1 mmol/l concentrations of the dibasic amino acids. This 25% inhibition of vesicle uptake of 0.27 mmol/l cystine by the dibasic amino acids again corresponded to cessation of that amount of entry expected from the low K_m component (29%) of total transport.

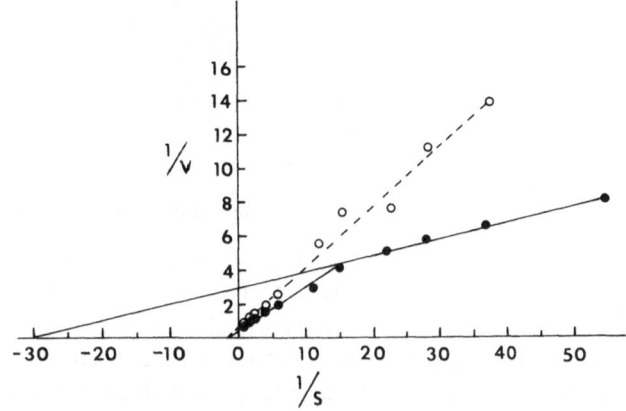

Figure 13.6 Influence of the L-cystine concentration and of 1 mmol/l L-lysine on the initial rate of cystine uptake by brush-border membrane vesicles. Solid circles represent uptake of L-[14C]cystine and open circles show its uptake in the presence of 1 mmol/l L-lysine. From Segal, S., McNamara, P. D. and Pepe, L. M. (1977). *Science*, **197**, 169–171. Copyright 1977 by the American Association for the Advancement of Science

DISCUSSION

Since Dent and Rose[1] postulated a common transport system for cystine and the dibasic amino acids, numerous *in vitro* attempts to confirm this hypothesis have been made. Cystine and the dibasic amino acids did appear to share a common transport system in studies with human jejunal mucosa[19]. With renal cortical slices from both humans[5] and rats[6], separate transport systems for cystine and the dibasic amino acids were observed.

TABLE 13.1   Effect of unlabelled amino acids on uptake of ^{14}C-labelled cystine by brush-border membrane vesicles

Additions	Concentration	Percentage of ^{14}C-cystine uptake (0.5 min) at	
	(mmol/l)	0.027 mmol/l	0.27 mmol/l
None		100.0 ± 4.3	100.0 ± 4.4
Arginine	1	45.8 ± 2.8*	72.6 ± 4.6*
	3	33.5 ± 4.8**	
Lysine	1	46.0 ± 2.8*	75.5 ± 3.0*
	3	33.2 ± 4.3**	
Ornithine	1	48.7 ± 3.7*	77.9 ± 3.6*
Glycine	1	88.1 ± 5.3	
Valine	1	102.9 ± 4.5	
α–Aminoisobutyric acid	1	102.2 ± 6.5	
Proline	1	85.6 ± 4.9	
Phenylalanine	1	88.0 ± 5.2	

Values given are means ± SE for 8–16 determinations
* $p < 0.01$ for differences from control
** $p < 0.05$ for differences between values with 3 mM and 1 mM of the same added amino acid
From Segal, S., McNamara, P. D. and Pepe, L. M. (1977). *Science*, **197**, 169–171.
Copyright 1977 by the American Association for the Advancement of Science

With the use of the isolated renal cortical tubule and the isolated renal brush-border membrane vesicle, a more complete picture of cystine and dibasic amino acid transport in the proximal tubule has emerged. Cystine uptake by the isolated cortical tubule occurred via two saturable transport systems. With the brush-border membrane preparation, two comparable (Table 13.2) transport systems for cystine were demonstrated. It would appear from these data that transport across the luminal side of the proximal tubule cell can be observed with the renal cortical tubule, although transport across the basal–lateral membrane, which does occur[20], may also be observed. With the renal cortical slice, only one component of cystine transport was demonstrated corresponding to the high K_m system observed with both the renal cortical tubule and brush-border membrane vesicle. Because only the high K_m system was observed in the slice, an interaction between cystine and the dibasic amino acids would not be expected since this interaction appeared to occur on the low K_m system. Similarly, the one K_m system that was demonstrated in human jejunal mucosa[19] seemed to correlate with the low K_m system observed with the tubule and the vesicle, since an interaction between cystine and the dibasic amino acids was demonstrated.

TABLE 13.2 K_m values for cystine uptake

Preparation	K_{m1} (mM)	K_{m2} (mM)
Renal cortical slice	—	0.80
Renal cortical tubule	0.012	0.55
Brush-border membrane vesicle	0.033	0.90

From this evidence for a common transport system for cystine and the dibasic amino acids, some aspects of human cystinuria may be explicable, and a model for cystine and dibasic amino acid transport is shown in Figure 13.7. At physiological concentrations in the glomerular ultrafiltrate, cystine uptake is nearly equally divided between the two K_m systems as determined from Figure 13.4. A defective low K_m system, which may occur in classical human cystinuria, would result in significant amounts of cystine appearing in the final urine. Because this low K_m system also interacts with the dibasic amino acids, hyperdibasic aminoaciduria in human cystinuria appears explicable. Increased cystine excretion after infusion of dibasic amino acids in normal dogs[4] and humans[2,3] also seems explicable.

Further extension of this model for cystine transport in the renal tubular cell to explain the defect in patients with other disorders of cystine and dibasic amino-acid transport can possibly be made. Cystinuric patients who do not have hyperdibasicaminoaciduria[8] may have a defect in the high K_m system that does not appear to interact with the dibasic amino acids. Similarly, dibasic amino acid uptake has been shown to be mediated by two saturable systems[6], and the possibility

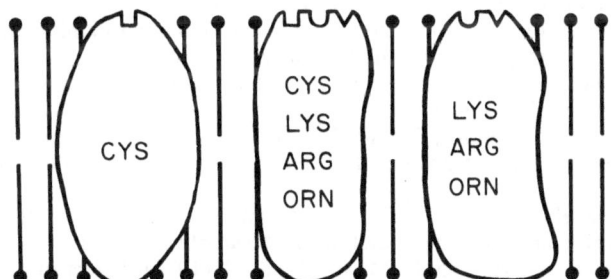

Figure 13.7 Schematic diagram of a membrane from the renal tubule cell showing the possible diversity of carrier proteins for cystine (cys), lysine (lys) and the other dibasic amino acids, arginine (arg) and ornithine (orn)

arises that cystine interacts with only one, explaining the isolated hyperdibasicaminoaciduria described in some patients[9,10]. Remaining to be explained, however, is the apparent secretion of cystine by humans[21,22] and dogs[11] with cystinuria, as well as the interaction of cysteine and the dibasic amino acids in the efflux transport process of renal tubule cells[23]. Although the nature of cystine reabsorption in the kidney is more complex than originally formulated, the common transport system for cystine and the dibasic amino acids proposed by Dent and Rose has been substantiated after many years of research.

References

1. Dent, C. E. and Rose, G. A. (1951). Amino acid metabolism in cystinuria. *Q. J. Med.*, **20,** 25
2. Robson, E. B. and Rose, G. A. (1957). The effect of intravenous lysine on the renal clearances of cystine, arginine, and ornithine in normal subjects, in patients with cystinuria and Fanconi syndrome and their relatives. *Clin. Sci.*, **16,** 75
3. Kato, T. (1977). Renal handling of dibasic amino acids and cystine in cystinuria. *Clin. Sci. Mol. Med.*, **53,** 9
4. Webber, W. A., Brown, J. L. and Pitts, R. F. (1961). Interaction of amino acids in renal tubular transport. *Am. J. Physiol.*, **200,** 380.
5. Fox, M., Thier, S., Rosenberg, L., Kiser, W. and Segal, S. (1964). Evidence against a single renal transport defect in cystinuria. *N. Engl. J. Med.*, **270,** 556
6. Rosenberg, L. E., Downing, S. J. and Segal, S. (1962). Competitive inhibition of dibasic amino acid transport in rat kidney. *J. Biol. Chem.*, **237,** 2265
7. Silbernagl, S. and Deetjen, G. (1972). The tubular reabsorption of L-cystine and L-cysteine: A common transport system with L-arginine or not? *Pflügers Arch.*, **337,** 277
8. Brodehl, J., Gellissen, K. and Kowelewski, S. (1967). Isolierte Cystinurie (ohne Lysin-, Ornithin-, and Arginin- urie) in einer Familie mit hypocalcamischer Tetanie. *Monatsschr. Kinderheil.*, **115,** 317
9. Whelan, D. T. and Scriver, C. R. (1968). Hyperdibasic aminoaciduria: An inherited disorder of amino acid transport. *Pediatr. Res.*, **2,** 525
10. Oyanagi, K., Muira, R. and Yamanouchi, T. (1970). Congenital lysinuria: A new inherited transport disorder of dibasic amino acids. *J. Pediatr.*, **77,** 259
11. Bovee, K. C., Thier, S. O., Rea, C. and Segal, S. (1974). Renal clearance of amino acids in canine cystinuria. *Metabolism*, **23,** 51
12. Roth, K. S., Hwang, S. M. and Segal, S. (1976). Effect of maleic acid on the kinetics of α-methyl-D-glucoside uptake by isolated rat renal tubules. *Biochim. Biophys. Acta*, **426,** 675
13. Foreman, J. W. and Segal, S. (1979). Hypoxanthine uptake in isolated rat renal cortex tubule fragments. *J. Clin. Invest.*, **63,** 765

14. Burg, M. B. and Orloff, J. (1962). Oxygen consumption and active transport in separated renal tubules. *Am. J. Physiol.*, **203**, 327
15. Crawhall, J. C. and Segal, S. (1967). The intracellular ratio of cysteine and cystine in various tissues. *Biochem. J.*, **105**, 891
16. Segal, S. and Smith, I. (1969). Delineation of cystine and cysteine transport systems in rat kidney cortex by developmental patterns. *Proc. Natl. Acad. Sci. USA*, **63**, 926
17. Booth, A. G. and Kenny, A. J. (1974). A rapid method for the preparation of microvilli from rabbit kidney. *Biochem. J.*, **142**, 575
18. McNamara, P. D., Ožegović, B., Pepe, L. M. and Segal, S. (1976). Proline and glycine uptake by rat kidney cortex brush border membrane vesicles. *Proc. Natl. Acad. Sci. USA*, **73**, 4521
19. Thier, S. O., Segal, S., Fox, M., Blair, A. and Rosenberg, L. E. (1965). Cystinuria: defective intestinal transport of dibasic amino acids and cystine. *J. Clin. Invest.*, **46**, 1162
20. Greth, W., Thier, S. O. and Segal, S. (1973). The cellular accumulation of L-cystine in rat kidney cortex *in vivo*. *J. Clin. Invest.*, **52**, 454
21. Crawhall, J. C., Scowen, E. F., Thompson, C. J. and Watts, R. W. E. (1967). The renal clearance of amino acids in cystinuria. *J. Clin. Invest.*, **46**, 1162
22. Morin, C. L., Thompson, M. W., Jackson, S. H. and Sass-Korsak, A. (1971). Biochemical and genetic studies in cystinuria: observations on double heterozygotes of genotype I/II. *J. Clin. Invest.*, **50**, 1961
23. Schwartzman, L., Blair, A. and Segal, S. (1966). A common renal transport system for lysine, ornithine, arginine, and cysteine. *Biochem. Biophys. Res. Commun.*, **23**, 220.

14

5-Oxoprolinuria and other inborn errors related to the γ-glutamyl cycle

A. Larsson

Glutathione (γ-L-glutamyl-L-cysteinyl-glycine) was isolated by Hopkins more than 50 years ago[1]. Initial analyses of the peptide indicated that it contained glutamic acid and cysteine, and the compound was therefore named glutathione. Its composition was revised and the correct structure was established in 1929[2]. Since then glutathione has been identified in virtually all cells, from micro-organisms to man.

The biosynthesis and degradation of glutathione occurs via a series of enzyme reactions called the γ-glutamyl cycle (Figure 14.1)[3]. Meister and Tate[4] have recently reviewed glutathione metabolism. Glutathione has been postulated to be involved in a variety of metabolic processes[5]. In addition to its potential role as a scavenger for free radicals in the cell, it has been suggested that glutathione participates in the active transport of amino acids across cell membranes[6]. A recent hypothetical function for glutathione is its participation in the synthesis of transmitters in the central nervous system[7].

Several inborn errors in glutathione metabolism have been described during the last decade. By mutual efforts in basic science and clinical medicine, patients with such genetic defects can help us to clarify the bio-

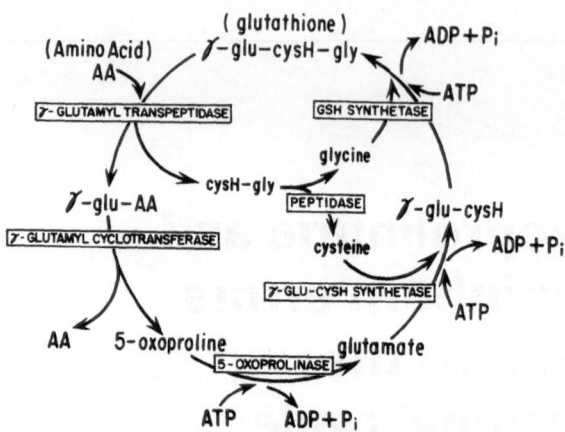

Figure 14.1   The γ-glutamyl cycle

logical role(s) of glutathione and in return they will be offered better diagnostic procedures, treatment and, hopefully, preventive measures. In the present chapter, emphasis will be placed on the possible role of glutathione in the active transport of amino acids, in the light of the present knowledge of human genetic defects in the metabolism of glutathione.

THE γ-GLUTAMYL CYCLE

Glutathione is located predominantly intracellularly. The concentrations range from 0.5 to 10 mmol/kg in several mammalian tissues and thus often exceed those of free amino acids in the cell. The glutathione molecule has two functional residues, the sulphydryl and the γ-glutamyl residues, by which it participates in a variety of metabolic reactions.

The biosynthesis and degradation of glutathione is catalysed by six enzymes interacting in the γ-glutamyl cycle (Figure 14.1). The formation of glutathione from its constituent amino acids is catalysed by two enzymes, γ-glutamyl-cysteine synthetase and glutathione synthetase. The initial step in the degradation is catalysed by γ-glutamyl transpeptidase. This enzyme transfers the γ-glutamyl residue of glutathione to amino-acid acceptors. This leads to the synthesis of γ-glutamyl dipeptides, which are subsequently hydrolysed by γ-glutamyl cyclotransferase into 5-oxoproline (pyroglutamic acid). 5-oxoproline is then cleaved by 5-oxoprolinase into glutamate. Cysteinyl-glycine, formed in the transpeptidase reaction, is split by dipeptidase. The constituents of glutathione are thus returned to the free pools of the corresponding amino acids and they can readily be utilized for the resynthesis of glutathione. For each turn in the γ-glutamyl cycle, three molecules of ATP are converted into ADP and Pi.

The enzymes of the γ-glutamyl cycle have been isolated and characterized[4]. The presence of these enzymes has been demonstrated in a number of different tissues and there is general agreement that the γ-glutamyl cycle plays a significant role in the turnover of glutathione. The location of the γ-glutamyl cycle enzymes within the cell is somewhat remarkable. One of the enzymes, γ-glutamyl transpeptidase, is bound to the membranes of a variety of epithelial cells, whereas the remaining enzymes are soluble in the cytoplasm[8]. An interesting observation with regard to the function of γ-glutamyl transpeptidase has recently been made by Tate and Orlando[9]. They studied a pure preparation of the enzyme from rat kidney and obtained evidence that the γ-glutamyl transpeptidase also has glutathione oxidase activity catalysing the conversion of glutathione to glutathione disulphide. Another catalytic property of one of the two subunits in γ-glutamyl transpeptidase is a peptidase activity[10]. The role of the newly discovered catalytic activities apparently inherent to γ-glutamyl transpeptidase remains to be clarified.

Regulation of glutathione biosynthesis is apparently exerted by means of feedback inhibition by glutathione exerted on the initial enzyme, γ-glutamyl-cysteine synthetase[11,12]. As discussed below, the function *in vivo* of the postulated regulation was confirmed by studies of one of the inborn errors of glutathione metabolism, 5-oxoprolinuria[13].

The lack of certain of the γ-glutamyl cycle enzymes in normal erythrocytes has challenged the functional role of the γ-glutamyl cycle[14]. For instance, erythrocytes lack 5-oxoprolinase[15] and also contain very little, if any, γ-glutamyl transpeptidase activity[16]. Such cells seem to have an incomplete enzyme content to allow an operating γ-glutamyl cycle. It would be possible to metabolize 5-oxoproline generated in erythrocytes if this metabolite were transported to some tissue with high 5-oxoprolinase activity, such as the kidney. It would be more difficult to visualize inter-organ cooperation substituting for the lack of γ-glutamyl transpeptidase in erythrocytes. As a matter of principle, the question about the absence of γ-glutamyl transpeptidase in erythrocytes is important. Glutathione in human erythrocytes has a half-life of approximately 4 days[17]. It has been postulated that transport of oxidized glutathione from the red cells accounts for a significant part of the glutathione turnover. This has recently seemed less likely since the rate of efflux of oxidized glutathione was found to be too low[18].

The inter-organ transport as a model for glutathione turnover has, however, recently gained new interest. Thus Griffith and Meister[19] postulated that glutathione is normally translocated from tissues with relatively low γ-glutamyl transpeptidase activity, such as liver, via the blood plasma to tissues with high activity, such as kidney. This would involve considerable instability in the small extracellular pool of gluta-thione, which remains to be established. It is remarkable, however, that the relative activities of the γ-glutamyl cycle enzymes are very variable in different tissues. Furthermore, there is considerable difference between fetal and adult tissue with respect to some of these enzymes. For instance in the rat, γ-glutamyl transpeptidase activity decreases markedly post-natally in the liver, but increases in the kidney[20].

Several enzymes are involved in the metabolism of glutathione outside the γ-glutamyl cycle. Glutathione reductase is one of these and the bio-logical role of this enzyme has recently been reviewed[21]. Others, such as glutathione peroxidase and glutathione transferases will, however, not be considered in the following presentation.

BIOLOGICAL ROLES OF GLUTATHIONE

Glutathione has been postulated to be involved in a variety of biological functions. Some of these processes have been considered in detail in a recent review[5]. Often glutathione participates by means of its sulphydryl group. This is illustrated by a number of fundamental processes such as the detoxification of reactive metabolites formed from acetaminophen and other xenobiotica, by metabolism in the liver[22], and the protection of cells against free radicals formed after high energy irradiation[23].

Two additional functions for glutathione have been recently postula-ted, one being of specific interest in the field of inborn errors of metab-olism. Lindblad et al.[24] have postulated an attractive model to account for the severe liver and kidney damage in hereditary tyrosinaemia. According to these authors, the primary enzymatic defect is localized to fumaryl acetoacetase. Consequently, fumaryl acetoacetate and maleyl acetoacetate accumulate and these compounds, which are highly reac-tive, will eventually lead to irreversible damage of the liver cell. It has been postulated that the sulphydryl groups of glutathione are able to protect the cells from such damage. This is in principle an extension of the model for acetaminophen detoxification mentioned above. An alter-native function for glutathione has recently been postulated. This is related to glutaredoxin, a protein which has been identified in *Escherichia coli*[25,26]. In the presence of glutaredoxin, glutathione acts as hydrogen donor in the synthesis of deoxyribonucleotides catalysed by ribonucleotide reductase. Glutathione and glutathione reductase thus work as an alternative to the thioredoxin system, which has previously been identified in *Escherichia coli* as well as in mammalian cells[27,28].

The involvement of the γ-glutamyl residue of glutathione in the active transport of amino acids was proposed by Meister and coworkers[3,6]. According to their model, the turnover of glutathione in the γ-glutamyl cycle is linked to the translocation of amino acids across cell membranes. The γ-glutamyl transpeptidase is membrane bound in many epithelial cells and is postulated to interact with free amino acids outside the cell and with glutathione inside the cell (Figure 14.1). The amino acid is then transferred across the cell membrane where it is released as a γ-glutamyl dipeptide. It is finally released from its γ-glutamyl carrier by the action of γ-glutamyl-cyclotransferase. The model was proposed on very little experimental evidence obtained *in vivo*. Activities of the γ-glutamyl cycle enzymes were ubiquitous and they were high especially in epithelial cells involved in active transport of amino acids. For instance, by histochemical techniques it could be demonstrated that γ-glutamyl transpeptidase was particularly abundant in the brush border of the proximal convolute tubule in the kidney, the choroid plexus, small intestinal mucosa and the ciliary body of the eye[29]. In addition to indirect evidence, the γ-glutamyl cycle model for amino-acid transport was supported by animal experiments using inhibitors to different enzymes in the γ-glutamyl cycle[29]. Meister and his co-workers have presented additional evidence that the γ-glutamyl cycle plays a significant role in the overall transport of amino acids. Their most recent contributions with animal experiments have substantiated their previous observations[30]. Although the γ-glutamyl cycle model for amino-acid transport has several attractive features, it still remains to be established.

Glutathione has been postulated to participate in a number of processes. *A priori* it might seem surprising that inborn errors of metabolism have indeed been recognized in clinical medicine with enzymatic defects localized to the γ-glutamyl cycle. More work on the biochemistry of glutathione in such patients, normal individuals and various experimental systems will be necessary in order to understand the clinical conditions concerned. And *vice versa*, careful studies of patients with different disorders in the metabolism of glutathione may be of help in determining which of the postulated functions of glutathione are of biological significance.

γ-GLUTAMYL CYSTEINE SYNTHETASE DEFICIENCY

Hereditary deficiency of γ-glutamyl cysteine synthetase has so far been reported in only two siblings[31,32]. Both suffered from increased rate of haemolysis since childhood, with intermittent episodes of anaemia and jaundice. At the age of 29 years one of the siblings, a woman, became psychotic and anaemic after treatment with sulphonamide. At 35 years of age they had developed mild ataxia, impaired coordination and dysmetria. The male had developed muscular weakness and ataxia at the age of 36 years and exhibited decreased vibratory and position sensation in the extremities, with dysmetria and dysdiadochokinesis. When examined one year later, he had developed irregular staccato speech and myoclonic spasms in one leg. An electromyogram indicated myopathy in the brother, and both patients had electrocardiograms with ST-segment and T-wave changes. So, in addition to haemolytic anaemia, both patients showed progressive degeneration of the neuromuscular system. They also had markedly decreased levels of γ-glutamyl cysteine synthetase in erythrocytes, i.e. 2–7% of the normal activity. The levels of glutathione were 3% in erythrocytes, 40% in leukocytes and 25% in muscle. In contrast, the levels of glutathione synthetase in erythrocytes were normal. This indicates that the enzymatic defect was localized to the initial step in the biosynthesis of glutathione and that it was expressed in several types of cells. A remarkable finding was a rather generalized aminoaciduria[32]. Both siblings had virtually identical patterns of excretion involving dibasic amino acids (lysine, arginine and cystine) and monobasic/monocarboxylic amino acids (alanine, valine, asparagine, glutamine and threonine). In serum, moderately increased levels were observed for alanine, valine, asparagine, threonine, glutamine and lysine. Unfortunately, no further reports of amino acid levels and transport have appeared concerning these or other patients with γ-glutamyl cysteine synthetase deficiency. It is, of course, tempting to consider renal aminoaciduria in the patients as evidence in favour of the involvement of the γ-glutamyl cycle in the active transport of amino acids in the kidney. However, the causal relationship between the lack of γ-glutamyl cysteine synthetase, deficiency of glutathione and the defective renal handling of several amino acids needs further clarification.

GLUTATHIONE SYNTHETASE DEFICIENCY
WITHOUT 5-OXOPROLINURIA

The first reports of patients with genetic defects in the synthesis of glutathione were published by Oort *et al.*[33] and Prins *et al.*[34]. Compensated haemolytic anaemia was the only symptom observed, and decreased levels of glutathione in erythrocytes occurred in several relatives. Deficiency of glutathione synthetase in red blood cells was demonstrated in two adult patients with haemolytic anaemia[35]. The same enzyme defect was later found in a 32-year-old man[36] and a 27-year-old woman[37]. Thus four patients with glutathione synthetase deficiency in erythrocytes have been reported; their common symptom being a haemolytic anaemia, which usually was well compensated. Splenomegaly has been observed in three of the patients and one of them[36] also had fever, lymphopenia and monocytosis and a diagnosis of Hodgkin's disease was entertained. This patient was splenectomized in connection with abdominal exploration and Hodgkin's disease was ruled out. There are no reports of neonatal jaundice in patients with erythrocyte glutathione synthetase deficiency[37]. Their neurological development is normal. In the three reported French patients there is no metabolic acidosis and no excretion of 5-oxoproline in the urine[37].

Unfortunately there are no reports of the levels of glutathione or glutathione synthetase in cells from these patients other than erythrocytes, but it has been speculated that their enzymatic defect is limited to red blood cells[38]. This could, for instance, involve a structural gene-mutation yielding decreased stability but normal catalytic activity. Erythrocytes which are unable to maintain continuous synthesis of new enzyme molecules would therefore express the defect, whereas nucleated cells could retain a sufficient amount of active enzyme molecules. This hypothesis could be tested experimentally. Although definite proof of this model is still lacking, it seems reasonable to assume that patients with glutathione synthetase deficiency without 5-oxoprolinuria have a defect localized to erythrocytes. They exhibit haemolytic anaemia as the only symptom to be recognized so far. Thus they show no neurological symptoms.

GLUTATHIONE SYNTHETASE DEFICIENCY WITH 5-OXOPROLINURIA

5-Oxoproline (pyroglutamic acid, pyrrolidone carboxylic acid) is an intermediate in the γ-glutamyl cycle (Figure 14.1). It is a cyclic amide of glutamate which is ninhydrin negative and usually not detected by conventional colorimetric reactions. The levels of 5-oxoproline in mammalian tissues and body fluid are very low[3].

The first case of 5-oxoprolinuria (pyroglutamic aciduria) was described in 1970[39]. The patient was then 19 years old and he developed a near-fatal metabolic acidosis after an operation for hiatus hernia[40]. In the subsequent examination he excreted massive amounts of 5-oxoproline in the urine. The patient suffered from a variety of signs of neurological damage including mental retardation, ataxia, impaired coordination and spastic tetraparesis. He was described as being jaundiced and seriously ill in the neonatal period, but recovered spontaneously. During childhood he presented neurological symptoms and there was a very definite progression of his neurological damage. Apparently he had a chronic metabolic acidosis which he had been able to compensate for until the operation at 19 years of age.

The first reported infants with 5-oxoprolinuria were two sisters who developed chronic metabolic acidosis during the first few days of life and have needed correction with bicarbonate continuously ever since[41,42]. So far twelve patients with 5-oxoprolinuria have been reported, some in more detail than others. Their clinical and biochemical characteristics are summarized in Table 14.1.

The typical clinical picture involves onset of symptoms during the first few days of life. A combination of metabolic acidosis, jaundice and haemolytic anaemia is frequent. This is a well-known triad which predisposes to bilirubin encephalopathy, and perhaps some of the neurological symptoms registered might in fact be the result of neonatal hyperbilirubinaemia. Acidosis correction is needed, and eventually exchange transfusions or phototherapy have to be performed. The need for continuous acidosis correction soon becomes apparent, and sodium bicarbonate or citrate are usually given orally. There is often, but apparently not always, an increased rate of haemolysis which is usually well compensated, but haemolytic crises can occur, and transfusions might then be needed. Viral infections have been suspected to precipitate such crises[43]. So far there is no evidence that specific drugs or foodstuffs can induce haemolytic episodes. As a precaution, however, our group has avoided treatment of patients with 5-oxoprolinuria with compounds which are known to cause haemolytic crises in individuals with glucose-6-phosphate dehydrogenase deficiency. Attacks of haemolytic anaemia usually subside spontaneously. Eventually the intake of bicarbonate or citrate has to be increased temporarily to compensate the acidosis. However, the acidosis may become complicated by secondary disturbance of the electrolyte homeostasis. The condition might then progress and at least one patient has, in fact, died in irreversible acidosis (Table 14.1).

The somatic development is usually uncomplicated but psychomotor development is not uniform (Table 14.1). Some patients are reported to be normal at 10 years of age, whereas others show signs of developmental delay already during infancy (Table 14.1). It is not yet possible to decide if this heterogeneity reflects varying degrees of enzyme deficiency, the timing of the start of acidosis correction therapy or some as yet unknown factor. It is notable that patient No. 1 showing the most advanced neurological symptoms was not given acidosis correction until the age of 19 years (Table 14.1). The same patient also exhibited progressive neurological involvement starting at school age. It is therefore difficult, at present, to speculate about the prognosis in young children with the same metabolic defect. Apparently there seems to be an over-representation of neurological damage among these patients.

The Norwegian patient (case 1, Table 14.1) showed progressive neurological deterioration. He died at 28 years of age and the immediate cause of death was pulmonary embolism. At autopsy a series of neuroanatomical abnormalities were found, including multiple infarctions and more specific cerebellar changes (E. Jellum, personal communication, 1979).

When increased rate of haemolysis was observed in two patients with 5-oxoprolinuria, studies of the glutathione metabolism in erythrocytes were started. Markedly decreased levels of glutathione were then observed[42] and the primary enzymatic defect was subsequently localized to the glutathione synthetase reaction of the γ-glutamyl cycle[44]. This has subsequently been confirmed in other patients (Table 14.1).

The mode of inheritance is autosomal recessive and heterozygotes for the defect can be identified by analysis of the levels of glutathione synthetase in erythrocytes[45]. A Swedish pedigree affected by 5-oxoprolinuria is shown in Figure 14.2. The five heterozygotes were clinically healthy.

The mechanism of over-production of 5-oxoproline is outlined in Figure 14.3. The primary metabolic error is the lack of glutathione synthetase in several, maybe all, tissues leading to a deficiency of glutathione which has a key role as a feedback inhibitor of the initial step in its own biosynthesis. The lack of the inhibitor results in excessive production of γ-glutamyl-cysteine which is converted to 5-oxoproline and cysteine by γ-glutamyl cyclotransferase. The excessive production of 5-oxoproline exceeds the endogenous 5-oxoprolinase activity. Thus 5-oxoproline accumulates in body fluids with concomitant renal overflow. This model has been substantiated by studies of erythrocytes[13] as well as purified γ-glutamyl cysteine synthetase from rat kidney[12]. The turnover of 5-oxoproline in vivo has been studied in patients 1 and 2 using ^{14}C-5- oxoproline[41,46]. These studies revealed that the rate of endogenous synthesis developmental milestones (Table 14.1). Some patients are reported to be normal at 10 years of age, whereas others show signs of development or delay already during infancy (Table 14.1). It is not yet possible to assess if this heterogeneity reflects varying degrees of enzyme deficiency, the timing of the stress periods, correction that over some as yet obscure factor. It is possible that patient 3, showing the least...

number of symptoms, may have... type of disease...

The Norwegian patient (no. 1, Table 14.1) showed glutathione accumulation downregulation of 16 and at 26 years of age and the normality...

symptoms of a complex symptoms include neurological retardation...

TABLE 14.1 Clinical and biochemical findings in 12 patients with glutathione synthetase deficiency associated with 5-oxoprolinuria

Patient no.	Country	Sex	Age at diagnosis	Age when last described	Neonatal onset of symptoms
1	Norway	M	19 y	24 y	+
2	Sweden	F	12 mon	7 y	+
3	Sweden	F	1 day	4 y	+
4	France	M	1 y	1 y	+
5	USA	M	1 week	2½ y	+
6	W. Germany	F	Post mortem	6 mon	+
7	W. Germany	M	4 y	7 y	+
8	France	M	?	10 y	+
9	France	M	?	8 y	+
10	France	F	9 mon	9 mon	+
11	Canada	?	2½ y	2½ y	+
12	USA	M	?	?	+

TABLE 14.1   (*continued*)

Chronic metabolic acidosis	Age when acidosis correction therapy was started	Neonatal jaundice	Haemolytic anaemia
+	19 y	+	−
+	3 days	+	+
+	1 day	+	+
+	neonatal period	−	−
+	2 days	+	+
+	1 day	+	+
+	2 h	+	+
−	—	+	+
−	—	+	+
+	neonatal period	+	+
+	1 day	+	+
+	?	?	+

TABLE 14.1 (continued)

Patient no.	Erythrocyte levels of glutathione (% of control)	Erythrocyte levels of glutathione synthetase (% of control)
1	0	1.4
2	16	1.6
3	8	2.0
4	10	0
5	9	1.7
6	not done	not done
7	< 10	2.0
8	7	0
9	8	0
10	16	0
11	25	5
12	?	—

TABLE 14.1 (*continued*)

Urinary 5-oxoproline excretion (mmol/24 h)	*Psychomotor development/Neurological symptoms/*
250	Severe mental retardation, spastic tetraparesis, ataxia, intentional tremor, epileptic seizures
60	Normal development quotients. No neurological symptoms
27	Normal psychomotor development. No neurological symptoms
70	No neurological symptoms at 1 year of age
40*	Normal psychomotor development at 1 year of age. No neurological symptoms
not done	Psychomotor development retarded. Nystagmus. Macular degeneration
110*	Mental retardation. DQ 51 at 4 years of age. Macular degeneration
12	Normal psychomotor development at 10 years of age. No neurological symptoms
9	Normal psychomotor development at 8 years of age. No neurological symptoms
30	No neurological symptoms at 9 months of age
increased	Delayed speech and psychomotor development. Ataxia. Abnormal sleep EEG
?	—

* mmol 5-oxoproline/mmol creatinine

TABLE 14.1 (*continued*)

Patient no.	Additional comments	References
1	Progressive course. The patient died 28 years old; pulmonary embolism immediate cause of death. Autopsy revealed a series of CNS changes, e.g. disseminated infarctions and cerebellar lesions (Jellum, personal communication).	39,52
2	—	41,53
3	Sibling of patient 2	42,53
4	—	37,75
5	Repeated episodes of suspected bacterial otitis media associated with neuropenia. Therapeutic trial with vitamin E	50,76
6	Several episodes of anaemia, vomiting, diarrhoea and sub-ileus. Died of therapy-resistant acidosis at 6 months of age. Diagnosis rests on clinical symptoms identical to those of the brother (patient 7). Parents are heterozygous for glutathione synthetase deficiency.	43
7	Episodes of anaemia. Aminoaciduria during periods of acidosis incompensation.	43
8	—	37
9	Sibling of patient 8	37
10	—	37
11	Therapeutic trial with vitamin E in progress. (Mendelson, personal communication)	
12	Sibling of case 5. Prophylactic treatment with vitamin E started neonatally	50

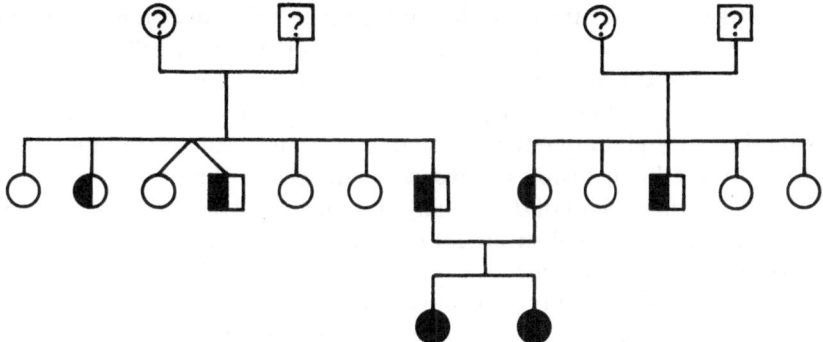

Figure 14.2 Swedish pedigree affected by 5-oxoprolinuria

was two to four times higher than the rate of excretion in the urine. In an adult patient this would mean a daily production of approximately 600 mmol (77 g) of 5-oxoproline.

Initially it was speculated[47,48] that the enzymatic defect was localized to the 5-oxoprolinase reaction. This hypothesis was rendered unlikely by the finding of normal levels of this enzyme activity in leukocytes[41] and definitely disproved by subsequent work which established a mechanism for 5-oxoproline over-production indicated in Figure 14.3.

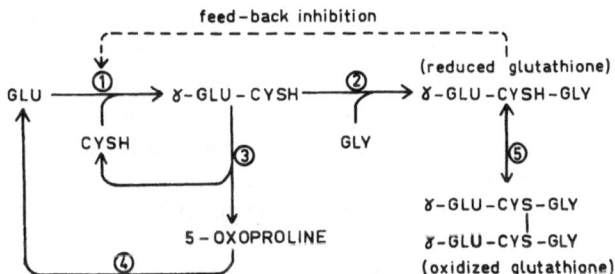

Figure 14.3 Enzymatic steps involved in the biosynthesis of glutathione. 1. γ-glutamyl-cysteine synthetase: 2 glutathione synthetase (deficient in 5-oxoprolinuria); 3. γ-glutamyl cyclotransferase; 4, 5-oxoprolinase; 5. glutathione reductase. Only the enzymatic reactions directly relevant to 5-oxoprolinuria are shown

This model offers several possible therapeutic approaches in this form of 5-oxoprolinuria. In theory, administration of glutathione to these patients would be attractive, but unfortunately this does not seem possible since the rate of transport of glutathione across cell membranes seems to be too slow. Various compounds have been shown to repress the excessive formation of γ-glutamyl-cysteine *in vitro*[13] and one potent inhibitor of γ-glutamyl-cysteine synthetase was found, cystamine[49] but it has not yet been tested *in vivo*. An alternative therapeutic approach involves replacement of the missing glutathione by some sulphydryl compound which could substitute for glutathione in a variety of fundamental processes without necessarily affecting the 5-oxoproline overproduction. Such compounds have still to be found. Recently, some 5-oxoprolinuria patients were involved in therapeutic trials with vitamin E[7,50,51]. The rationale is to minimize the need for glutathione by supplying a compound which also participates in the protection of vital cellular functions against oxidative stress. The clinical parameters monitored have mainly been haemolysis and granulocyte function. The results presented so far are very promising[50,51]. Whether vitamin E will also have an effect on neurological symptoms in 5-oxoprolinuria remains to be established. Until the role of vitamin E has been further elucidated the therapy of choice for patients with this form of 5-oxoprolinuria will be acidosis correction with bicarbonate or citrate and avoidance of patients' exposure to drugs or foods known to precipitate haemolytic crises in individuals with glucose-6-phosphate-dehydrogenase deficiency.

An observation by Marstein et al.[52] in their patient with 5-oxoprolinuria challenged the role of glutathione in amino-acid transport[14]. The plasma levels of amino acids were found to be normal, except for a two-fold increase in the level of proline, but the corresponding levels in isolated erythrocytes were grossly abnormal. The patient's erythrocytes were found to be loaded with free amino acids, mostly in concentrations of 5–100 times normal. The observation by Marstein et al.[52] questioned the generally accepted principle that the levels of amino acids in plasma essentially reflect those in the erythrocytes. The abnormal concentrations in erythrocytes could be documented repeatedly. In skeletal muscle from the same patient there was considerably less deviation from the normal situation, but increased levels of proline, threonine, asparagine and glycine were observed in combination with decreased levels of glutamate, tyrosine and aspartate. Marstein et al.[52] had thus made the first observation of a disturbance in amino-acid transport in a patient with 5-oxoprolinuria, due to glutathione synthetase deficiency. This indicated some involvement of the γ-glutamyl cycle in the transport of amino acids in erythrocytes, but how this could be explained by the model proposed by Orlowski and Meister[3] is not apparent. A study by Hagenfeldt *et al.*[53] of the levels of free amino acids in erythrocytes and plasma from two patients with the same disease did not confirm the previous observation. Compared with Marstein *et al.*[52] only minor deviations were found, and they differed qualitatively and quantitatively from those reported by Marstein *et al.*[52] In essence three amino acids, namely, threonine, proline and tyrosine, were found to accumulate in both plasma and erythrocytes and this is unlikely to reflect a defective active transport across the erythrocyte membrane. Such a defect would involve a changed concentration ratio between plasma and erythrocytes; a relative increase of glycine, however, was observed. The decreased erythrocyte level of glutamate could be explained by the excessive loss of 5-oxoproline from the intracellular compartment according to the model in Figure 14.2. The increased level of glycine in red blood cells might be due to decreased utilization of this amino acid in the biosynthesis of glutathione. Thus the findings of Hagenfeldt *et al.*[53] did not support the view that 5-oxoprolinuria is associated with some general defect in the active transport of amino acids in erythrocytes. It should be of interest to further elucidate this question by analyses of amino acids in erythrocytes from other patients with 5-oxoprolinuria or other enzyme defects in the γ-glutamyl cycle.

It is possible that the findings in the patient of Marstein *et al.*[52] are completely unrelated to his defective glutathione metabolism. A remarkable finding in the Norwegian patient has subsequently been made[54] (E. Jellum, personal communication, 1979). When studied a year later his erythrocytes had completely normal amino-acid concentrations. It was suggested that the patient could have a cyclical disease, and depending on the glutathione concentration which had been found to vary between 0 and 10% of the normal level, the amino-acid transport might be defective or adequate. This needs to be further substantiated.

The finding of markedly decreased levels of glutathione in several tissues in patients with 5-oxoprolinuria[44] does not necessarily exclude that the γ-glutamyl cycle is of significance in the active transport of amino acids. It is possible that even a low level of glutathione is sufficient to keep the γ-glutamyl cycle going. Another explanation might be that there are multiple genes for glutathione synthetase so that the enzyme levels in critical tissues are normal even in patients with 5-oxoprolinuria. Wellner *et al.*[44] suggested that a modified γ-glutamyl cycle might be responsible for active amino-acid transport in patients with 5-oxoprolinuria. This was based on the finding in cell-free systems that γ-glutamyl-cysteine could replace glutathione as substrate in the γ-glutamyl transpeptidase reaction. This does not seem likely, at least not in erythrocytes, since the levels of γ-glutamyl-cysteine are not significantly increased in patients with glutathione synthetase deficiency associated with 5-oxoprolinuria[53]. Apparently γ-glutamyl-cysteine is rapidly degraded by the γ-glutamyl cyclo-transferase.

If the levels of free amino acids in erythrocytes of 5-oxoprolinuria patients were drastically increased as reported by Marstein et al.[52] also in the neonatal period, it would be expected that they were identified during the routine screening for PKU and other amino-acid disorders. The patients could, however, easily be missed in a follow-up investigation if amino-acid levels in plasma were analysed and found to be normal.

So far routine laboratory and clinical studies of the active amino-acid transport in additional patients with 5-oxoprolinuria (Table 14.1) have not yielded evidence of any consistent abnormality except for increased proline levels. General aminoaciduria has been reported in one patient only (patient 6, Table 14.1)[43]. Aminoaciduria was, however, only present during episodes of extreme acidosis and could, therefore, be caused by a number of factors other than the specific defect in glutathione metabolism. Direct studies of the handling of amino acids in vivo have so far only been reported for one patient with 5-oxoprolinuria[48]. By infusion of a mixture of 18 amino acids the serum levels were markedly increased, and this was followed by massive aminoaciduria. It is not possible to decide, however, if the patient was more prone to develop renal overflow of amino acids than normal individuals. In parallel with the amino-acid load, and urinary overflow, there was a doubling in the urinary excretion of 5-oxoproline. Whether this reflects a similar increase in the rate of production or simply competitive inhibition of renal uptake remains to be established.

Based on rough clinical correlates of amino-acid transport there is very little to indicate a derangement in processing of amino acids. Only one patient (case 7, Table 14.1) was reported to show some growth retardation. The weight at birth, on the other hand, seemed to indicate an impairment of the intrauterine weight gain; five patients born at term had a mean weight of 2850 g (range 2450–3600 g).

In conclusion there is, at present, only circumstantial evidence in favour of a defect in the active transport of amino acids in patients with glutathione synthetase deficiency and simultaneous 5-oxoprolinuria. The intriguing observation by Marstein et al.[52] that erythrocytes from one such patient accumulated amino acids only when the glutathione levels become extremely low needs to be further investigated. The findings cannot be explained by the γ-glutamyl cycle model[3], but they hint at some relationship between the intracellular glutathione concentration and the translocation of amino acids across cell membranes.

γ-GLUTAMYL TRANSPEPTIDASE DEFICIENCY WITH GLUTATHIONURIA

The association in man between increased glutathione excretion in the urine and decreased levels of γ-glutamyl transpeptidase was established by Goodman et al.[55]. So far three patients with this inborn error have been recognized. The first patient was a child suffering from a psychiatric disorder not specified further[56]. The patient was unfortunately reported very briefly. The child was found to excrete markedly increased amounts of glutathione in the urine. The enzymatic defect was not investigated, but it is interesting that the author in fact proposed a defect in γ-glutamyl transpeptidase as a possible explanation for the finding.

A moderately retarded 33-year-old man was discovered by Goodman et al.[55] during routine screening of institutionalized patients for disorders of amino-acid metabolism. Increased urinary levels of glutathione were detected in this patient. The daily amount excreted was approximately 3 mmol. The patient also exhibited a moderately increased level of glutathione in plasma; 8 μmol/l compared to 1–2 μmol/l in control subjects. The level of γ-glutamyl transpeptidase in serum was only 6% of the normal level. The enzyme deficiency could also be demonstrated in cultured skin fibroblasts[57]. The serum concentrations of amino acids were within normal limits and so was the estimated renal tubular resorption of amino acids. Studies were also extended to cultured fibroblasts from the patient[58]. In spite of the fact that the patient's cells contained less than 0.5% of normal γ-glutamyl transpeptidase activity, the intracellular levels of 16 amino acids were normal and increased approximately twofold for cystine, cysteine and phenylalanine. Uptake kinetics for four amino acids were also normal. These amino acids were glutamine, methionine, cystine and alanine, i.e. those amino acids which are the best γ-glutamyl acceptors for purified γ-glutamyl transpeptidase from rat kidney[59]. The authors therefore concluded that amino-acid transport appeared to proceed normally even in the absence of active γ-glutamyl transpeptidase, at least in human fibroblasts in culture.

A third patient with glutathionuria and generalized γ-glutamyl transpeptidase deficiency was recently reported by Wright et al.[60]. She was a 23-year-old woman, mentally retarded with a mean IQ of 61–62 when tested at 14–16 years of age. The main psychiatric problem of the patient was, however, a very severe behavioural disorder dominated by aggression and self-destruction. Her plasma levels and renal tubular reabsorption of amino acids were considered to be normal, the only exception was the reabsorption of cystine which appeared somewhat impaired. The findings in this patient were similar to those obtained in another patient with γ-glutamyl transpeptidase deficiency. Furthermore, the enzymatic defect recurred to be transmitted by autosomal recessive inheritance[60].

Although the main clinical symptoms of the three patients were mental retardation and/or behaviour problems, it is not yet known if this is caused by the lack of γ-glutamyl transpeptidase. More patients have to be studied before this can be decided.

Griffith and Meister[19] have recently used inhibitors of γ-glutamyl transpeptidase in vivo in mice to reproduce a model system for the metabolic disorder of the three patients discussed above. Inhibition of the enzyme in vivo resulted in extensive glutathionuria and there was evidence that a substantial fraction of the glutathione in the urine arose from the kidney. Unfortunately, no data were reported on the transport of amino acids in these animals. There is at present no way to establish, with certainty, that amino-acid transport is normal in patients with markedly decreased levels of γ-glutamyl transpeptidase. Likewise, the distribution of the enzymatic defect is difficult to establish. But assuming that it is expressed in all tissues, the observations made in patients tend to argue against the involvement of γ-glutamyl transpeptidase in amino-acid transport in man. The lack of increased excretion of proteins and peptides in urine of the patients renders it unlikely that the γ-glutamyl transpeptidase is involved in the degradation of filtered proteins in the renal tubules. The mechanism by which glutathione is excreted from the cells to the extracellular fluid as a result of γ-glutamyl transpeptidase deficiency is to be established.

5-OXOPROLINASE DEFICIENCY
WITH 5-OXOPROLINURIA

Recently two siblings with 5-oxoprolinuria were discovered in Holland[61]. The older brother had had episodes of diarrhoea, vomiting and abdominal pain since infancy. He was subjected to extensive investigations but no organic cause could be identified for his gastrointestinal symptoms, and these continued throughout adolescence. At the age of 13 years he had an episode of haematuria which was found to be due to a renal stone which had to be removed surgically. The stone consisted of calcium oxalate and calcium carbonate. In the follow-up of this patient, markedly elevated excretion of L-5-oxoproline was found in the urine with an average of 33 mmol/day. The serum level of 5-oxoproline was 0.8 mmol/l. In the urine the level of glycolic acid was elevated in some samples, but except for 5-oxoproline, the pattern of amino acids and other organic acids was normal. In serum there was a twofold increase in the level of lysine, but other amino acids were in the normal range. The patient was not acidotic and there was no evidence of increased rate of haemolysis. Anaemia was noted once, but it was ascribed to salzopyrine treatment. After withdrawal of this treatment anaemia has not recurred. The psychomotor as well as the somatic development in the patient was normal.

A younger brother of this patient also has gastrointestinal symptoms of a similar nature. This boy has been investigated carefully but no aetiology has been established. When 5-oxoprolinuria was established in the elder brother, investigation of the urine of the younger sibling showed that he also excreted 5-oxoproline, corresponding to 42 mmol/day. In urine samples of the parents, 5-oxoproline could not be detected. The father of the two boys and several paternal relatives had urolithiasis of unknown aetiology. In erythrocytes from the two brothers with 5-oxoprolinuria, normal levels of glutathione as well as γ-glutamyl-cysteine synthetase, glutathione synthetase, γ-glutamyl cyclotransferase, and glutathione reductase were detected. Several possibilities for increased synthesis of 5-oxoproline were considered (Figure 14.3). One involved defective feedback regulation of the γ-glutamyl cysteine synthetase, with retained catalytic activity of the enzyme. This was considered to be unlikely since the enzyme present in erythrocytes was found to be inhibited by glutathione in a normal way. A defect in the 5-oxoprolinase step was then considered. This enzyme was studied in leukocytes and cultured fibroblasts. In cells from the two brothers significantly decreased levels of 5-oxoprolinase were demonstrated. Thus hereditary deficiency of this enzyme is the explanation offered to account for 5-oxoprolinuria in this family. To our knowledge this is the first time a deficiency in this enzyme has been demonstrated.

5-Oxoprolinuria of two types must be considered. One is due to a primary hereditary deficiency of glutathione synthetase and secondary 5-oxoproline overproduction (Figure 14.3). The second type is due to lack of 5-oxoprolinase with inability to metabolize the amount of 5-oxoproline which is normally turned over. The excretion of 5-oxoproline in the two siblings with the latter type of 5-oxoprolinuria is approximately 40 mmol (5 g)/day. The site of production of this amount of 5-oxoproline remains to be established. The clinical symptoms in the two brothers with 5-oxoprolinase deficiency are distinct from those of patients with 5-oxoprolinuria due to glutathione synthetase deficiency (Table 14.1). There are no signs of metabolic acidosis which needs correction or of haemolytic anaemia or neurological damage. The common denominator in the two brothers with 5-oxoprolinase deficiency is gastrointestinal symptoms. At present it is not clear if those symptoms are related to the defect in the degradation of 5-oxoproline.

An alternative source of urinary 5-oxoproline is certain artificial diets[62]. Significantly increased levels of 5-oxoproline were detected in plasma (40 μmol/l v. 5 μmol/l in control subjects) and urine (4.7 mmol/ mmol creatinine v. 0.1 mmol/mmol creatinine in control subjects). These levels are considerably lower than those reported in patients with 5-oxoprolinuria caused by genetic defects in either glutathione synthetase or 5-oxoprolinase. It is, of course, necessary to consider a dietary origin of 5-oxoproline whenever this compound is identified in body fluids.

In summary there is, so far, no evidence for any disturbance in the active transport of amino acids in patients with 5-oxoprolinase deficiency.

GLUTATHIONE REDUCTASE DEFICIENCY

Glutathione reductase is an enzyme not immediately involved in the γ-glutamyl cycle (Figure 14.1). The maintenance of glutathione in the reduced state is, however, important for the function of the cycle. Several patients have been reported to have decreased levels of glutathione reductase in erythrocytes, but the deficiency has apparently been due to inadequate riboflavin intake in the diet[63]. A family with inherited deficiency of glutathione reductase was described recently[64]. The index case was a 22-year-old woman who had attacks of haemolysis after ingestion of fava beans. In addition, the patient had bilateral cataracts. She was one of three siblings in a consanguineous marriage. A brother suffered from juvenile cataracts and a sister also had eye symptoms which were not described in detail. All three siblings were found to have very low levels of glutathione reductase in erythrocytes and the levels could not be corrected by addition of FAD to *in vitro* incubation mixtures or by supplying 5 mg of riboflavin per day to the patients. The levels of glutathione reductase in erythrocytes were less than 8%, and in isolated leukocytes approximately 15%, of the activity in cells from control subjects.

Intermediate enzyme levels were found in cells from the parents. The level of glutathione, the reduced form, was normal in erythrocytes of the patients, indicating that they are able to keep their glutathione reduced under normal conditions. On the other hand, if there is markedly increased rate of glutathione oxidation a glutathione-deficient state might be precipitated in erythrocytes and other types of cells. There are no reports of amino-acid transport studies in patients with glutathione-reductase deficiency or in cellular model systems obtained from such patients. It is remarkable that two of three patients with glutathione-reductase deficiency had developed cataracts. The role of glutathione in maintaining the lens-protein structure intact is recognized from other lines of work[21].

GENETIC γ-GLUTAMYL CYCLE DEFECTS
IN ANIMALS AND MICRO-ORGANISMS

Young and coworkers[65] have explored a very interesting animal model system to elucidate the role of glutathione in the active transport of amino acids in erythrocytes. They have studied two types of inherited erythrocyte glutathione deficiency in sheep. One is a variant of the Tasmanian Merino sheep, where the primary defect was found to be a lack of γ-glutamyl-cysteine synthetase[66]. The other type of glutathione deficiency is a mutation in the Finnish Landrace sheep. Decreased levels of glutathione in erythrocytes have been ascribed to the lack of available cysteine needed for the bio-synthesis of glutathione, and this is due to the absence of a specific amino-acid transport system[67]. The lack of this membrane transport function is associated with increased intracellular levels of certain amino acids, particularly lysine and ornithine[68]. Apparently ornithine is derived from arginine by the action of arginase present in sheep erythrocytes[69]. It is interesting that increased levels of several amino acids in erythrocytes were observed in a patient with glutathione-synthetase deficiency and 5-oxoprolinuria[52]. Arginine, lysine and ornithine also accumulated in this patient, as did a number of neutral and acidic amino acids. On the basis of studies with thiol-reactive agents, Young[70] has recently postulated that there are three distinct classes of cellular sulphydryl groups, the integrity of which are required for normal amino-acid transport in sheep erythrocytes. Young and coworkers have not obtained any experimental support for the involvement of the γ-glutamyl cycle in the amino-acid transport of erythrocytes from sheep. It would be of interest to know if the two mutants that they studied had generalized glutathione deficiency affecting tissues such as liver, kidney and brain, and also if the mutants presented aminoaciduria, neurological symptoms and other signs observed in patients with γ-glutamyl cycle defects. The Tasmanian Merino mutant would perhaps represent a model of human γ-glutamyl-cysteine synthetase deficiency[31,32]. One difference, however, is that the enzyme activity in erythrocytes of the sheep mutant was approximately 50% of normal[66] but in the human mutant it was 4–14% of normal[31]. Young and coworkers[65] have utilized rabbit red-cells to test the hypothesis that the γ-glutamyl cycle is involved in the active transport of amino acids in erythrocytes[15]. Even in the absence of glucose in the medium the cells were capable of large net transport of alanine, phenylalanine and lysine without decreasing the level of glutathione. It is therefore unlikely that the amino-acid transport studied depended on an active γ-glutamyl cycle, which is highly energy requiring.

Mutants of *Escherichia coli* defective in the γ-glutamyl cycle have been isolated. Cells lacking glutathione synthetase have been characterized[71,72]. This mutant is analogous to the corresponding human mutant associated with 5-oxoprolinuria. One apparent difference, however, is that the *E. coli* mutant accumulates γ-glutamyl cysteine[72], whereas the human mutant does not[53]. Bacterial mutants deficient in γ-glutamyl-cysteine synthetase were identified by Apontoweil and Berends[71]. Such mutants cannot replace glutathione by a γ-glutamyl dipeptide. They were more sensitive than the parental strain to exposure to a variety of chemical compounds, but they did not exhibit increased sensitivity to X-ray.

Further studies are needed to clarify the role of glutathione in microorganisms, especially with the recently discovered involvement of glutathione in the biosynthesis of deoxyribonucleotides[25]. At present there is no evidence that glutathione is involved in the active transport of amino acids in micro-organisms.

CONCLUSIONS

The involvement of the γ-glutamyl cycle in the turnover of glutathione seems to be uncontroversial. The role of the γ-glutamyl cycle in the active transport of amino acids across cell membranes is still highly speculative, however attractive the model proposed by Orlowski and

Meister[3] might appear from a theoretical point of view.

A series of inborn errors in the γ-glutamyl cycle have been identified and the enzymatic defects have been established. The clinical histories and biochemical findings in such patients have been examined with emphasis on possible disturbance in the active transport of amino acids. In fact very little evidence has been obtained in favour of Meister's model. The strongest support is the finding of generalized aminoaciduria in two patients with γ-glutamyl cysteine synthetase deficiency[32]. Furthermore, the massive accumulation of amino acids in erythrocytes of a patient with glutathione synthetase deficiency associated with 5-oxoprolinuria[52] indicates some relationship between amino-acid transport and the γ-glutamyl cycle, but it is not apparent how the finding can be explained by Meister's model. On the other hand, there are several pieces of evidence, unfortunately also circumstantial, which tend to exclude a role of the γ-glutamyl cycle in amino-acid transport. The model offers no explanation for the group of well known genetic defects of amino-acid transport in the renal tubule such as cystinuria, iminoglycinuria and Hartnup's disease. The γ-glutamyl transpeptidase is a critical enzyme in the cycle. Its specificity is another matter of concern since the enzyme does not utilize all amino acids as γ-glutamyl acceptors. Proline, threonine and aspartate are examples of amino acids which do not work or work very poorly as substrates. The apparent K_m of purified γ-glutamyl transpeptidase for amino acid acceptors, such as methionine, is two orders of magnitude higher than the physiological extracellular concentrations[73].

Studies of patients with genetic defects in the γ-glutamyl cycle provide very little support for the model proposed by Orlowski and Meister[3]. Such data must be interpreted with great care. One reason is that the mutations are often leaky and that even a few per cent of the normal enzyme activity might be sufficient to keep the γ-glutamyl cycle rolling. The great potential of using human mutants is the possibility of establishing model systems in culture and employ extreme conditions to test the amino-acid transport and other hypothetical glutathione-dependent functions in mutant and normal cells, respectively. It was recently emphasized by Meister[74] that the γ-glutamyl cycle was not proposed as the only amino-acid transport system. The cycle may be functional only in certain tissues and may be more active with certain amino-acids than with others. It is obvious that additional experiments are needed before it can be concluded that the γ-glutamyl cycle has any significance in amino-acid transport. Studies of inborn errors of metabolism have a definite role in this work.

Acknowledgements

This work was supported by grants from the Swedish Medical Research Council (4792, 4930), the Karolinska Institute and Svenska livförsäkringsbolagsnämnd för medicinsk forskning. The secretarial assistance of Miss Eivor Erkas is gratefully acknowledged.

References

1. Hopkins, F. G. (1921). An autoxidable constituent of the cell. *Biochem. J.*, **15**, 286
2. Hopkins, F. G. (1929). On glutathione: a reinvestigation. *J. Biol. Chem.*, **84**, 269
3. Orlowski, M. and Meister, A. (1970). The γ-glutamyl cycle: a possible transport system for amino acids. *Proc. Natl. Acad. Sci. USA*, **67**, 1248
4. Meister, A. and Tate, S. S. (1976). Glutathione and related γ-glutamyl compounds: biosynthesis and utilization. *Ann. Rev. Biochem.*, **45**, 559
5. Arias, I. M. and Jakoby, W. B. (eds.) (1976). *Glutathione: Metabolism and Function*. Kroc Foundation Series, Vol. 6. (New York: Raven Press)
6. Meister, A. (1973). On the enzymology of amino acid transport. *Science*, **180**, 33.
7. Mendelson, I. S., Zaleski, W. A., Casey, R. E., Christie, E. J., Wellner, V. P. and Meister, A. (1979). Ataxia in 5-oxoprolinuria: is there a connection between the γ-glutamyl cycle and GABA function? Abstract *XIth International Congress of Biochemistry*, Ottawa, Canada, July 1979.
8. Meister, A., Tate, S. S. and Ross, L. L. (1976). Membrane bound γ-glutamyl transpeptidase. In A. Martinosi (ed.). *Membrane-Bound Enzymes*, Vol. 3, pp. 315–347. (New York: Plenum Press)
9. Tate, S. S. and Orlando, J. (1979). Conversion of glutathione to glutathione disulfide, a catalytic function of γ-glutamyl transpeptidase. *J. Biol. Chem.*, **254**, 5573
10. Gardell, S. J. and Tate, S. S. (1979). Latent proteinase activity of γ-glutamyl transpeptidase light subunit. *J. Biol. Chem.*, **254**, 4942
11. Jackson, R. C. (1969). Studies on the enzymology of glutathione metabolism in human erythrocytes. *Biochem. J.*, **111**, 309
12. Richman, P. G. and Meister, A. (1975). Regulation of γ-glutamyl-cysteine synthetase by nonallosteric feedback inhibition by glutathione. *J. Biol. Chem.*, **250**, 1422
13. Larsson, A. and Mattsson, B. (1976). On the mechanism of 5-oxoproline over-production in 5-oxoprolinuria. *Clin. Chim. Acta*, **67**, 245
14. Beutler, E. (1976). Glutathione deficiency, pyroglutamic acidemia and amino acid transport. *N. Engl. J. Med.*, **295**, 441
15. Palekar, A. G., Tate, S. S. and Meister, A. (1974). Formation of 5-oxoproline from glutathione in erythrocytes by the γ-glutamyltranspeptidase – cyclotransferase pathway. *Proc. Natl. Acad. Sci. USA*, **71**, 293
16. Srivastava, S. K., Awasthi, Y. C., Miller, S. P., Yoshida, A. and Beutler, E. (1976). Studies on γ-glutamyl transpeptidase in human and rabbit ery-

throcytes. *Blood,* **47,** 645
17. Dimant, E., Landsberg, E. and London, I. M. (1955). The metabolic behavior of reduced glutathione in human and avian erythrocytes. *J. Biol. Chem.,* **213,** 769
18. Prchal, J., Srivastava, S. K. and Beutler, E. (1975). Active transport of GSSG from reconstituted erythrocyte ghosts. *Blood,* **46,** 111
19. Griffith, O. W. and Meister, A. (1979). Translocation of intracellular glutathione to membrane-bound γ-glutamyl transpeptidase as a discrete step in the γ-glutamyl cycle: glutathionuria after inhibition of transpeptidase. *Proc. Natl. Acad. Sci. USA,* **76,** 268
20. James, S. P. and Pheasant, A. E. (1978). Glutathione conjugation and mercapturic acid formation in the developing rat *in vivo* and *in vitro. Xenobiotica,* **8,** 207
21. Roos, D., Weening, R. S. and Loos, J. A. (1979). The protective role of glutathione. The effect of congenital defects of glutathione metabolism on the function of erythrocytes, eye lens cells and phagocytic leukocytes. A review and some personal observations. In F. Güttler, J. W. T. Seakins and R. A. Harkness (eds.). *Inborn Errors of Immunity and Phagocytosis,* pp. 261–286. (Lancaster: MTP)
22. Mitchell, J. R., Jollow, D. J., Potter, W. Z., Gillette, J. R. and Brodie, B. B. (1973). Acetaminophen-induced hepatic necrosis. IV. Protective role of glutathione. *J. Pharmacol. Exp. Ther.,* **187,** 211.
23. Edgren, M., Larsson, A., Nilsson, K., Révész, L. and Scott, O. C. A. (1980). Lack of oxygen-effect in glutathione deficient human cells in culture. *Int. J. Radiat. Biol.,* **37,** 299
24. Lindblad, B., Lindstedt, S. and Steen, G. (1977). On the enzymatic defects in hereditary tyrosinemia., *Proc. Natl. Acad. Sci, USA,* **74,** 4641.
25. Holmgren, A. (1979). Glutathione dependent synthesis of deoxyribonucleotides. Purification and characterization of glutaredoxin from *Escherichia coli. J. Biol. Chem.,* **254,** 3664
26. Luthman, M., Eriksson, S., Holmgren, A. and Thelander, L. (1979). Glutathione dependent hydrogen donor system for calf thymus ribonucleosidediphosphate reductase. *Proc. Natl. Acad. Sci. USA,* **76,** 2158
27. Laurent, T. C., Moore, E. C. and Reichard, P. (1964). Enzymatic synthesis of deoxyribonucleotides. IV. Isolation and characterization of thioredoxin, the hydrogen donor from *Escherichia coli* B. *J. Biol. Chem.,* **239,** 3436
28. Engström, N. E., Holmgren, A., Larsson, A. and Söderhäll, S. (1974). Isolation and characterization of calf liver thioredoxin. *J. Biol. Chem.,* **249,** 205
29. Meister, A. (1974). The γ-glutamyl cycle. Diseases associated with specific enzyme deficiencies. *Ann. Intern. Med.,* **81,** 247
30. Griffith, O. W., Anderson, M. E. and Meister, A. (1979). Inhibition of glutathione biosynthesis by prothionine sulfoximine (S-*n*-propyl homocysteine sulfoximine) a selective inhibitor of γ-glutamyl cysteine synthetase. *J. Biol. Chem.,* **254,** 1205
31. Konrad, P. N., Richards, F. H., Valentine, W. N. and Paglia, D. E. (1972). γ-Glutamyl cysteine synthetase deficiency: a cause of hereditary hemolytic anemia. *N. Engl. J. Med.,* **286,** 557

32. Richards, F. II, Cooper, M. R., Pearce, L. A., Cowan, R. J. and Spurr, C. L. (1974). Familial spinocerebellar degeneration, hemolytic anemia and glutathione deficiency. *Arch. Intern. Med.*, **134**, 534

33. Oort, M., Loos, J. A. and Prins, H. K. (1961). Hereditary absence of reduced glutathione in the erythrocytes – a new clinical and biochemical entity? *Vox Sanguinis*, **6**, 370

34. Prins, H. K., Oort, M., Loos, J. A., Zürcher, C. and Beckers, T. (1966). Congenital nonspherocytic hemolytic anemia associated with glutathione deficiency of the erythrocytes. *Blood*, **27**, 145

35. Boivin, P. and Galand, C. (1965). La synthèse du glutathion au cours de l'anémie hémolytique congénitale avec deficit en glutathion réduit. Déficit congénital en glutathion-synthétase érythrocytaire? *Nouv. Rev. Fr. Hematol.*, **5**, 707

36. Mohler, D. N., Majerus, P. W., Minnich, V., Hess, C. E. and Garrick, M. D. (1970). Glutathione synthetase deficiency as a cause of hereditary hemolytic disease. *N. Engl. J. Med.*, **283**, 1253

37. Boivin, P., Galand, C. and Schaison, G. (1978). Déficit en glutathion-synthétase avec 5-oxoprolinurie. Deux nouveaux cas et revue de la littérature. *Nouv. Presse Méd.*, **7**, 1531

38. Meister, A. (1978). 5-Oxoprolinuria (pyroglutamic aciduria) and other disorders of glutathione biosynthesis. In J. B. Stanbury, J. B. Wyngaarden and D. S. Fredrickson (eds.). *The Metabolic Basis of Inherited Disease*, 4th Edn., pp. 328–335. (New York: McGraw-Hill).

39. Jellum, E., Kluge, T., Börresen, H. C., Stokke, O. and Eldjarn, L. (1970). Pyroglutamic aciduria – a new inborn error of metabolism. *Scand. J. Clin. Lab. Invest.*, **26**, 327

40. Kluge, T., Börresen, H. C., Jellum, E., Stokke, O., Eldjarn, L. and Fretheim, B. (1972). Esophageal hiatus hernia and mental retardation: life threatening postoperative metabolic acidosis and potassium deficiency linked with a new inborn error of nitrogen metabolism. *Surgery*, **71**, 104

41. Hagenfeldt, L., Larsson, A. and Zetterström, R. (1974). Pyroglutamic aciduria. Studies in an infant with chronic metabolic acidosis. *Acta Paediatr. Scand.*, **63**, 1

42. Larsson, A., Zetterström, R., Hagenfeldt, L., Andersson, R., Hörnell, H. and Dreborg, S. (1974). Pyroglutamic aciduria (5-oxoprolinuria) an inborn error in glutathione metabolism. *Pediatr. Res.*, **8**, 852

43. Porath, U. and Schreier, K. (1978). Eine Familie mit Pyroglutaminacidurie. *Dtsch. Med. Wochenschr.*, **103**, 939

44. Wellner, V. P., Sekura, R., Meister, A. and Larsson, A. (1974). Glutathione synthetase deficiency, an inborn error of metabolism involving the γ-glutamyl cycle in patients with 5-oxoprolinuria (pyroglutamic aciduria). *Proc. Natl. Acad. Sci. USA*, **71**, 2505

45. Larsson, A., Zetterström, R., Hörnell, H. and Porath, U. (1976). Erythrocyte glutathione synthetase in 5-oxoprolinuria: kinetic studies of the mutant enzyme and detection of heterozygotes. *Clin. Chim. Acta*, **73**, 19

46. Eldjarn, L., Jellum, E. and Stokke, O. (1973). Pyroglutamic aciduria: rate of formation and degradation of pyroglutamate. *Clin. Chim. Acta*, **49**, 311

47. Eldjarn, L., Stokke, O. and Jellum, E. (1972). Pyroglutamic aciduria. A new inborn error of metabolism possibly in the γ-glutamyl cycle proposed

for amino acid transport. In J. Stern and C. Toothill (eds.), *Organic Acidurias*, pp. 113–120. (Edinburgh: Churchill Livingstone)

48. Eldjarn, L., Jellum, E. and Stokke, O. (1972). Pyroglutamic aciduria. Studies on the enzyme block and on the metabolic origin of pyroglutamic acid. *Clin. Chim. Acta*, **40**, 461

49. Griffith, O., Larsson, A. and Meister, A. (1977). Inhibitor of γ-glutamyl cysteine synthetase by cystamine: an approach to a therapy of 5-oxoprolinuria (pyroglutamic aciduria). *Biochem. Biophys. Res. Commun.*, **79**, 919

50. Boxer, L. A., Oliver, J. M., Spielberg, S. P., Allen, J. M. and Schulman, J. D. (1979). Protection of granulocytes by vitamin E in glutathione synthetase deficiency. *N. Engl. J. Med.*, **301**, 901

51. Spielberg, S.P., Boxer, L. A., Corash, L. M. and Schulman, J. D. (1979). Improved erythrocyte survival with high-dose vitamin E in chronic hemolyzing G6PD and glutathione synthetase deficiencies. *Ann. Intern. Med.*, **90**, 53

52. Marstein, S., Jellum, E., Halpern, B., Eldjarn, L. and Perry, T. L. (1976). Biochemical studies of erythrocytes in a patient with pryoglutamic acidemia (5-oxoprolinemia). *N. Engl. J. Med.*, **295**, 406

53. Hagenfeldt, L., Larsson, A. and Andersson, R. (1978). The γ-glutamyl cycle and amino acid transport. Studies of free amino acids, γ-glutamyl cysteine and glutathione in erythrocytes from patients with 5-oxoprolinuria (glutathione synthetase deficiency). *N. Engl. J. Med.*, **299**, 587

54. Perry, T. L. (1978). Discussion of disorders of nitrogenous compounds. Related genetic and animal studies. *Adv. Neurol.*, **21**, 347

55. Goodman, S. I., Mace, J. W. and Pollak, S. (1971). Serum gammaglutamyl transpeptidase deficiency. *Lancet*, **1**, 234

56. O'Daly, S. (1968). An abnormal sulphydryl compound in urine. *Ir. J. Med. Sci.*, **7**, 578

57. Schulman, J. D., Goodman, S. I., Mace, J. W., Patrick, A. D., Tietze, F. and Butler, E. J. (1975). Glutathionuria: inborn error of metabolism due to tissue deficiency of gamma-glutamyl transpeptidase. *Biochem. Biophys. Res. Commun.*, **65**, 68

58. Pellefigue, F., Butler, J. D., Spielberg, S. P., Hollenberg, M. D., Goodman, S. I. and Schulman, J. D. (1976). Normal amino acid uptake by cultured human fibroblasts does not require γ-glutamyl transpeptidase. *Biochem. Biophys. Res. Commun.*, **73**, 997

59. Tate, S. S. and Meister, A. (1974). Interaction of γ-glutamyl transpeptidase with amino acids, dipeptides, and derivatives and analogs of glutathione. *J. Biol. Chem.*, **249**, 7593

60 Wright, E. C., Stern, J., Ersser, R. and Patrick, A. D. (1979). Glutathionuria: γ-glutamyl transpeptidase deficiency. *J. Inherited Metabol. Dis.*, **2**, 3

61. Larsson, A., Mattsson, B., Wadman, S. K., van der Heiden, C., Duran, M., Wauters, E. A. K., van Gool, J. D., Beemer, F. A. and van Sprang, F. J. (1981). 5-oxoprolinuria caused by hereditary deficiency of 5-oxoprolinase. *Acta. Paediatr. Scand.* (In press)

62. Oberholtzer, V. G., Wood, C. B. S., Palmer, T. and Harrison, B. M. (1975). Increased pyroglutamic acid levels in patients on artificial diets. *Clin. Chim. Acta*, **62**, 299

63. Löhr, G. W., Blume, K. G., Rüdiger, H. W. and Arnold, H. (1974). Genetic variability in the enzymatic reduction of oxidized glutathione. In L. Flohé, H. C. Benöhr, H. Sies, H. D. Waller and A. Wendel (eds.) *Glutathione*, pp. 165–172. (Stuttgart: Georg Thieme)

64. Loos, H., Roos, D., Weening, R. and Houwerzijl, J. (1976). Familial deficiency of glutathione reductase in human blood cells. *Blood*, **46**, 53

65. Young, J. D., Ellroy, J. C. and Wright, P. C. (1975). Evidence against the participation of the γ-glutamyltransferase–γ-glutamylcyclotransferase pathway in amino acid transport by rabbit erythrocytes. *Biochem. J.*, **152**, 713

66. Young, J. D. and Nimmo, I. A. (1975). GSH biosynthesis in glutathione deficient erythrocytes from Finnish landrace and Tasmanian merino sheep. *Biochim. Biophys. Acta*, **404**, 132

67. Young, J. D., Ellroy, J. C. and Tucker, E. M. (1976). Amino acid transport in normal and glutathione-deficient sheep erythrocytes. *Biochem. J.*, **154**, 43

68. Tucker, E. M. and Kilgour, L. (1970). An inherited glutathione deficiency and a concomitant reduction in potassium concentration in sheep red cells. *Experientia*, **26**, 203

69. Tucker, E. M., Wright, P. C. and Young, J. D. (1977). Influence of arginase deficiency on amino acid concentrations in sheep erythrocytes with a normal and with a defective transport system for amino acids. *J. Physiol.*, **271**, 47P

70. Young, J. D. (1978). The role of thiol groups in erythrocyte amino acid transport. *Biochem. Soc. Trans.*, **7**, 683

71. Apontoweil, P. and Berends, W. (1975). Isolation and initial characterization of glutathione deficient mutants of *Escherichia coli* K12. *Biochim. Biophys. Acta*, **399**, 10

72. Fuchs, J. A. and Warner, H. (1975). Isolation of an *Escherichia coli* mutant deficient in glutathione synthesis. *J. Bacteriol.*, **124**, 140

73. Elce, J. S. and Broxmeyer, B. (1976). γ-Glutamyl transferase of rat kidney. Simultaneous assay on the hydrolysis and transfer reactions with (glutamate-14C) glutathione. *Biochem. J.*, **153**, 223

74. Meister, A. (1978b). Relation between ataxia and defects of the γ-glutamyl cycle. *Adv. Neurol.*, **21**, 289

75. Boivin, P., Saudubray, J. M., Pousset, J. L. and Galand, C. (1975). Glutathione synthetase deficiency and pyroglutamic aciduria. *Internat. Soc. Haematol. Third Meeting of European African Division*, London, Abstract 1:20

76. Spielberg, S. P., Kramer, L. I., Goodman, S. I., Butler, J., Tietze, F., Quinn, P. and Schulman, J. D. (1977). 5-Oxoprolinuria: biochemical observations and case report. *J. Pediatr.*, **91**, 237

SECTION FIVE

Transport in Red Blood Cells

15

Anion transport
in red blood cells
B. Deuticke

INTRODUCTION: PHYSIOLOGICAL ROLE
OF CHLORIDE–BICARBONATE EXCHANGE

Red cells play an important role in the convective transport of O_2, CO_2, H^+ and other ions, substrates and metabolites between the organs of their uptake, utilization and excretion. For many of the 'passengers' this importance is due only to the fact that the intracellular aqueous space of the red cells contributes about 35% of the total solvent space of the blood. For others, the erythrocyte provides a particular vehicle at a high concentration (haemoglobin for O_2 and H^+), or a catalyst and subsidiary mechanisms for temporary conversion into a form more suitable for transportation. This applies to CO_2. It is well-known that CO_2 is transported in the blood to about 80% as HCO^-_3, which is formed almost exclusively inside the erythrocyte (Figure 15.1, upper) in a reaction catalysed by carbonic anhydrase and requiring haemoglobin as a H^+-acceptor. In order to reach its full efficiency, this reaction has to be followed by the distribution of the newly formed HCO^-_3 between erythrocytes and plasma. This requires an exchange for extracellular Cl^-, the well-known 'Hamburger shift'. It can easily be calculated that of the total CO_2 output in resting man (about 12 mmol/min), 60% are transported in the plasma and thus have to pass the erythrocyte membrane as HCO^-_3.

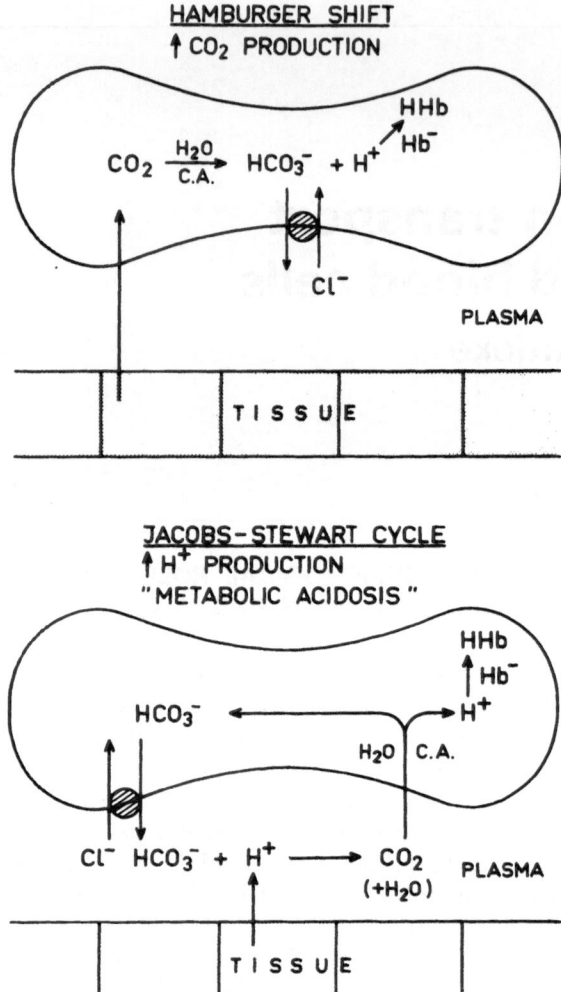

Figure 15.1   Schematic representation of the role of erythrocytes in the transport of CO_2 and the handling of H^+ ions in blood. C.A. = carbonic anhydrase

Movements of HCO^-_3 are also required for making accessible the high buffer capacity of the red cell interior (65% of the total capacity of the blood) to H^+ ions entering the plasma from the tissue, e.g. in metabolic acidosis. In the so-called Jacobs–Stewart cycle (Figure 15.1, lower) H^+ combines with HCO^-_3 in the plasma, H_2CO_3 is dehydrated (uncatalysed) to form CO_2 which rapidly enters the red cell and is rehydrated (catalysed by carbonic anhydrase) to $H^+ + HCO^-_3$ The former is buffered by haemoglobin, while HCO^-_3 leaves the cells in exchange for Cl^- and re-enters the cycle, which in balance has promoted a net uptake of $H^+ + Cl^-$ into the erythrocyte[1].

Anion movements across the erythrocyte membrane are thus of paramount importance in the disposal of CO_2 and of fixed acids. It seems possible that the discharge of CO_2 in the lung could be limited by this anion exchange, which may have the slowest half time of all reactions shown in Figure 15.1, upper. At least under conditions of physical exercise, or after partial blockage of the exchange mechanism, the pulmonary transit time[2] might be too short to warrant alveolar-capillary equilibration of CO_2.

PROPERTIES OF THE INORGANIC ANION-EXCHANGE SYSTEM

Kinetic data and models

Attempts to characterize the system mediating anion exchange go back half a century (see reference 3 for references). They have been hampered by the formidable difficulties of analysing Cl^-/HCO^-_3 exchange under physiological conditions. Only very recently, techniques[4] have been developed for measuring fluxes of ^{14}C-labelled HCO^-_3. These will hopefully soon provide the answer as to whether Cl^-/HCO^-_3 exchange can become rate limiting for CO_2 transport. The general characterization in kinetic and molecular terms, however, of the transfer system mediating Cl^-/HCO^-_3 exchange is well advanced. This was possible due to the fact that this system also catalyses anion movements other than Cl^-/HCO^-_3 exchange, in particular a self-exchange of Cl^- and various other anions (for reviews see references 3, 5 and 8). All movements via this system are passive, which already follows from the Donnan distribution of anions between cells and plasma.

Furthermore, anion movements in the system are electrically silent and occur in a tightly coupled mode. This became clear from comparisons of Cl^- fluxes under two different experimental conditions. Measurements of *self-exchange* of labelled against non-labelled Cl^- yield an extremely high apparent permeability of $5.4 \cdot 10^{-4}$ cm/s (38°C, pH 7.35), corresponding to a half time for the exchange[9] of approximately 0.05 s. The *net efflux* of chloride (and potassium) – into media free of anions able to use this system – is slower by four orders of magnitude[10], indicating that the lack of an external exchange partner for internal anions almost abolishes anion movements. The calculation of ion conductivities or resistances revealed that the Cl⁻ resistance obtained from net flux permeability[3,6,10] corresponds to the total electric resistance of the membrane, as measured by microelectrodes in erythrocytes of the giant salamander, *Amphiuma means*[11]. The Cl⁻ resistance calculated from the exchange flux is five orders of magnitude lower. Anion exchange, which accounts for almost all of the anion movement, is thus electrically silent.

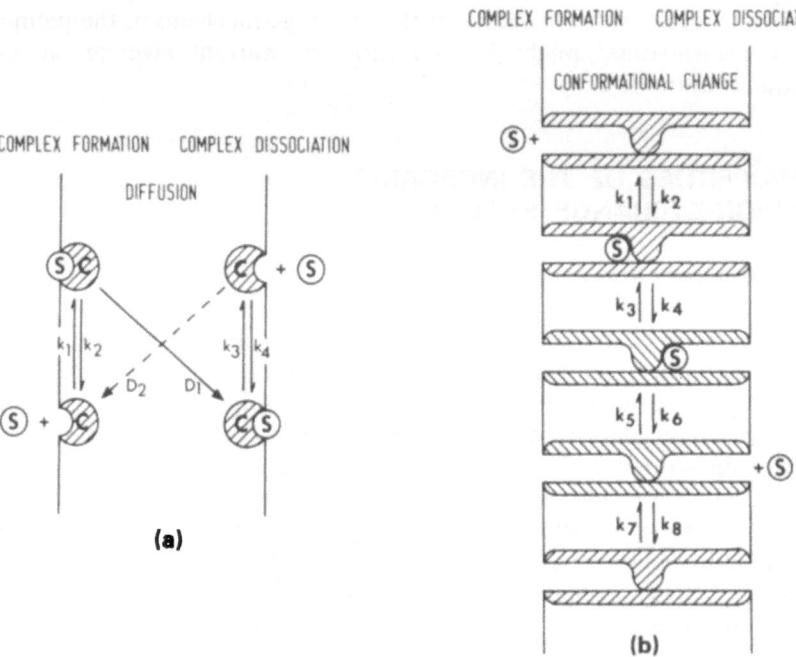

Figure 15.2 Models of carriers for the facilitated diffusion in biomembranes. (a) Classical ferry boat model. C = carrier, S = substrate, k_1–k_4 = rate coefficients of on- and off-reaction, D_1, D_2 = diffusion coefficient of loaded and empty carrier. (b) Gated-pore model with conformation changes, k_1–k_8 rate coefficients of on- and off-reaction and of the conformation change

The most reasonable explanation for a tightly coupled, electrically silent anion exchange is reversible binding of the transported anions to a membrane-constituent mediating the exchange, i.e. a carrier. By definition, a carrier, in contrast to an open pore, is a constituent which exposes a binding site for a transport substrate alternating to the solutions on either side of the membrane, but is never accessible from both sides at the same time. The classical physical model of such a carrier (Figure 15.2) was that of a mobile ferry boat, linking both membrane surfaces by a diffusion process. While being realized in case of ionophorous antibiotics, e.g. valinomycin, carriers in biomembranes are most likely to be represented by a different model. Intrinsic membrane-spanning proteins, forming 'gated pores' (Figure 15.2) could act as carriers if a conformational change in the protein following the binding of substrate translocates the binding site from the *cis*- to the *trans*-side of the membrane. Kinetically, the two models are essentially indistinguishable, therefore the term 'mobile carrier' seems justified for both of them.

The evidence that inorganic anion exchange is in fact mediated by a carrier is as follows[3,6]. Anion self-exchange measured at ion equilibrium exhibits saturation kinetics (Figure 15.3A) and even self-inhibition at high substrate concentrations[12,13]. This demonstrates that only a limited number of sites is available for transport. This limitation also leads to marked competition among anions (Figure 15.3B): sulphate exchange, e.g. is diminished when increasing concentrations of chloride are added to the system.

Furthermore, anion exchange depends on pH in a way consistent with the assumption that titratable positive (e.g. $-NH^+_3$) groups are present at or near the binding site[3,14] and that only the protonated form is transporting.

Protonation of these groups occurs according to a reaction of the general form

$$C + H^+ \rightleftharpoons CH^+$$
$$\text{(inactive)} \qquad \text{(active)} \tag{1}$$

The equilibrium is defined by

$$K_1 = \frac{[C] \cdot [H^+]}{[CH^+]}, \text{ or } CH^+ = \frac{[C] \cdot [H^+]}{K_1} \tag{2}$$

The transported anions (A^-) react with the active binding site (CH^+) according to

$$CH^+ + A^- \rightleftharpoons CHA, \tag{3}$$

$$K_2 = \frac{[CH^+] \cdot [A^-]}{[CHA]} \tag{4}$$

Anion exchange can thus be modelled by the scheme shown in Figure 15.4 in which the anion is translocated across a diffusion barrier by a

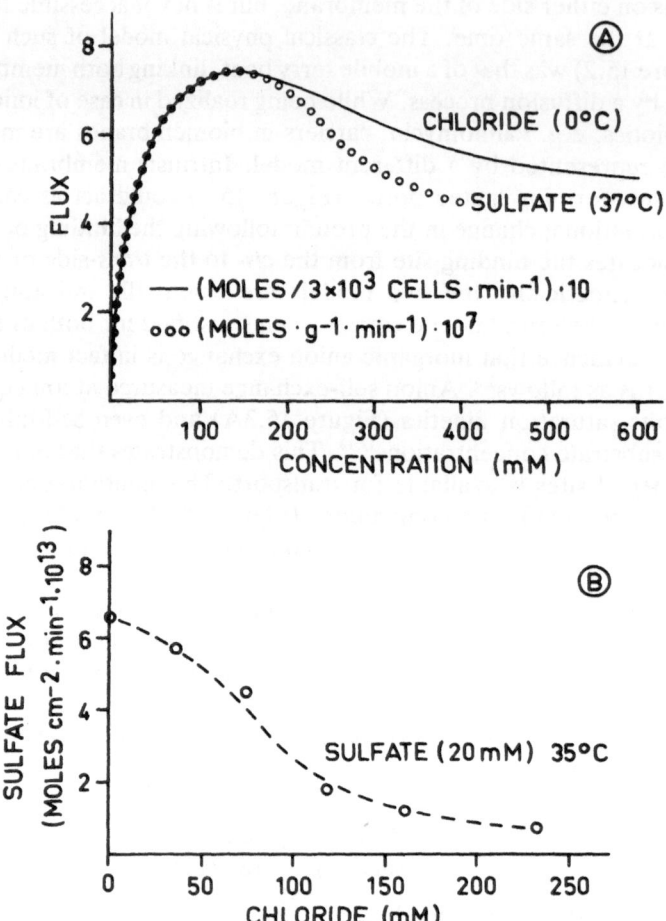

Figure 15.3 Kinetic characteristics of anion self-exchange in human erythrocytes. (A) Saturation kinetics and self-inhibition (from reference 12 for Cl⁻ and reference 13 for sulphate): (B) Anion competition: chloride inhibition of sulphate self-exchange

change of the conformation in the carrier protein which has to be protonated. The model assumes one binding site which reciprocates and mediates in sequence the coupled exchange of the two anions, since it can only re-orient when an anion is bound. In alternative to this 'sequential model' a simultaneous translocation of two anions bound to *two* opposite binding sites would also lead to tight coupling. The kinetic data of anion exchange, however, are not compatible with such a simultaneous model[6,15].

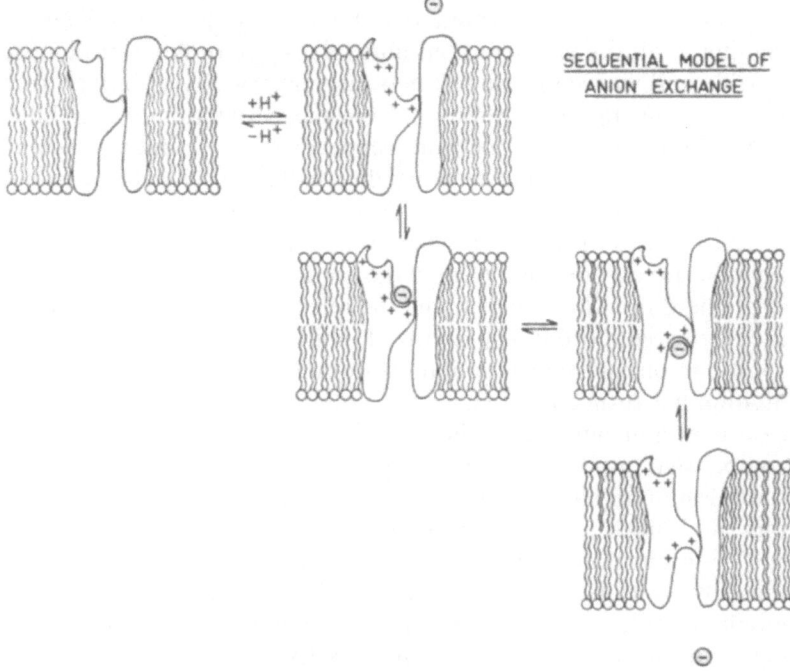

Figure 15.4 Model of anion exchange by a gated-pore mechanism with a titratable binding site in the erythrocyte membrane

The aforementioned protonation equilibria induce an asymmetric distribution of the binding sites between the two surfaces of the membrane. This interesting feature of the system rests on the following consideration[12]. At ion equilibrium the unidirectional fluxes (J) arising at the two surfaces are equal. Moreover, they are proportional to the concentration of the loaded carrier: $\overrightarrow{J} = P \cdot [CHA]_i = \overleftarrow{J} = P \cdot [CHA]_e$. Consequently, $[CHA]_i = [CHA]_e$. From equation (4) it then follows that $[CH^+]_i \cdot [A^-]_i = [CH^+]_e \cdot [A^-]_e$ or $[CH^+]_i/[CH^+]_e = [A^-]_e/[A^-]_i$. Since at equilibrium anions are distributed between a red cell and its environment according to a pH-dependent Donnan equilibrium governed by the intracellular concentration of impermeant anions, the ratio $[A^-]_i/[A^-]_e$ usually differs from 1. Consequently, the binding sites (CH^+_i, CH^+_e) will also be distributed asymmetrically between the two membrane surfaces at ion equilibrium. This prediction assumes identical values of the equilibrium constant K_2 at both surfaces, not a very realistic assumption since K_{2i} pertains to different conformations of the carrier protein. As a consequence of this, and of the inherently asymmetric nature of proteins, an even higher degree of asymmetry of the binding sites might be expected leading to different kinetic constants (K_m, V_{max}) for fluxes from inside to outside and vice versa. Such kinetic asymmetries have, in fact, recently been demonstrated[15]. Moreover, from the assumption of a mobile reciprocating transfer site, one would expect a marked, but non-symmetric dependence of each unidirectional flux on the concentration of anions at the *opposite* membrane surface. This has also been shown[15,16].

The kinetics of anion exchange thus indicate the involvement of an asymmetric carrier, able to undergo conformational changes upon substrate binding. This concept, and the relevance of carrier conformation, are further supported by patterns of inhibition. As was shown in Figure 15.3B, anion exchange is inhibited by other small anions present. This inhibition has turned out to have two components, a competitive one due to a common binding to the transfer site on the carrier, and a noncompetitive one[17]. The latter component can be rationalized by the assumption of an allosteric modifier site on the carrier. Anion binding to this site, which has a much lower affinity for anions than the transfer site[17], inhibits transfer by decreasing the turnover rate of the carrier and thus lowering its V_{max} value (Figure 15.5a). Anion binding to such a modifier site also accounts for the self-inhibition of anion exchange at high concentrations shown in Figure 15.3A.

Inhibitors

Anion exchange can be blocked by a host of structurally unrelated amphiphilic organic compounds[5] (Table 15.1). They can be grouped into three classes. First, agents bound non-covalently to the membrane. This group comprises, besides simple organic compounds, numerous drugs which inhibit noncompetitively at low concentrations. Some of them are impermeable and can therefore be used to study the 'sidedness' of the inhibitory binding site. In passing it should be noted that it does not seem altogether impossible that some of these compounds may inhibit Cl^-/HCO_3^- exchange *in vivo* at plasma levels obtained with therapeutical doses[18]. The symptoms would be similar to those observed after treatment or poisoning with inhibitors of carbonic anhydrase, namely respiratory, or mixed-type acidosis and hyperventilation.

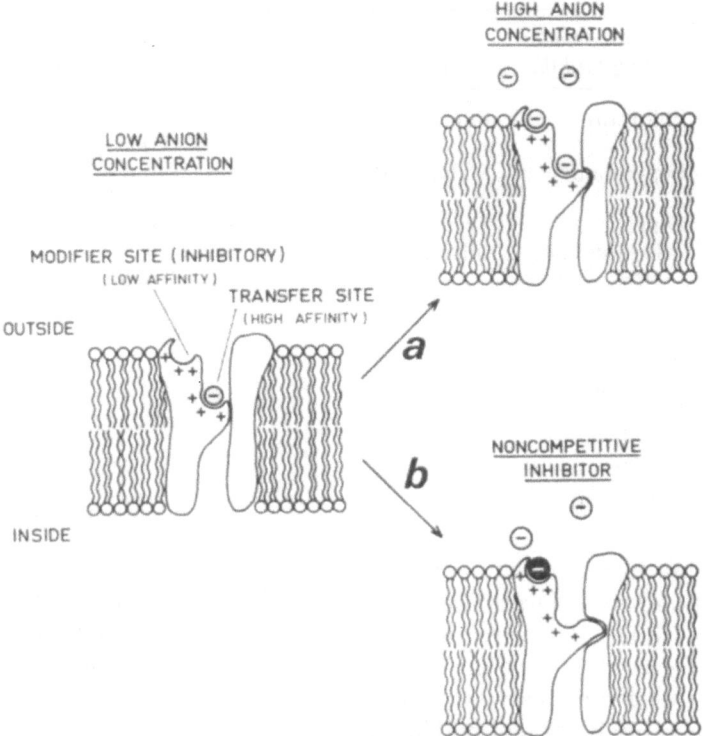

Figure 15.5 Model of an (allosteric) modifier site on the anion carrier responsible for non-competitive inhibition of anion exchange by (a) high concentrations of transported anions and (b) amphiphilic inhibitors. This inhibition is illustrated by the increasing interlocking of the 'gate' with the opposite wall

A second class of the inhibitors comprises agents which bind covalently to specific side-groups of the carrier protein and thus perturb its structure. Strong inhibition is observed with most amino reagents while SII reagents are ineffective.

The third class comprises what we have termed 'bimodal inhibitors', compounds which primarily inhibit by reversible non-covalent interaction due to their specific structural properties, but can be converted into irreversible inhibitors by minor changes of their structure or the experimental conditions[5-7,19]. This bimodal nature allows the characterization of the binding site in mechanistic terms (competitive inhibition indicates binding to the transfer site, non-competitive inhibition binding to an allosteric modifier site), and its molecular identification by virtue of the irre-

TABLE 15.1 Inhibitors of anion exchange

Non-covalent, amphiphilic	Covalent, sidegroup-specific	'Bimodal' non-covalent → covalent
Phloretin	Fluodinitrobenzene	Stilbene disulphonates ('DIDS', 'SITS', 'DNDS')
Dipyridamole	Maleic anhydride	N-azido-nitrophenyl taurine (NAP-taurine)
Diuretics furosemide, ethacrynic acid	Trinitrobenzene sulphonate	
		Diazo-sulphanilate
Local anaesthetics		Pyridoxalphosphate/BH$_4^-$
Anti-inflammatory drugs salicylate, niflumic acid, phenylbutazone		

versible attachment of the inhibitor to the carrier. Among the compounds used for these purposes, derivatives of stilbene disulphonic acids (SITS, DIDS*)[6,20] and a photoreactive organic monosulphonate (NAP-taurine)[21] have proven most useful, particularly since they have a very low permeability and can be used to study sidedness and transmembrane reorientation of binding sites.

Two points of information relevant to the mechanism of anion exchange have recently been obtained with the aid of impermeable inhibitors. First, some of the modifier sites, as defined above, seem to be located only at the exofacial membrane surface. This follows from the observation that certain impermeable inhibitors are highly effective when added to the extracellular medium, but ineffective from the cytoplasmic membrane surface when introduced into erythrocytes by certain tricks (Figure 15.6)[21–33]. These inhibitors compete, however, at their exofacial binding sites with inorganic anions[22] that act as inhibitors via these sites (Figure 15.5b), a complex situation, underlining once more the marked asymmetry of the system.

Secondly, the concept of reciprocating (= mobile) binding sites on the

* Abbreviations: SITS, 4-acetamido-4'isothiocyano-2,2'-stilbene-disulphonate; DIDS, 4,4'-diisothiocyano stilbene-2,2'-disulphonate; PCMBS, p-chloromercuriphenylsulphonate; PCMB, p-chloromercuribenzoate; NAP-taurine, N-(4-azido-2-nitrophenyl)-2-aminoethylsulphonate; HEPES, N-2-hydroxyethylpiperazin-N'-2-ethanesulphonic acid; SDS, sodium dodecylsulphate.

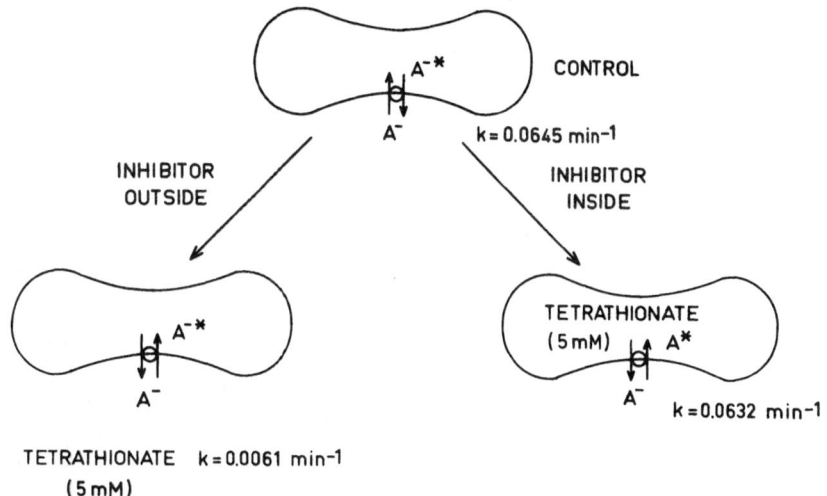

Figure 15.6 Asymmetric inhibition of anion self-exchange by tetrathionate and other inhibitors as an indication for the exofacial localization of the modifier site on the erythrocyte membrane. Impermeability prevents equilibration of inhibitor, k = rate coefficient of self-exchange

anion-exchange carrier could be substantiated using impermeable bimodal inhibitors which bind to the transfer site. If an inhibitor of this type is first reacted with the membrane from one surface (Figure 15.7), subsequent binding of a second inhibitor of the same type to the opposite membrane surface is considerably reduced[23]. This finding is taken to indicate that the reaction of the carrier with inhibitor 1 from one side recruits and sequesters binding sites to this surface and makes them unavailable for a reaction with inhibitor 2 from the opposite surface, a valuable point of evidence for binding sites able to undergo transmembrane reorientation.

Structural data and models

Kinetic and mechanistic properties of the inorganic anion-exchange system are thus known to a point justifying the question of its molecular identity. This problem could be attacked successfully due to the conjunction of some lucky circumstances. One of the most potent impermeable

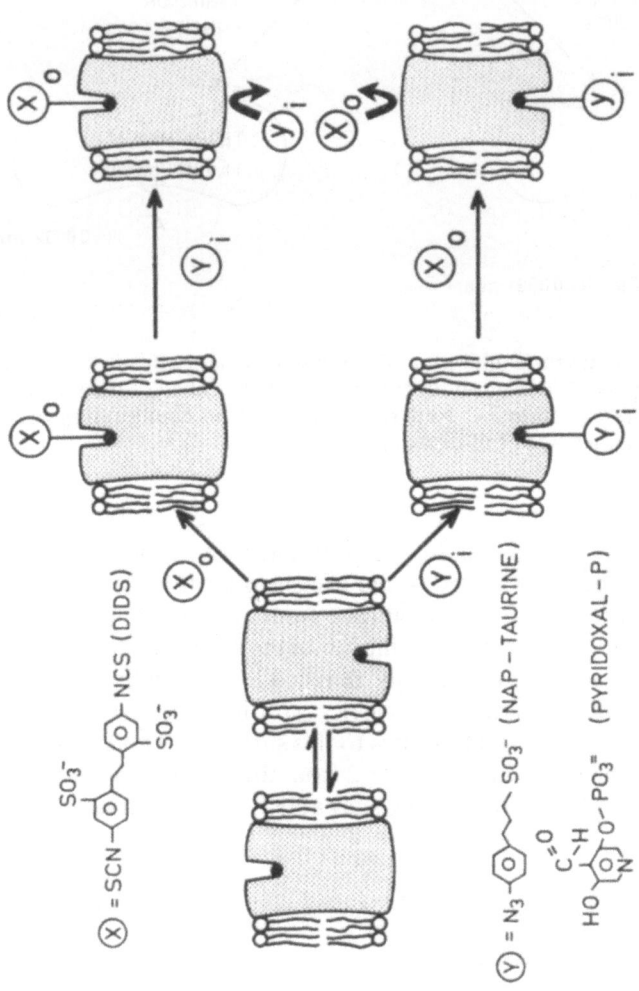

Figure 15.7 Recruitment of mobile binding sites of the anion-exchange system to one face of the erythrocyte membrane by impermeable, covalent inhibitors reacting with the binding site. Reaction of the membrane from one side with inhibitor X (or Y) reduces subsequent binding of inhibitor Y (or X) from the opposite side of the membrane. Schematic representation based on data compiled by Grinstein et al.[23]

bimodal inhibitors of anion exchange, DIDS, binds highly selectively to one of the most abundant peptide fractions of the erythrocyte membrane, usually called Band 3, according to its position on SDS–polyacrylamide electrophoretic gels[19,20]. DIDS binding to this fraction strictly parallels inhibition. The maximum is reached upon binding of one DIDS molecule for each copy of Band 3 (i.e. about 1.2×10^6 per cell). Peptides in Band 3 (see reference 21 for a recent review) constitute 25% of the total membrane protein, have a molecular weight of about 95 000 and are highly, although not completely, homogeneous. They are membrane-spanning intrinsic proteins present in their native environment as dimers or even tetramers. A minor amount of carbohydrate bound to the exofacial domain of the protein constitutes the I-antigen and the concanavalin A binding site[25] of the erythrocyte membrane. Numerous data are available in favour of Band 3 being the purported anion-exchange carrier. The most convincing piece of evidence is the successful reconstitution of a DIDS-sensitive anion transport by inserting purified Band 3 into artificial phospholipid membranes, which was reported by Cabantchik et al.[6]. We have been able to confirm this important result (Köhne and Deuticke, *Biochim. Biophys. Acta,* in press).

We may thus proceed to the question of *how* Band 3 mediates anion exchange. In this context the structural details of the protein are of interest. The present state of information is compiled in Figure 15.8, and has recently been reviewed[24]. The monomer consists of three domains, a hydrophobic one (41 K Dalton) protruding into the cytoplasma, a very hydrophilic one (17 K Dalton) spanning the bilayer in at least one loop and a third one (38 K Dalton) accessible from the outside but firmly integrated into the membrane and interacting with the 17 K fragment even after proteolysis. Anion exchange seems to involve the central 17 K fragment since (1) the 41 K fragment can be clipped off without destroying anion exchange[26] (2) the 17 K fragment bears the DIDS binding site[27] and (3) incorporation of the 17 K fragment (plus a piece of the 38 K fragment?) conveys DIDS-sensitive anion permeability to artificial lipid vesicles[28].

In the light of these data and the intensive work on Band 3 in numerous laboratories it may not seem overoptimistic to predict that the inorganic anion-exchange system of the erythrocyte may be one of the first transport processes understood on a molecular basis, although this may still take quite a time.

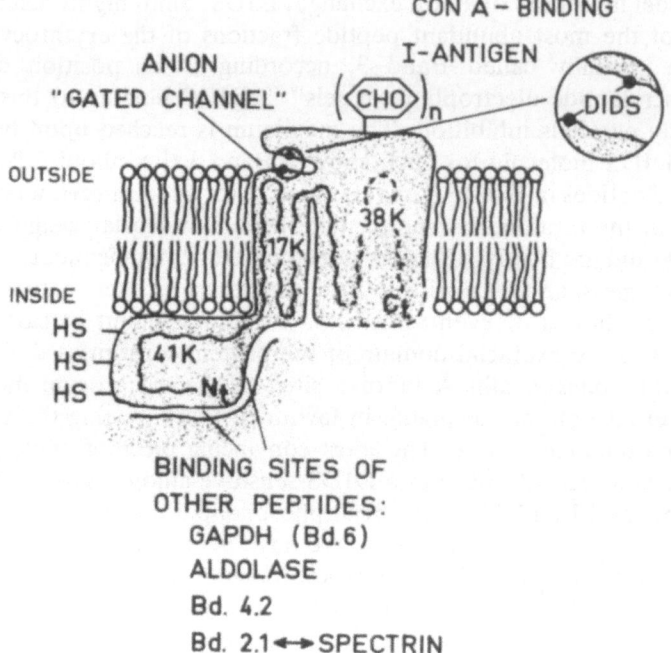

Figure 15.8 Present views on the disposition and some structural details of Band 3, the alleged anion-exchange protein in the human erythrocyte membrane. CHO = carbohydrate, N_t, C_t = NH_2 and COO^- terminal of the peptide chain. For references underlying this scheme see reference 24

PROPERTIES OF THE MONOCARBOXYLATE TRANSFER SYSTEM IN THE ERYTHROCYTE MEMBRANE

The problem of anion transfer across the erythrocyte membrane is not only one of the characterization of the function of Band 3. Recent studies in a number of laboratories have provided clear evidence that in many, although not all, mammalian species a second anion-transfer system is present, specialized on monocarboxylate anions such as lactate, pyruvate, β-hydroxybutyrate. These anions are also transported by the classical exchange system, however only at low rates.

Kinetic data and models

The claim of an additional, independent transfer system for monocarboxylate anions is based mainly on the observation that lactate self-exchange is almost insensitive to potent disulphonate inhibitors of inorganic anion-exchange, but strongly inhibited by SH-reagents, which do not affect inorganic anion exchange (Figure 15.9). The SH-dependent transfer system discriminates L- and D-enantiomers, in contrast to the classical system, and apparently operates by a different mechanism. Justification for this claim stems from the marked differences in the mode of coupling of the fluxes between the two sides of the membrane. As in case of inorganic anion transfer[4,15] the fluxes of monocarboxylate anions are enhanced in a concentration-dependent saturating fashion by monocarboxylates present on the opposite side of the membrane. This 'trans-acceleration' (Figure 15.10) and the related phenomenon of uphill countertransport, which could also be demonstrated[31], indicate that in this case, too, a mobile carrier is involved. In contrast to the inorganic anion-exchange system, however, lactate net fluxes can also proceed at a considerable rate in the absence of anions on the trans-side of the membrane (Table 15.2). In order to meet the requirements of electroneutrality, we must conclude from this finding that the monocarboxylate carrier mediates net movements of its substrates, either in exchange for hydroxyl anions or by a cotransport with protons (Figure 15.11). In essence this means that a transfer of lactic acid is catalysed by this system. Experimental evidence for such a model comes from studies on the pH-dependency of monocarboxylate net movements[32,34] and from the observation of pH changes accompanying lactate net transfer[34].

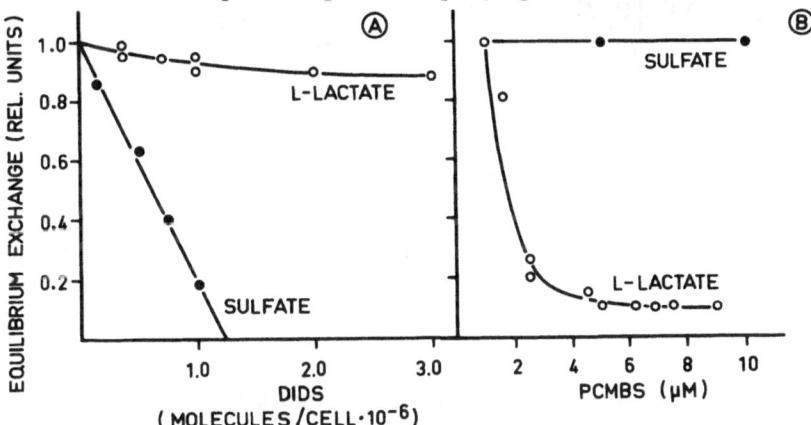

Figure 15.9 Discrimination of the inorganic anion-exchange system and the monocarboxylate-transfer system by their different sensitivities to disulphonate and mercurial inhibitors. Measurements of equilibrium exchange of sulphate and L-lactate in the presence of the inhibitors

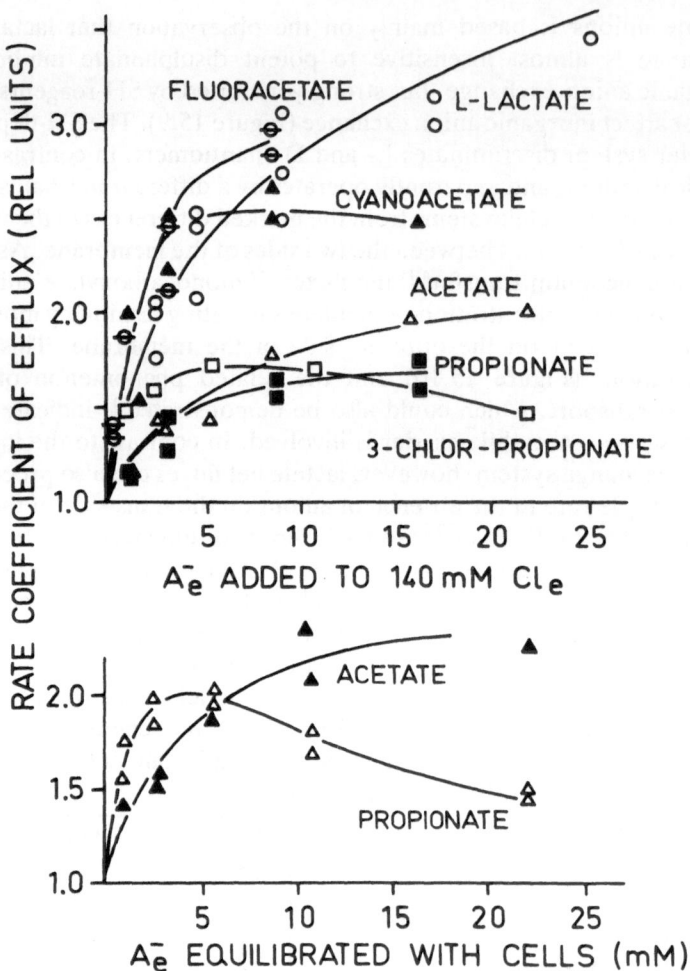

Figure 15.10 Trans-acceleration of L-lactate net efflux by extracellular mono-carboxylates as an indicator for the presence of a 'mobile' carrier for mono-carboxylates in the human erythrocyte membrane (from reference 32). A_e^- = extracellular organic monocarboxylate anion

Possible physiological role of the monocarboxylate carrier

A parallel movement of protons and monocarboxylate anions is, of course, a very suitable mechanism of transport since both are formed in stoichiometric amounts in glycolytic and other metabolic reactions. In

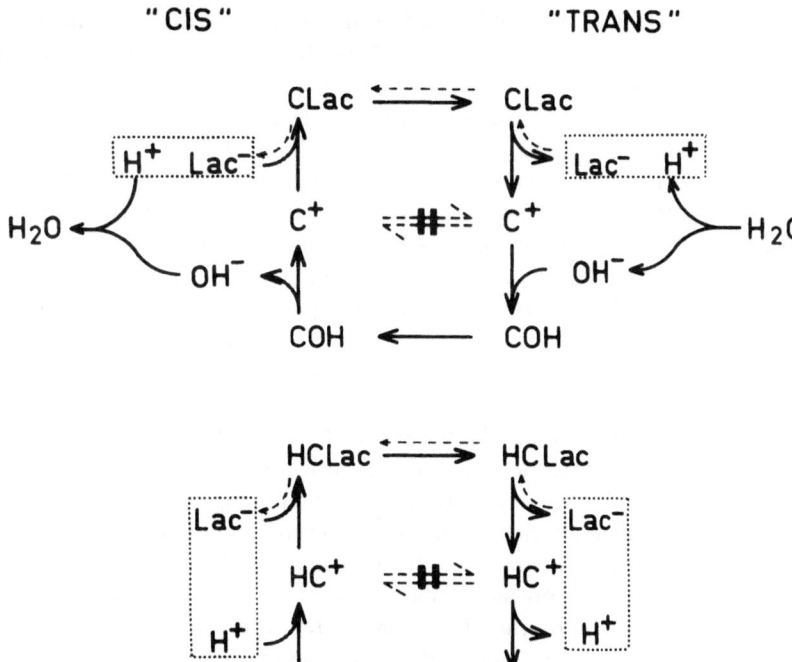

"CIS" "TRANS"

Figure 15.11 Operational scheme of lactic acid net movements (from *cis* to *trans*) across the human erythrocyte membrane by a lactate/OH⁻ antiport (upper panel) or a lactate–H⁺ symport (lower panel). In both models the movement of charged carrier (C^+, HC^+) is not allowed

TABLE 15.2 L-Lactate efflux into anion-free
media

Extracellular medium		Rate coefficient of L-lactate efflux
NaCl	135 mmol/1*	0.0417
Sucrose	270 mmol/1*	0.0449

Cells pretreated with DIDS (3×10^6 molecules/cell) $pH_i = 7.3$, $pH_e = 8.00$, 10°C, $Lac_i = 3.8$ mmol/l
* Plus 15 mmol/l impermeable buffer (HEPES)

fact, passive monocarboxylate-carrier systems of this type are most likely present in a number of membrane systems, e.g. the plasma membranes of striated muscle[35,36] and ascites tumour cells[37], in the blood–brain barrier[38] and in mitochondria[39]. In these systems the requirement for an effective transport of monocarboxylic acids is quite evident. What is it needed for, however, in red cells? The small amounts of lactate formed in these cells ($2\,\mu$mol/ml cells per hour at 37°C) could easily be disposed of by a lactate$_i$/Cl$_e^-$ exchange followed by an OH$_e^-$/Cl$_i^-$ exchange, via the inorganic anion-exchange system. Alternatively, one might consider an involvement of this system in the removal of monocarboxylic acids from metabolizing tissues. In order to proceed with minimal perturbation of blood pH, this process requires haemoglobin for buffering. The entry of protons into the erythrocytes, prior to their binding to haemoglobin, is mediated by the Jacob–Stewart cycle (Figure 15.1, lower). Its rate is limited by the slowest reaction of this sequence, namely the uncatalysed dehydration of HCO$_3^-$ to CO$_2$ in plasma. It would seem conceivable that a direct movement of protons across the membrane by a lactate–H$^+$ cotransport system (Figure 15.12) might be a more effective mechanism. The data presently available, however, do not bear out this assumption. Protons react with haemoglobin with a half-time of 0.3 s when lactic acid is added to blood samples *in vitro* at 37°C[40], as indicated by the liberation of O$_2$ in the subsequent Bohr shift. Lactate net movements across the erythrocyte membrane, on the other hand, occur with an estimated half-time of about 10–20 s as can be con-

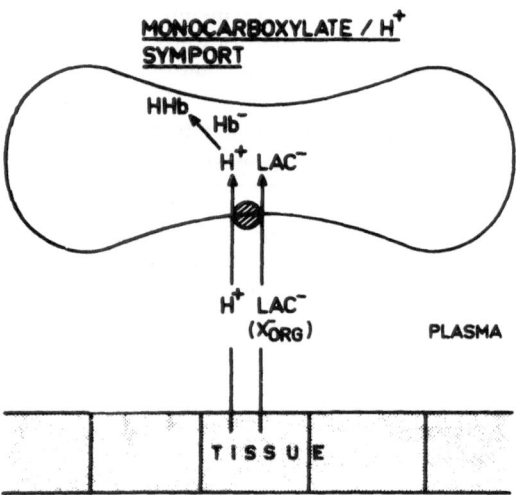

Figure 15.12 Monocarboxylate-H$^+$ cotransport as a mechanism of proton uptake into erythrocytes, e.g. in metabolic acidosis

cluded from measurements of this process at lower temperatures (Deuticke, unpublished data).

Thus, the biological importance of the monocarboxylate carrier of the erythrocyte membrane remains to be elucidated. It might, of course, also just be a remnant from the earlier developmental stages of that cell.

Molecular properties of the carrier

The molecular characterization of the monocarboxylate carrier is still at its beginning. Using trans-acceleration of lactate efflux by various types of anions as an indicator we could establish[32] that the system accepts, besides hydroxy- and keto-acids, many of their substituted analogues as well as simple fatty acids (Table 15.3). In contrast, aromatic monocarboxylates, amino acids, dicarboxylates and, notably, inorganic anions are not accepted. A provisional 'negative structure' of the binding-site has been constructed from this pattern.

TABLE 15.3 Specificity of the monocarboxylate carrier

Accepted
Fatty acids (C_2–C_4), except: formate
Hydroxy-acids, except: glyoxylate
                       glycerate
                       α-hydroxy isobutyrate
Keto-acids
Halogeno-acids
Cyano-, azido-acids

Not accepted
Amino acids
Aromatic monocarboxylates
Dicarboxylates
Sulphonates
Inorganic anions

A tightly bound, impermeable mercurial inhibitor of lactate transport, *p*-chloromercuribenzoate, has been used to estimate the maximal number of transfer sites. The number obtained, $1.5 \cdot 10^5$/cell, is 10 times lower than that found for inorganic anion exchange sites, but almost certainly still too high, since SH-groups not involved in monocarboxylate transfer are also present on the erythrocyte surface. The same SH-inhibitor has also been used for attempts to localize the protein involved

(Deuticke, unpublished results). While only minor amounts were bound to the Band 3 region, most of the inhibitor was located in the region of the intrinsic protein bands 4.5 and 7. Band 4.5 contains a very heterogeneous population of membrane-spanning (glyco)-peptides (45–65 K Dalton)[43] including, probably, the alleged glucose-transport protein of the erythrocyte membrane[41,42]. If the monocarboxylate carrier is located in this fraction, the total number of copies per cell is likely to be very low. Band 7 (approximately 30 K Dalton)[43] is almost uncharacterized, except that it spans the membrane. Further progress in its molecular identification will probably have to await the availability of more specific, covalently bound inhibitors of the monocarboxylate carrier.

CONCLUDING REMARKS

The physiological and biochemical evidence summarized above indicates the presence, in the human erythrocyte membrane, of two anion transfer systems operating by different mechanisms and probably located in different proteins. One serves an important task in the transport of acid equivalents in blood and the maintenance of acid–base homeostasis. The biological relevance of the other one is still open.

In a conference devoted to the study of genetic defects of biocatalytical functions, the question should be raised whether such defects are also known for the two transport systems discussed here. To my knowledge, this has not been described. The clinical symptoms expected to result from a deficiency of the Cl^-/HCO_3^- exchange system are rather unspecific – respiratory or mixed acidosis, hyperventilation – and will probably only become evident under conditions of physical exercise. It might be worthwhile, in unexplainable cases of acidosis or hyperventilation, to think at least of a deficit or defects in one of these transport systems.

Acknowledgement

Work from the author's laboratory reported here was supported by the Deutsche Forschungsgemeinschaft (Sonderforschungsbereich 160).

References

1. Jacobs, M. H. and Stewart, D. R. (1941). The role of carbonic anhydrase in certain ionic exchanges involving the erythrocyte. *J. Gen. Physiol.*, **25**, 539
2. Swenson, E. R. and Maren, Th. H. (1978). A quantitative analysis of CO_2 transport at rest and during maximal exercise. *Respir. Physiol.*, **35**, 129

3. Gunn, R. B. (1979). Transport of anions across red cell membranes. In *Membrane Transport in Biology*. G. Giebisch, D. C. Tosteson and H. H. Ussing (eds.). Vol. II, p. 59. (Berlin: Springer)

4. Wieth, J. O. (1979). Bicarbonate exchange through the human red cell membrane determined with [^{14}C] bicarbonate. *J. Physiol. (London)*, **294**, 521

5. Deuticke, B. (1977). Properties and structural basis of simple diffusion pathways in the erythrocyte membrane. *Rev. Physiol. Biochem. Pharmacol.*, **78**, 1

6. Cabantchik, Z. I., Knauf, Ph. A. and Rothstein, A. (1978). The anion transport system of the red blood cell. The role of membrane protein evaluated by the use of 'probes'. *Biochim. Biophys. Acta*, **515**, 239

7. Fortes, P. A. G. (1977). Anion movements in red blood cells. In *Membrane Transport in Red Cells*. J. C. Ellory and V. L. Lew (eds.), p. 175. (London: Academic Press)

8. Motais, R. (1977). Organic anion transport in red blood cells. In *Membrane Transport in Red Cells*. J. C. Ellory and V. L. Lew (eds.). P. 197. (London: Academic Press)

9. Brahm, J. (1977). Temperature-dependent changes of chloride transport kinetics in human red cells. *J. Gen. Physiol.*, **70**, 283

10. Hunter, M. J. (1976). Human erythrocyte anion permeabilities measured under conditions of net charge transfer. *J. Physiol. (London)*, **268**, 35

11. Lassen, U.V. (1977). Electrical potential and conductance of the red cell membrane. In *Membrane Transport in Red Cells*. J. C. Ellory and V. L. Lew (eds.), p. 37. (London: Academic Press)

12. Dalmark, M. (1975). Chloride transport in human red cells. *J. Physiol. (London)*, **250**, 39

13. Schnell, K. F., Gerhardt, S. and Schöppe-Fredenburg, A. (1977). Kinetic characteristics of the sulfate self-exchange in human red blood cells and red blood cell ghosts. *J. Membr. Biol.*, **30**, 319

14. Gunn, R. B. (1978). Considerations of the titratable carrier model for sulfate transport in human red blood cells. In *Membrane Transport Processes*. J. F. Hoffman (ed.). Vol. I, p. 61. (New York: Raven Press)

15. Gunn, R. B. and Fröhlich, O. (1979). Asymmetry in the mechanism for anion exchange in human red blood cell membranes. *J. Gen. Physiol.*, **74**, 351

16. Jennings, M. L. (1979). Some experimental tests of the carrier model of red cell anion exchange. Alfred Benzon Symposium 14: *Membrane Transport in Erythrocytes*. U. Lassen, II. H. Ussing and J. O. Wieth (eds.), p. 450 (Copenhagen: Munksgaard)

17. Dalmark, M. (1976). Effects of halides and bicarbonate on chloride transport in human red blood cells. *J. Gen. Physiol.*, **67**, 223

18. Wieth, J. O. and Brahm, J. (1979). Kinetics of bicarbonate exchange in human red cells: Physiological implications. U. Lassen, H. H. Ussing and J. O. Wieth (eds.). Alfred Benzon Symposium 14: *Membrane Transport in Erythrocytes*, p. 467. (Copenhagen: Munksgaard)

19. Rothstein, A., Cabantchik, Z. I. and Knauf, P. (1976). Mechanism of anion transport in red blood cells: role of membrane proteins. *Fedn. Proc. Fedn. Socs. Exp. Biol.*, **35**, 3

20. Lepke, S., Fasold, H., Pring, M. and Passow, H. (1976). A study of the relationship between inhibition of anion exchange and binding to the red blood cell membrane of 4,4'-diisothiocyano stilbene-2,2'-disulfonic acid (DIDS) and its dihydro-derivative (H$_2$DIDS). *J. Membr. Biol.*, **29**, 147

21. Knauf, P. A., Ship, S., Breuer, W., McCulloch, L. and Rothstein, A. (1978). Asymmetry of the red cell anion exchange system: Different mechanisms of reversible inhibition by N-(4-azido-2-nitrophenyl)-2-aminoethylsulfonate (NAP-Taurine) at the inside and outside of the membrane. *J. Gen. Physiol.*, **72**, 607

22. Deuticke, B., v. Bentheim, M., Beyer, E. and Kamp, D. (1978). Reversible inhibition of anion exchange in human erythrocytes by an inorganic disulfonate, tetrathionate. *J. Membr. Biol.*, **44**, 135

23. Grinstein, S., McCulloch, L. and Rothstein, A. (1979). Transmembrane effects of irreversible inhibitors of anion transport in red blood cells. *J. Gen. Physiol.*, **73**, 493

24. Steck, Th. L. (1978). The Band 3 protein of the human red cell membrane: A review. *J. Supramolec. Struct.*, **8**, 311

25. Findlay, J. B. C. (1974). The receptor proteins for concanavalin A and Lens culinaris phytohemagglutinin in the membrane of the human erythrocyte. *J. Biol. Chem.*, **249**, 4398

26. Lepke, S. and Passow, H. (1976a). Effects of incorporated trypsin on anion exchange and membrane proteins in human red blood cell ghosts. *Biochim. Biophys. Acta*, **455**, 353

27. Grinstein, S., Ship, S. and Rothstein, A. (1978). Anion transport in relation to proteolytic dissection of Band 3 protein. *Biochim. Biophys. Acta*, **507**, 294

28. Rothstein, A., Ramjeesingh, M. and Grinstein, S. (1979). The arrangement of transport and inhibitory sites in Band 3 protein. Alfred Benzon Symposium 14: Membrane transport in erythrocytes. U. Lassen, H. H. Ussing and J. O. Wieth (eds.), p. 329. (Copenhagen: Munksgaard)

29. Halestrap, A. P. (1976). Transport of pyruvate and lactate into human erythrocytes. Evidence for the involvement of the chloride carrier and a chloride independent carrier. *Biochem. J.*, **156**, 193

30. Deuticke, B., Rickert, I. and Beyer, E. (1978b). Stereoselective, SH-dependent transfer of lactate in mammalian erythrocytes. *Biochim. Biophys. Acta*, **507**, 137

31. Deuticke, B., v. Bentheim, M. and Schneege, B. (1978c). Properties of the monocarboxylate transfer system in the human erythrocyte membrane. *Hoppe-Seylers's Z. Physiol. Chem.*, **359**, 1463

32. Deuticke, B. (1979). Kinetic properties and substrate specificity of the monocarboxylate carrier in the human erythrocyte membrane. Alfred Benzon Symposium 14: Membrane transport in erythrocytes. U. Lassen, H. H. Ussing and J. O. Wieth (eds.), p. 359. (Copenhagen: Munksgaard)

33. Dubinsky, W. P. and Racker, E. (1978). The mechanism of lactate transport in human erythrocytes. *J. Membr. Biol.*, **44**, 25

34. Regen, D. M. and Tarpley, H. J. (1978). Effects of pH on β-hydrocybutyrate transport in rat erythrocytes and thymocytes. *Biochim. Biophys. Acta*, **508**, 539

35. Foulkes, E. C. and Paine, C. M. (1961). The uptake of monocarboxylic

acids by rat diaphragm. *J. Biol. Chem.*, **236**, 1019

36. Hirche, Hj., Hombach, V., Langohr, H. D., Wacker, U. and Busse, J. (1975). Lactic acid permeation rate in working gastrocnemii of dogs during metabolic alkalosis and acidosis. *Pflügers Arch.-Eur. J. Physiol.*, **356**, 209

37. Spencer, T. L. and Lehninger, A. L. (1976). L-Lactate transport in Ehrlich ascites-tumor cells. *Biochem. J.*, **154**, 405

38. Oldendorf, W. H. (1973). Carrier-mediated blood–brain barrier transport of short-chain monocarboxylic organic acids. *Am. J. Physiol.*, **224**, 1450

39. Paradies, G. and Papa, S. (1977). On the kinetics and substrate specificity of the pyruvate translocator in rat liver mitochondria. *Biochim. Biophys. Acta*, **462**, 333

40. Forster, R. E. and Steen, J. B. (1968). Rate limiting processes in the Bohr shift in human red cells. *J. Physiol. (London)*, **196**, 541

41. Kasahara, M. and Hinkle, P. (1977). Reconstitution and purification of the D-glucose transporter from human erythrocytes. *J. Biol. Chem.*, **252**, 7384

42. Kahlenberg, A. and Zala, C. A. (1977). Reconstitution of D-glucose transport in vesicles composed of lipids and intrinsic protein (Zone 4,5) of the human erythrocyte membrane. *J. Supramolec. Struc.*, **7**, 287

43. Steck, Th. L. (1974). The organization of proteins in the human red blood cell membrane. *J. Cell Biol.*, **62**, 1

16

Inherited disorders of
red-cell cation transport

G. W. Stewart

INTRODUCTION

This review is intended firstly, to enumerate the red-cell sodium and
potassium transporting systems with some · of their properties, then
secondly, to present an account of the inherited primary disorders of red-
cell cation transport, with an emphasis on those most recently reported.
A section is devoted to some recent work on cation transport in essential
hypertension. Many clinical conditions which exhibit abnormal red-cell
cation transport secondary to a more fundamental defect, such as pyruvate kinase deficiency, are omitted.

PATHWAYS OF SODIUM AND POTASSIUM TRANSPORT
ACROSS THE RED-CELL MEMBRANE

The principal functions of the red cell are to carry oxygen and carbon
dioxide to and fro between lungs and tissues. The haemoglobin within
the red cell exerts an osmotic pressure under which water tends to enter
the cell. To counteract this force, the red cell maintains a low total
cation-concentration relative to plasma. Internal Na ($[Na]_i$), is normally
kept low at approximately 8 mmol/l cells, while internal K ($[K]_i$) is kept
up at 100 mmol/l cells, creating an overall cation deficit within the cell. If

these gradients are allowed to dissipate to equilibrium with plasma, the cell swells and ultimately bursts.

At least four pathways have been described for Na and K transport: (1) the Na–K pump; (2) the cotransport system; (3) the 'linear leak'; (4) the Ca-sensitive K channel.

The Na–K pump

The pump has been intensively studied for 20 years and much is known about its behaviour. While hydrolysing one molecule of ATP to ADP and inorganic phosphate, the pump uses this chemical energy to actively transport three sodium ions out of the cell while moving two potassium ions in the reverse direction, against the respective electrochemical gradients[1]. The pump rate is stimulated by internal Na and by external K. Although virtually saturated by external K at physiological concentrations, it is only about 25% saturated by internal Na. Small variations in internal [Na], therefore, provide one control over the pumping rate and the determination of intracellular cation content. The pump is inhibited by low concentrations (10^{-8} M) of digitalis glycosides, e.g. ouabain, and by micromolar amounts of vanadate[2]. Since vanadate is present at these concentrations physiologically, it is tempting to infer that it may have a regulatory role[3]. Ouabain-sensitive Na–K pumps are widely distributed throughout the body. The number of pumping sites per red cell can be measured using a labelled ouabain method.

The cotransport system

If the influxes of Na and K are measured as functions of $[Na]_0$ and $[K]_0$ respectively, while the pump is suppressed by ouabain, both fluxes can be resolved into saturable (carrier mediated) and non-saturable components. The situation for K is shown in Figure 16.1. The non-saturable, linear component will be dealt with below. The saturable system will be called here the 'cotransport' system. It is a puzzle, because a reason for its existence in the red cell has not yet been demonstrated. Its major features are:

(i) Mutual inter-dependence of the cations on each other. The saturable ouabain-insensitive influxes of Na or K can be abolished by substituting, say, choline for the complementary cation. This

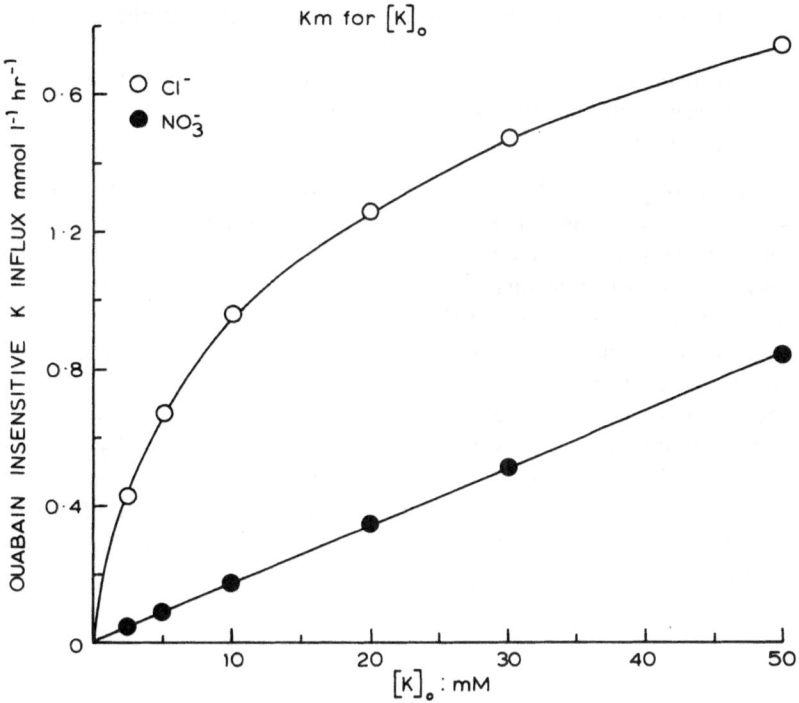

Figure 16.1 Ouabain-insensitive K influx as a function of external [K], measured using a rubidium tracer. Open circles denote fluxes measured in the presence of chloride; closed circles, chloride replaced by nitrate. The saturable (cotransport) component is abolished by the anion substitution

mutual inter-dependence led Wiley and Cooper[4] to call the system 'cotransport', the parallel movement of two species across the membrane by a system.

(ii) Operation of Na–Na and K–K exchange under physiological conditions of external Na and K. Wiley and Cooper[4] showed that, for both Na and K, the cotransport influxes and effluxes balanced each other. The fluxes of K exceed those of Na.

(iii) Inhibition by 'loop diuretics'. Furosemide[5], piretanide[6], and Mk 196 (personal observation) all inhibit Na and K cotransport influx and efflux. Ethacrynic acid[5] inhibits Na efflux, but for some reason stimulates Na influx.

(iv) Dependence on chloride. We[28] have shown that the cotransport influxes and effluxes of Na and K are abolished if chloride is replaced by another anion, such as methyl sulphate or nitrate (Figure 16.1). It would be interesting to determine whether Cl is transported by the red-cell cotransport system, but the very rapid anion-exchange mechanism in the red cell precludes such a measurement.

Interesting parallels can be drawn between this red cell system and similar mechanisms in other cells. Burg *et al.*[7] identified in renal tubules an active transport of Cl inhibited by furosemide. Nellans *et al.*[8], working on rabbit ileum, demonstrated a coupled Cl and Na transport across the membrane. They proposed that the active Cl transport here was energized by the simultaneous dissipation of the parallel Na gradient, which was itself set up by the Na–K pump splitting ATP at the opposite side of the cell (Figure 16.2). Zeuthen *et al.*[9] in marine teleost intestine, presented evidence for the inhibition of active Cl transport by piretanide. The model of Nellans *et al.* – active transport of the species at the expense of the dissipation of the Na or K gradient – is likely to prove fruitful in the eventual elucidation of the role of the cotransport system in the red cell.

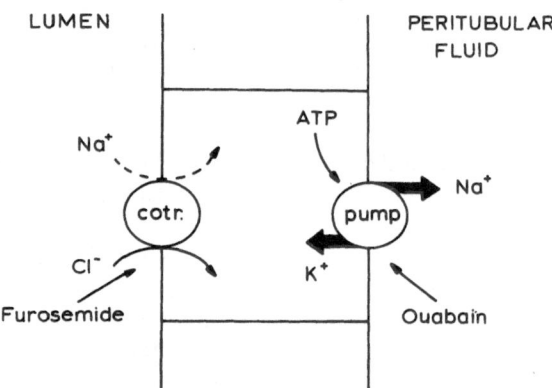

Figure 16.2 Diagrammatic representation of epithelial cell to show energy coupling between active Cl⁻ transport and the Na–K pump, after Nellans *et al.*[8]. The Na–K pump on one side of the cell generates an intracellular Na deficit using chemical energy; a cotransport-like system on the opposite side dissipates this Na gradient to provide energy for active Cl⁻ transport

The linear leak

The non-saturable fluxes of Na and K have a rate constant of approximately 0.012/h[4]. If the linear leak influx of a cation is known, the efflux rate constant can be predicted using Ussing's flux ratio equation[10].

The Ca-sensitive K channel

Gardos[11] and later Lew[12] have shown that, if cells are depleted of intracellular ATP, the powerful Ca extrusion pump, which normally maintains intracellular Ca at micromolar levels, fails. If the cells are incubated in a Ca-containing medium, Ca leaks in and accumulates within the cell. This high intracellular [Ca] triggers a specific K channel which mediates a large K efflux. Although this channel does not operate in the red cell in life (except possibly during the final demise of the cell), it is of importance not only in the understanding of some haemolytic states, but also in the understanding of Ca control of membrane permeability throughout the body.

CLINICAL CONDITIONS

Disorders of red-cell membrane Na and K transport are fairly numerous[13], but primary membrane lesions are rare. Three such conditions will be considered, then some recent work on hypertension will be described.

Hereditary stomatocytosis

Lock et al.[14] coined the term 'stomatocytosis' to describe swollen, bowl-shaped cells which they saw in a case of congenital haemolytic anaemia. The osmotic fragility was increased and they were surprised not to see spherocytes on the film. Some disorder of Na and K transport was suspected, but it was Zarkowsky et al.[15], studying a similar congenital haemolytic anaemia, who first demonstrated with isotopically measured fluxes the increased Na and K transport rates which are the hallmark of this disease. They found that both ouabain-sensitive ('pump') and ouabain-insensitive (loosely called 'leak' at that time: the term embraced both linear leak and cotransport fluxes) were increased. It was felt that the increased pumping rate was secondary to some increase in the 'leak'. No distinction was made into linear leak and cotransport fluxes at that time.

Seven further reports[16-22] appeared, detailing families and individual patients with haemolytic anaemias having in common a primary-membrane Na and K permeability problem. All show autosomal dominant inheritance, and increased ouabain-binding sites, where measured, consistent with the universal increase in pumping rate. However, in many important respects the group is heterogeneous: the severity of the anaemia is very variable, the osmotic fragility may be normal, increased or even decreased, and the isotopic fluxes are variably increased. Two broad groups, which are not well separated emerge: (i) 'overhydrated' and (ii) 'dehydrated'. The overhydrated variety shows predominantly stomatocytes on smear, has increased osmotic fragility and increased cell water. The original cases described by Lock et al.[14] fall into this category. In the dehydrated variety, the cells are shrunken in appearance, have low cell water levels, and tend to have decreased osmotic fragility. One explanation for this difference could lie in the relative severity of the Na and K transport defects: a greater Na 'leak' than K would result in ion gain (and by osmosis water gain) leading to swollen cells; whereas a dominant K 'leak', following the K gradient out of the cell, would render the cell dehydrated. The bulk of the available data does not distinguish linear leak and cotransport components and therefore it is difficult to draw conclusions. Wiley[23], however, has performed these measurements on two patients, one of each variety. In his review, he does not quote the data in detail, but broadly, in the overhydrated variety, while the linear leak fluxes of Na and K were increased, the cotransport Na and K influxes were absent. In the dehydrated variety, both the linear leak and cotransport fluxes were abnormally high. Quantitative efflux data were not quoted, so the picture remains unclear. Perhaps some slight differences in Na and K linear leak permeability somehow influence the cotransport system response via the internal cation levels. Although the linear leak fluxes are influenced by few factors other than the applied cation concentration gradient and pH, the various fluxes of the cotransport system may well be under complex control. Much further work is obviously required to unravel the complexities of this multi-flux situation.

Two abnormalities of membrane structure have been found in some cases of hereditary stomatocytosis: Shohet et al.[19] and Wiley et al.[21] both reported increased phosphatidyl choline in the membrane stroma.

Mentzer *et al.*[22] found the phospholipids in his cases to be normal, but noted a deficiency in the incorporation of labelled ^{32}P from ATP into the membrane protein, spectrin. The relationship of these two abnormalities to the fluxes is not known.

Glader *et al.*[20] and later, Wiley *et al.*[24] have reported low levels of the glycolytic intermediate 2–3 diphosphoglycerate (2–3 DPG) in all cases where the measurement was made. This was attributed by Wiley *et al.* to the diversion of the glycolytic process away from 2–3 DPG synthesis towards ATP production which is demanded by the increased Na–K pump activity. Wiley *et al.*[24] further reported an increased whole-blood oxygen affinity, which would be the natural consequence of the low 2–3 DPG level.

Familial pseudohyperkalaemia

In 1979, we reported a family[25], none of whom was anaemic, who had a temperature-dependent net red-cell K loss. The propositus presented with an artefactual hyperkalaemia related to the storage of her blood in plasma at room temperature for up to 6 h prior to centrifugation and separation (Figure 16.3). Family studies revealed 15 similarly affected individuals, all well, linked by an autosomal dominant pattern of inheritance (Figure 16.4). Affected members have a mild compensated haemolytic state, a slight reticulocytosis and mildly abnormal blood films showing a few target cells. The erythrocyte potassium concentration was mildly reduced at 80 mmol/l cells, but the internal [Na] was normal. Flux studies are in progress, and it seems probable that this condition will ultimately be classified as a mild form of dehydrated stomatocytosis.

Microcytic haemolytic anaemia with Ca leak

Given existing evidence quoted above regarding the Ca-sensitive K channel, it could be predicted that if a red cell was invested with either an inward Ca leak with which its Ca extrusion pump could not cope, or with a deficient Ca pump, then such a cell would lose K, and therefore water, to become very shrunken. Wiley and Gill[26] described such a case, where the MCV was as low as 30 fl. Both Ca and K fluxes were abnormal, while Na fluxes were not. Tests of intracellular glycolytic enzymes and haemoglobin were normal. The osmotic fragility was increased: one might expect such shrunken cells to show decreased osmotic fragility. The

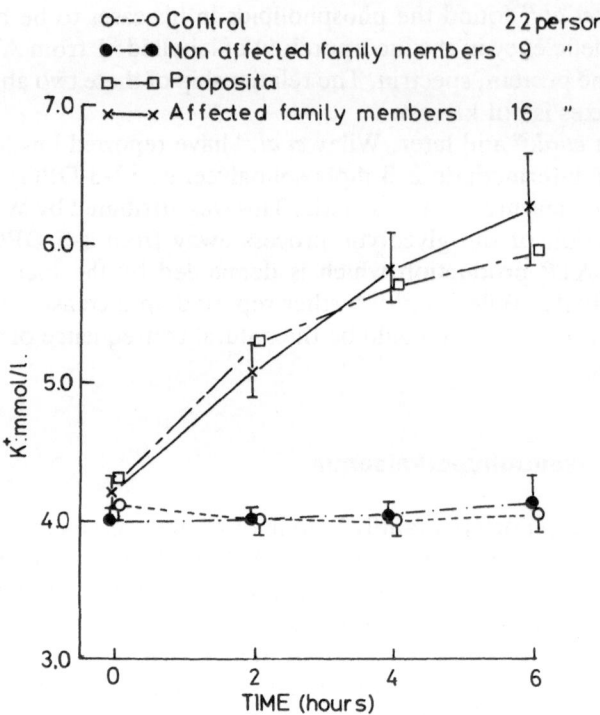

Figure 16.3 Familial pseudohyperkalaemia. Blood from normal volunteers and family members was withdrawn and divided between four lithium heparin tubes. These were stored at room temperature and spun and separated at 0, 2, 4 and 6 h. Plasma [K] was determined by flame photometry

patient, a small boy, was well apart from some complications of haemolytic anaemia. There were no manifestations of abnormal calcium metabolism in other systems.

ESSENTIAL HYPERTENSION

In 1979, Garay and Meyer[27] reported some interesting abnormalities of red-cell Na and K transport in essential hypertensives. Their technique was to load the cells with Na and deplete them of K to levels of 100 mM and 5 mM, respectively, using the PCMBS technique, and then to

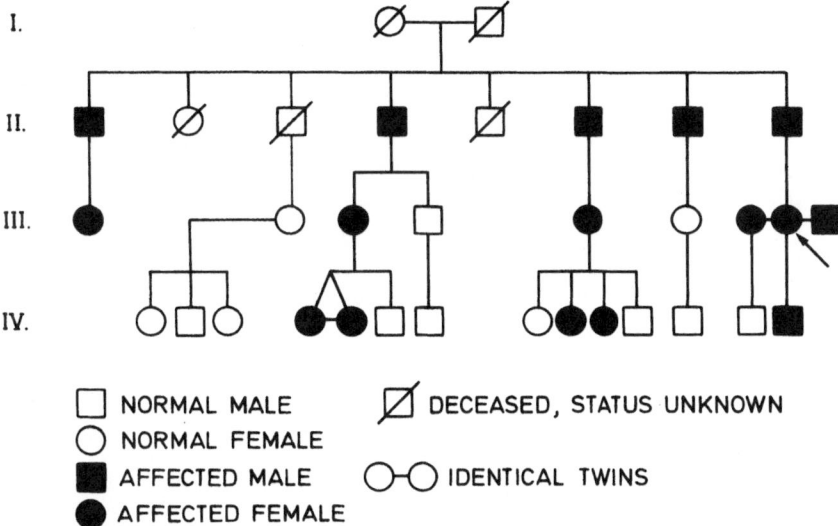

I.

II.

III.

IV.

NORMAL MALE   DECEASED, STATUS UNKNOWN
NORMAL FEMALE
AFFECTED MALE   IDENTICAL TWINS
AFFECTED FEMALE

Figure 16.4 Familial pseudohyperkalaemia: family tree. Arrow indicates propositus

follow, with flame photometry, the net Na and K fluxes which ensued when the cells were incubated at 37°C in a 145 mM Na, 5 mM K solution. From existing knowledge of the behaviour of red cells, such cells would be expected to show a net loss of Na via the pump, while the linear leaks would almost balance out. The cotransport system would probably mediate a net Na loss due to the increased internal Na, although the effect of the low internal K is impossible to predict. A net K gain is expected, again via the pump, the linear leaks cancelling out. The situation is illustrated diagrammatically in Figures 16.5 and 16.6. Normal cells exhibited such net fluxes, but in the cells of essential hypertensives, the expected net Na loss was less than in normals, while the K gain was greater. They found that the ratio between the two net fluxes (net Na efflux/net K influx) was a sensitive discriminator between normal subjects and essential hypertensives. Three patients with 'renal' hypertension had normal net flux ratios. A small family with essential hypertensive members were studied: all three hypertensives were abnormal, and one member of the next generation, whose blood pressure at that time was normal, showed a decreased flux ratio. This test may, therefore, be able to predict susceptible subjects.

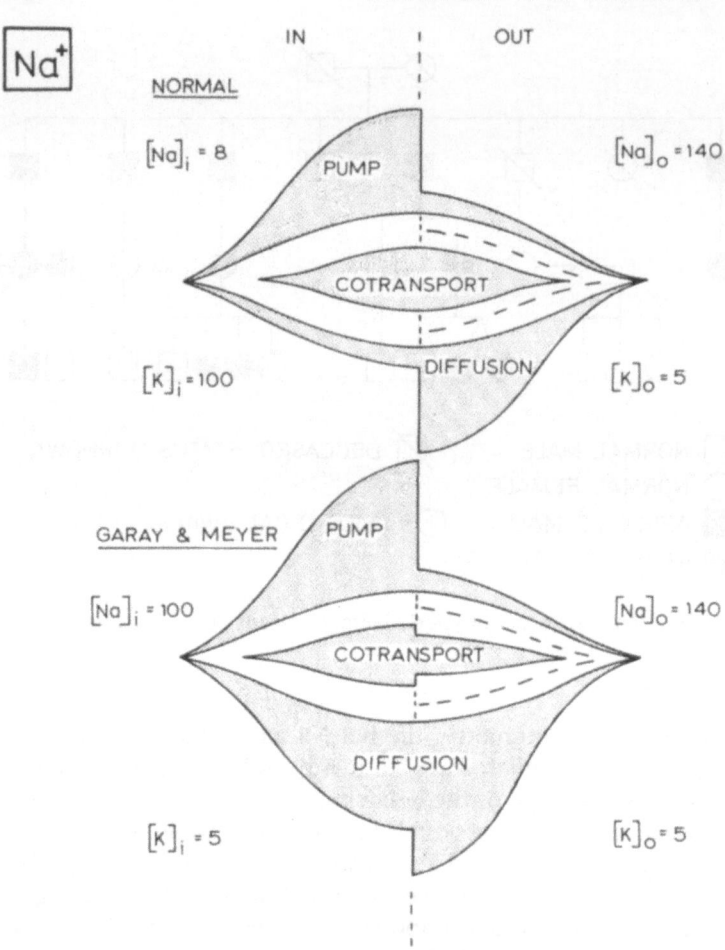

Figure 16.5 Diagrammatic representation of Na balance in normal (upper figure) and probable situation in Na loaded cells (lower figure). In non-loaded cells, there is no net flux owing to the equal and opposite Na fluxes through the linear leak and Na–K pump. The cotransport system merely mediates Na–Na exchange. In Garay and Meyer's[27] Na loaded cells, the linear leak fluxes will almost cancel and a major net efflux will occur via the Na–K pump, which will be stimulated by the high internal Na. The behaviour of the cotransport system is difficult to predict, probably being influenced by not only the increased $[Na]_i$, but also the reduced $[K]_i$. The dotted lines indicate the proposed abnormality in cotransport Na influx which, in conjunction with the K data presented by Garay and Meyer, best explains the net flux changes

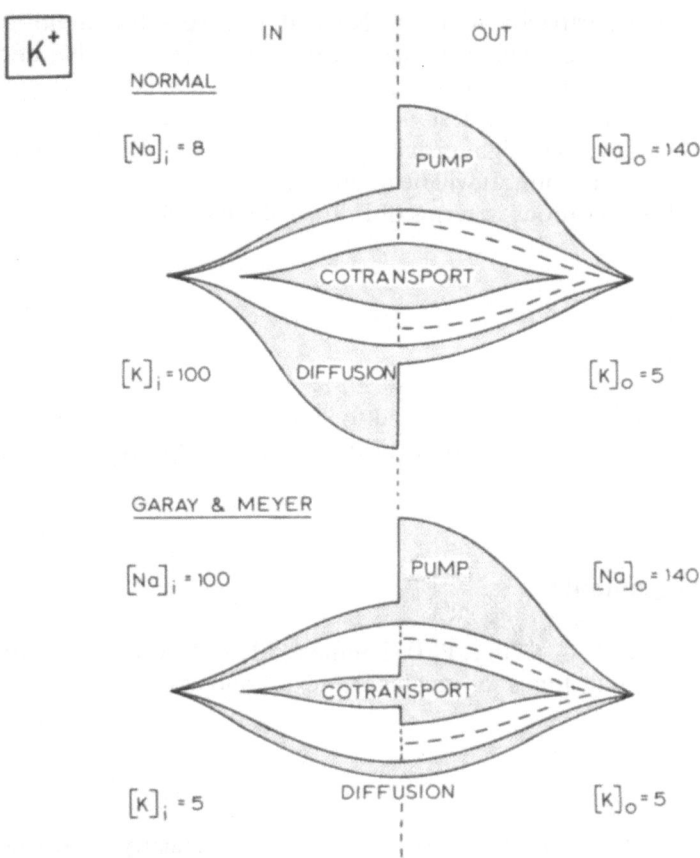

Figure 16.6 Diagrammatic representation of the K balance of non-depleted and K-depleted red cells. As for Na, the linear leak fluxes balance each other, while a net efflux is expected to occur via the pump. Again, there is insufficient existing experimental evidence to confidently predict the response of the cotransport system. The proposed cotransport increase in K influx in hypertensives is depicted by the dotted lines

The particular pattern of net flux abnormality seen here is best explained by an abnormality of the cotransport system. An increased activity on the part of the Na–K pump would give rise to the increased Na net flux which was seen in hypertensives, but would *not* give the observed reduction in net K efflux which was quoted: the reverse, in fact. The linear leak is unlikely to be involved because there will be little net flux through this pathway in Garay and Meyer's cells, the concentrations of Na and K across the membrane being roughly equal. The cotransport system, with its capacity to move Na and K across the membrane together, is the most likely candidate. Either an increase in Na and K cotransport influx or a decrease in efflux, would explain Garay and Meyer's data. If a similar lesion existed in the furosemide-sensitive systems in kidney, this might provide a cellular basis for the mechanism of essential hypertension. It will be interesting to see the development of these initial observations in terms of isotopically measured fluxes.

SUMMARY

Existing knowledge of the four red-cell Na and K transporting mechanisms has been reviewed and related to a number of clinical conditions exhibiting pathological alterations of the normal erythrocyte Na and K balance.

Acknowledgements

I am indebted to J. C. Ellory, P. B. Dunham, M. J. Wolowyk, Elisabeth Simonsen and Sian Jones for invaluable advice and assistance.

References

1. Garrahan, P. J. and Glynn, I. M. (1967). The stoichiometry of the sodium pump. *J. Physiol. (London)*, **192**, 217
2. Beauge, L. A. and Glynn, I. M. (1978). Commercial ATP containing traces of vanadate alters the response of $(Na^+ + K^+)$ATPase to potassium. *Nature (London)*, **272**, 551
3. Cantley, L. C., Josephson, L., Warner, R., Yanagisawa, M., Lechene, C. and Guidotti, G. (1977). Vanadate is a potent (Na, K)-ATPase inhibitor found in ATP derived from muscle. *J. Biol. Chem.*, **252**, 7421
4. Wiley, J. S. and Cooper, R. A. (1975). A furosemide sensitive cotransport of sodium and potassium in the human red cell. *J. Clin. Invest.*, **53**, 745
5. Dunn, M. J. (1973). Ouabain-uninhibited sodium transport in human erythrocytes: evidence against a second pump. *J. Clin. Invest.*, **52**, 658
6. Brooks, B. A. and Lant, A. F. (1978). The use of the human erythrocyte as a model for studying the action of diuretics on sodium and chloride transport. *Clin. Sci. Molec. Med.*, **54**, 679
7. Burg, M., Stoner, L., Cardinal, J. and Green, N. (1973). Furosemide effect on isolated perfused tubules. *Am. J. Physiol.*, **225**, 119
8. Nellans, H. N., Frizell, R. A. and Schultz, S. G. (1973). Coupled sodium-

chloride influx across the brush border of rabbit ileum. *Am. J. Physiol.*, **225** (2), 467

9. Zeuthen, T., Ramos, M. and Ellory, J. C. (1978). Inhibition of active chloride transport by piretanide. *Nature (London)*, **273**, 678

10. Ussing, H. H. (1949). Transport of ions across biological membranes. *Acta Physiol. Scand.*, **29**, 127

11. Gardos, G. (1958). The function of calcium in the potassium permeability of human erythrocytes. *Biochim. Biophys. Acta*, **30**, 653

12. Lew, V. L. (1970) Effect of intracellular calcium on the potassium permeability of human red cells. *J. Physiol. (London)*, **306**, 35P

13. Parker, J. C. and Welt, L. G. (1972). Pathological alterations of cation movements in red blood cells. *Arch. Intern. Med.* **129**, 320

14. Lock, S. P., Sephton-Smith, R. and Hardisty, R. M. (1961). Stomatocytosis: A hereditary, red cell anomaly associated with haemolytic anaemia. *Br. J. Haematol.*, **7**, 303

15. Zarkowsky, H. S., Oski, F. A., Sha'afi, R., *et al.* (1968). Congenital haemolytic anaemia with high sodium, low potassium red cells. I. Studies of membrane permeability. *N. Engl. J. Med.*, **278**, 573

16. Oski, F. A., Naiman, J. L., Blum, S. F., Zarkowsky, H. S., Whaun, J., Shohet, S. B., Green, A. and Nathan, D. G. (1969). Congenital haemolytic anaemia with high sodium, low potassium red cells. *N. Engl. J. Med.*, **280**, 909

17. Honig, G. R., Lacsow, P. S. and Maurer, H. S. (1971). A new familial disorder with abnormal erythrocyte morphology and increased permeability of the erythrocytes to sodium and potassium. *Pediatr. Res.*, **5**, 159

18. Miller, D. R., Rickles, F.-R. and Lichtmann, M. A. (1971). A new variant of hereditary haemolytic anaemia with stomatocytosis and erythrocyte cation abnormality. *Blood*, **38**, 184

19. Shohet, S. B., Nathan, D. G., Livermore, B. M., Feig, S. A. and Jaffe, E. A. (1973). Hereditary haemolytic anaemia associated with abnormal membrane lipid. II. Ion permeability and transport abnormalities. *Blood*, **42**, 1

20. Glader, B. E., Nathan, D. G., Albala, M. M. and Fortier N. (1974). Congenital haemolytic anaemia with potassium loss. *N. Engl. J. Med.*, **291**, 491

21. Wiley, J. S., Ellory, J. C., Schuman, M. A., Shaller, C. C. and Cooper, R. A. (1975). Characteristics of the membrane defect in the hereditary stomatocytosis syndrome: *Blood*, **46**, 337

22. Mentzer, W. C., Byron-Smith, W., Goldstone, J. and Shohet, S. (1975). Hereditary stomatocytosis: membrane and metabolism studies. *Blood*, **46**, 659

23. Wiley, J. S. (1977). Genetic abnormalities of cation transport in the human erythrocyte. In J. C. Ellory and V. L. Lew (eds). *Membrane Transport in Red Cells*, pp. 337–362. (London: Academic Press)

24. Wiley, J. S., Cooper, R. A., Adachi, K. and Asakura, T. (1979) Hereditary stomatocytosis: Association of low 2,3 diphosphoglycerate with increased pumping by the red cell. *Br. J. Haematol.*, **41**, 133

25. Stewart, G. W., Corrall, R. J. M., Fyffe, J. M. and Stockdill, G. (1979). Familial pseudohyperkalaemia – a new syndrome, *Lancet*, **2**, 175

26. Wiley, J. S. and Gill, F. M. (1976). Red cell calcium leak in congenital

hemolytic abnormality with extreme microcytosis. *Blood*, **47**, 197

27. Garay, R. P. and Meyer, P. (1979) A new test showing abnormal net Na$^+$ and K$^+$ fluxes in erythrocytes of essential hypertensive patients. *Lancet*, **1**, 349.

28. Dunham, P. B., Stewart, S. W. and Ellory, J. C. (1980). Chloride-activated passive potassium transport in human erythrocytes. *Proc. Natl. Acad. Sci. USA*, **77**, 1711

Red-cell amino
acid and nucleoside transport:
inherited lesions and
related enzyme deficiencies
in sheep

J. D. Young and S. M. Jarvis

INTRODUCTION

Amino acids and nucleosides, important intermediates in many biochemical reactions, are transported across cell membranes by specific translocation mechanisms which accommodate a diverse range of
intracellular requirements. Although considerable progress has been
made over the last few years, as yet little is understood of the detailed
mechanisms, control and physiological significance of these transport
systems (see for example refs. 1–3 for recent reviews). One way to study
translocation systems and their interaction with intracellular metabolism
is to make use of inborn errors of metabolism. Biochemical lesions of
both amino acid and nucleoside metabolism have been described in
man[4,5], and a number of the amino-acid defects attributed to transport
lesions. Their occurrence, however, is rare, and samples are sometimes
difficult to obtain. We have chosen to investigate inherited amino-acid

and nucleoside transport variation and related enzyme deficiencies in sheep erythrocytes, not only for their intrinsic interest in this species, but also because they might provide information leading to a better understanding of transport mechanisms in man. This paper reviews some of these studies. In the case of amino-acid transport, we pay particular attention to the metabolism of glutathione (GSH), a tripeptide essential for normal cell function, and a molecule previously proposed to play a direct role in amino-acid transport. We discuss the possible role of nucleoside transport in erythrocyte energy metabolism.

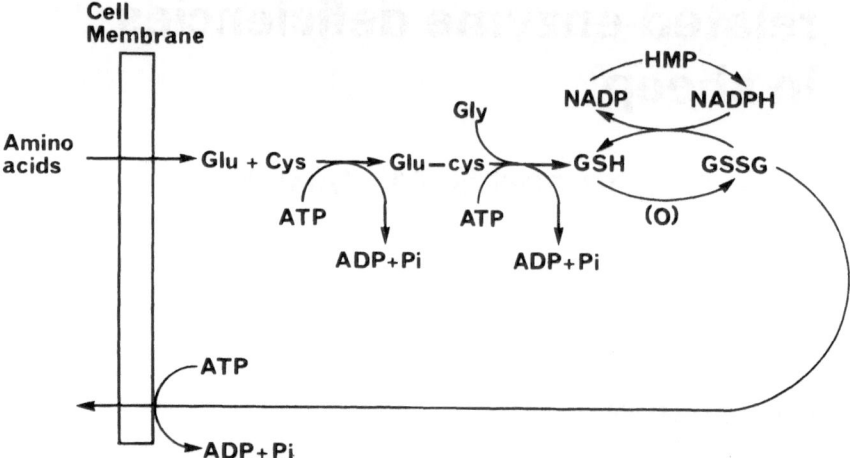

Figure 17.1 Erythrocyte GSH metabolism. GSH is synthesized in two enzymic steps catalysed by γ-glutamyl cysteine synthetase (GC-S) and GSH synthetase (GSH-S). GSH protects the cells against oxidative damage by being converted to the disulphide GSSG. One of the enzymes involved in these protective reactions is glutathione peroxidase. GSSG is converted back to GSH by the action of glutathione reductase. GSSG is also transported out of the cell by an active transport mechanism. HMP, hexose monophosphate pathway

AMINO-ACID TRANSPORT

Almost all cells possess membrane-transport systems for amino acids, and kinetic studies over the last 30 years have led to the definition of a number of discrete transport systems common to a wide range of cell types[1,2]. Interest in sheep erythrocyte amino-acid transport originated from the discovery of a recessive GSH-deficiency associated with high intracellular levels of a number of amino acids, notably ornithine and lysine – GSH approximately 30% of normal with up to 20 mmol amino acid/l cells[6,7]. The biochemical pathway leading to GSH synthesis in erythrocytes from its constituent amino acids is shown in Figure 17.1. Subsequent transport studies have established that GSH-deficient cells have a markedly diminished permeability to a number of amino acids, notably cysteine, its non-sulphur analogue α-amino-*n*-butyrate and alanine (Figure 17.2)[8,9]. Concentration dependence experiments demonstrated that while alanine and cysteine transport in normal cells was saturable, in GSH-deficient erythrocytes it was slow and linear with concentration (Figure 17.3)[10,11].

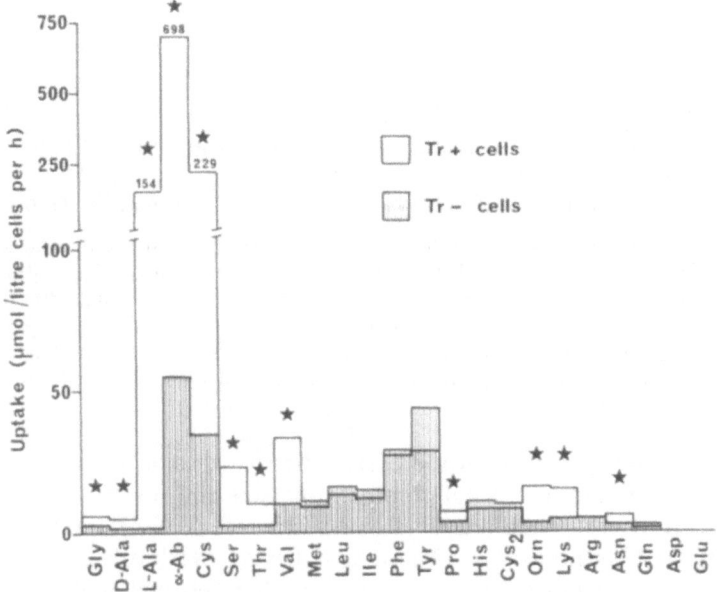

Figure 17.2   Amino-acid transport in normal (Tr+) and GSH-deficient (Tr−) sheep erythrocytes. Initial amino-acid uptake rates were determined at 37°C and an extracellular concentration of 0.2 mmol/l. Data are the means for four animals of each type. Standard errors (not shown) were typically 10% of mean values. Significant differences are indicated by stars. Results from Young *et al.*[10]

It is clear that normal sheep erythrocytes possess an amino-acid transport system selective for cysteine (the C-system) which is functionally absent from GSH-deficient cells. This system also has a low, but significant affinity for dibasic amino acids[10,11]. Thus, the absence of the C-system from GSH-deficient erythrocytes can explain the GSH-deficiency and is presumably also responsible for the accumulation of ornithine and lysine. Erythrocytes heterozygous for the transport lesion have an intermediate transport activity, significantly diminished GSH levels, but essentially normal amino acid concentrations (Young and Tucker, unpublished observations).

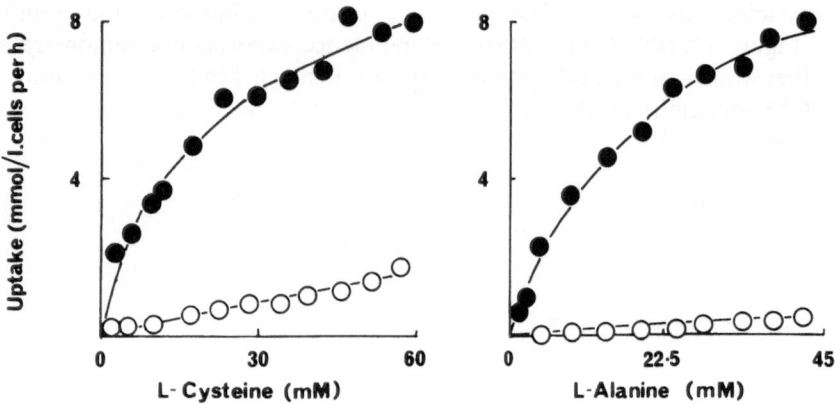

Figure 17.3 Concentration dependence of L-cysteine and L-alanine transport by normal (Tr+) and GSH-deficient (Tr−) sheep erythrocytes. Initial uptake rates were determined at 37°C. Analysis of the Tr+ uptake data (●) following subtraction of the Tr− (O) linear uptake gave apparent K_m and V_{max} values of 13.7 mmol/l and 8.0 mmol/l cells per h for L-cysteine respectively and 20.4 mmol/l and 11.0 mmol/l cells per h for L-alanine respectively. Data redrawn from Young et al.[11]

A second type of inherited GSH-deficiency also occurring in sheep, is inherited in an autosomal dominant manner and results from a diminished activity of γ-glutamyl cysteine synthetase (GC-S), the first enzyme of GSH biosynthesis[12-14]. These cells have GSH levels comparable to those of transport-deficient erythrocytes, have normal amino-acid transport properties and do not accumulate dibasic amino acids[6,8]. The combined study of transport deficient and GC-S deficient cells has allowed us to probe a number of important aspects of erythrocyte amino-acid transport and metabolism. In the next three sections information gained from the study of these lesions is discussed.

Physiological significance of erythrocyte amino-acid transport

GSH is synthesized in the erythrocyte from its constituent amino acids[15] and removed from the cell by a GSSG transport mechanism[16]. There is, therefore, a continuous requirement for GSH-precursor amino acids. The transport lesion studies suggest, first, that this requirement is met, at least for cysteine, by transport from the plasma, and second, that GSH-biosynthesis is limited by cysteine availability. The low GSH concentrations of sheep cells with a diminished activity of GC-S demonstrates that GSH biosynthesis is regulated further by the activity of this enzyme which is also subject to feedback inhibition by GSH[14].

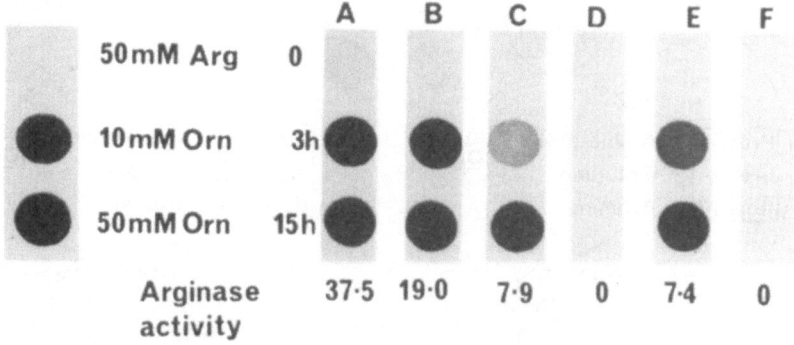

Figure 17.4 Arginase spot test. Sheep erythrocyte lysates, incubated with 50 mM L-arginine, were deproteinized with chloroform–ethanol, and the extracts applied to Whatman 3 MM filter paper. Samples, including appropriate standards, were stained for ornithine by a specific alkaline-vanillin reagent. Arginase activities (μmmol/g Hb per min) were determined by an automated spectrophotometric method. Samples D and F are arginase-deficient. From Young and Wright[18] (with permission)

The massive accumulation of amino acids in transport-deficient erythrocytes suggests a second, previously unsuspected, role of amino-acid transport in these cells, namely the removal of endogenous amino acids. We still do not know the origin of the amino acids, particularly ornithine and lysine, which accumulate in transport-deficient erythrocytes. One obvious possibility is that these amino acids are breakdown products of reticulocyte maturation which are normally transported out of the cell. One difficulty with this proposal is that ornithine is not a normal constituent of protein. However, many cells, including erythrocytes from most sheep, possess arginase, an enzyme which converts arginine to ornithine. It is therefore possible that the ornithine seen in transport-deficient cells was originally derived from arginine. To test this, use was made of an inherited arginase-deficiency which occurs independently in the erythrocytes of some sheep[17]. This deficiency can be readily detected by conventional enzyme assay or by a simple spot-test (Figure 17.4)[18].

Transport-deficient erythrocytes which were also arginase-deficient, accumulated arginine plus lysine instead of ornithine and lysine[19]. One interpretation of the results is summarized diagrammatically in Figure 17.5.

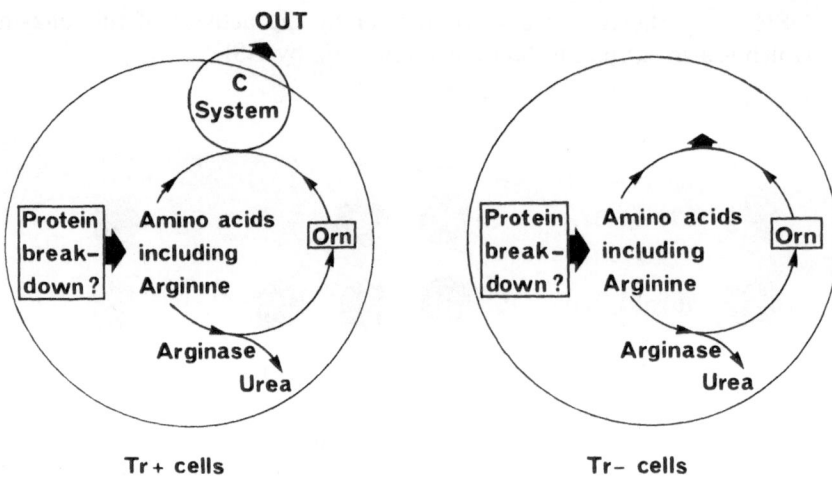

Figure 17.5 Mechanism of amino-acid accumulation in GSH-deficient (Tr−) sheep erythrocytes

Physiological role of GSH in erythrocytes

A major role of GSH in erythrocytes is the protection of the cell against oxidative damage, the GSH:GSSG couple acting as a redox buffer (Figure 17.1). Sheep erythrocytes with the GC-S lesion have a normal potential life span[20], demonstrating that the high intracellular GSH concentration usually found in erythrocytes is substantially in excess of that required, at least under normal circumstances. Transport-deficient sheep erythrocytes, on the other hand, have a markedly diminished life span (Figure 17.6)[21], despite having similar intracellular GSH concentrations and GSH:GSSG redox potentials to GC-S deficient cells[22]. It is likely that the diminished viability of these cells is not a direct consequence of their low GSH status, although they do show evidence of oxidative damage as indicated by Heinz body inclusions (unpublished observations). Perhaps some product of the transport lesion (for example the intracellular amino acids) interferes with the GSH protective mechanism or potentiates endogenous oxidative reactions. Sheep which have inherited both the transport and GC-S lesions have lower erythrocyte GSH concentrations than cells with either lesion alone (approximately 6-fold lower than normal). Erythrocytes from such sheep tend to have a shorter life span than cells with only the transport lesion (unpublished observations) and these animals have a higher mortality as lambs[13].

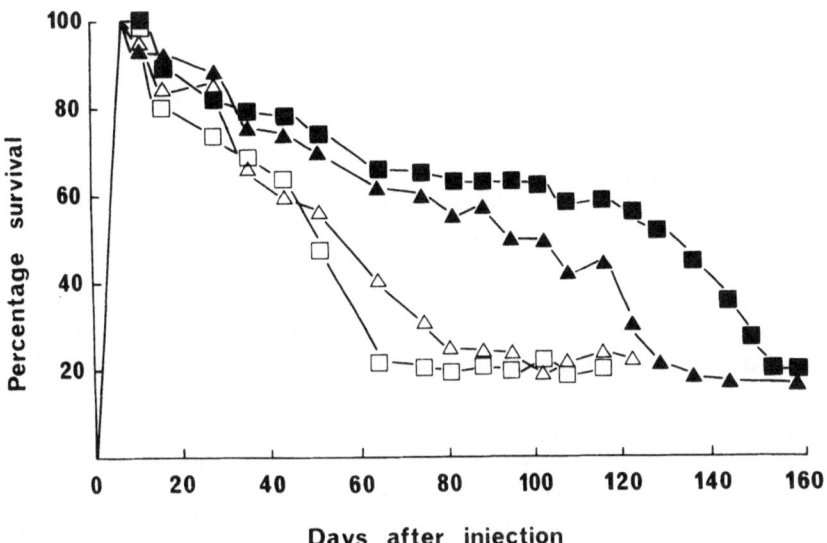

Figure 17.6 Life span of normal (Tr+) and GSH-deficient (Tr−) sheep erythrocytes. Erythrocyte survival was monitored using ^{59}Fe. Two normal (■ ▲) and two Tr − sheep (□ △) were used. Redrawn from Tucker[21]

Erythrocyte GSH deficiency also occurs in man, and as in sheep, is attributed to a diminished ability to synthesize GSH[23-28]. Cases of GC-S[26] and GSH synthetase (GSH-S)[23-25,27] deficiency have been described. Such cells have GSH levels similar to, or lower than, those found in sheep with combined transport and GC-S deficiency. As a result, the human lesions are usually associated with clinical symptoms of well compensated non-spherocytic haemolytic anaemia. Exposure of both GSH-deficient humans and sheep to oxidative stress resulting from the administration of oxidant drugs or the ingestion of certain food stuffs (for example, fava beans in man and kale in sheep) can precipitate a severe haemolytic crisis[23,29].

Human disorders of the GSH:GSSG protective mechanism are not restricted to simple GSH-deficiency. Other enzyme lesions occur, some of which, like glucose-6-phosphate dehydrogenase deficiency, are relatively common[30,31]. Patients with these enzyme deficiencies are also susceptible to oxidative stress[30,31], and one direct use of GSH-deficient sheep, particularly those which have inherited both lesions, would be to screen drugs and food stuffs for potential oxidant side effects. Dietary deficiency of selenium, resulting in reduced glutathione peroxidase activities[32], would further increase the oxidant sensitivity of these animals.

Mechanism and control of erythrocyte amino-acid transport

The importance of amino-acid transport to sheep erythrocyte function led to a detailed examination of amino-acid transport in human erythrocytes. Surprisingly, human cells lack the C-system, but instead have four additional transport routes, none of which occur in sheep[11,33-38]. The first, and most important in the present context, is a high-affinity, low capacity system for cysteine and alanine. This system is Na^+-dependent and its apparent K_m for cysteine (20μm) is close to physiological plasma levels of this amino acid. Second, there is a high-capacity, medium-affinity system with a specificity broadly directed towards large neutral amino acids, the L-system. Small neutral amino acids, including cysteine, are transported by this route, but with a low affinity. A further system for large neutral amino acids, but selective for aromatic amino acids, has also been found (T-system). Finally, there is a specific dibasic amino-acid transport system (Ly$^+$-system). Amino-acid transport in human and sheep erythrocytes therefore provides an interesting example of different mechanisms having evolved to fulfil the same physiological functions.

An important conclusion from detailed kinetic studies of the sheep C-system is that its properties are unlike those of previously characterized amino-acid transport systems[1,2,8-11]. Its substrate specificity closely resembles that of the widespread ASC-system known to occur in rabbit reticulocytes[39], but the C-system, unlike the ASC-system, does not require Na^+. In contrast, alanine transport in sheep reticulocytes is Na^+-dependent[40], and it is possible that the C-system represents a modified ASC-system which has lost its Na^+ requirement during reticulocyte maturation[1,10,41,42]. This transformation coincides with the appearance of the transport lesion, since reticulocytes from normal and transport-deficient sheep have similar transport characteristics (unpublished observations). The Na^+-dependent transport route in mature human erythrocytes resembles the ASC-system both in its substrate specificity and Na^+ requirement. Thus the human and sheep cysteine transport systems may be end products of two different reticulocyte maturation routes for the ASC-system.

Enzymes of GSH biosynthesis and degradation together constitute the γ-glutamyl cycle. Operation of this cycle involves the uptake and release of free amino acids. It has been suggested that the γ-glutamyl cycle may participate directly in amino-acid transport by a number of cell types, including the erythrocyte[43-45]. Striking evidence in support of this hypothesis comes from the study of Marstein et al.[25], who found an 8-fold increase in the total free amino acids of erythrocytes taken from a patient with GSH-S deficiency. As in the case of sheep with the transport lesion, ornithine and lysine were amongst the amino acids whose concentrations were elevated. However, a number of observations rule out any participation of the γ-glutamyl cycle in erythrocyte amino-acid transport. First, with the possible exception of the Na^+-dependent alanine and cysteine transport in human cells, the erythrocyte cannot accumulate amino acids. The γ-glutamyl cycle predicts active amino-acid transport. Second, γ-glutamyl transpeptidase, a key enzyme of the cycle, is absent from erythrocytes[46], previously reported enzyme activity[45,47] arising from white cell contamination of the erythrocyte preparation[46]. Third, direct attempts to demonstrate a consumption of GSH during amino-acid transport have failed[48,49]. Fourth, subsequent studies of GSH-S deficient human erythrocytes have failed to find substantially elevated intracellular amino acid concentrations[27]. In the case of sheep, any possibility that the defective amino-acid transport seen in cells with the transport lesion is the result of GSH deficiency (as would be predicted by the γ-glutamyl cycle theory) is eliminated by finding normal transport and intracellular levels of amino acids in GSH deficient erythrocytes containing the GC-S lesion[8]. Therefore, the high amino-acid concentrations seen by Marstein et al.[25] were probably not a consequence of a γ-glutamyl cycle coupled amino-acid transport defect. Experiments with sheep have found that several classes of membrane thiol are essential for normal transport activity[49]. If amino-acid transport in human erythrocytes has a similar membrane thiol dependence, and if, as seems likely, GSH-deficient human cells cannot always support these thiols in the reduced state, then perturbed amino-acid transport and hence amino acid accumulation would result.

The γ-glutamyl cycle and its role in amino-acid transport is further discussed in this volume by Larsson[28].

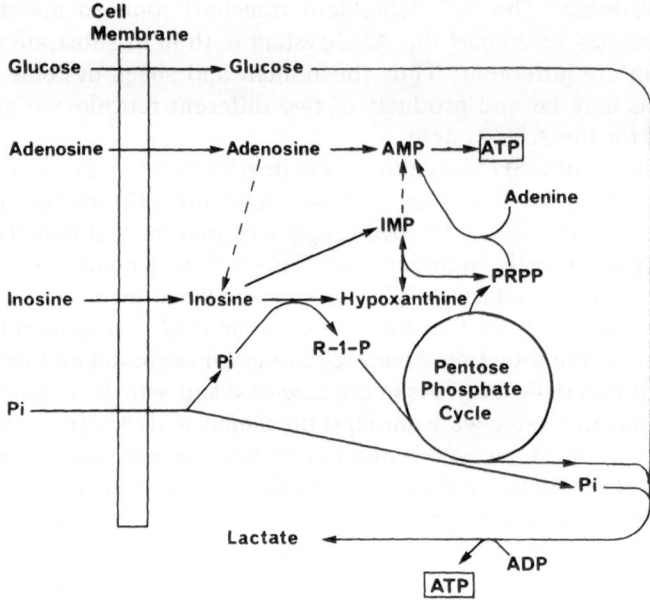

Figure 17.7   Metabolic reactions involved in the synthesis of erythrocyte ATP from adenosine, phosphate, inosine and glucose. Inosine is metabolized to hypoxanthine and ribose-1-phosphate (R-1-P) by nucleoside phosphorylase. R-1-P subsequently enters the pentose phosphate cycle as ribose-5-phosphate. Adenosine is phosphorylated initially by adenosine kinase to yield AMP which is converted to ADP by adenylate kinase. Both these enzymes require ATP. Sheep erythrocytes do not have adenosine deaminase and cannot convert adenosine to inosine[51]. Rabbit, but not mature human erythrocytes, have the additional ability to convert IMP to AMP due to the presence of adenylosuccinate synthetase[85]. The conversion of adenine and phosphoribosylpyrophosphate (PRPP) to AMP is catalysed by adenine phosphoribosyltransferase. Although not directly relevant to the synthesis of AMP from adenosine, this enzyme has been considered to be important for adenine nucleotide biosynthesis *in vivo* (see text)

NUCLEOSIDE TRANSPORT

Nucleosides cross cell membranes by facilitated diffusion[3] and studies of the human erythrocyte have revealed a single broad specificity system for both purine and pyrimidine nucleoside transport (see reference 50 for references). In 1972 McManus and Lamb[51] reported that erythrocytes from some sheep synthesized ATP when incubated with adenosine, inosine and inorganic phosphate, whereas cells from other sheep were unable to do so. Since erythrocytes from the two types of animal were equally capable of synthesizing ATP when inosine was replaced by glucose, and since haemolysates from the two types of sheep metabolized inosine at the same rate, it was considered probable that the erythrocytes differed in their permeability to inosine (see Figure 17.7 for a summary of the metabolic reactions involved). Experiments from our laboratory demonsrated subsequently that sheep erythrocytes are divisible into two distinct types on the basis of their permeability to inosine[50, 52, 53]. The majority of animals were virtually impermeable to this nucleoside (nucleoside-impermeable type) whereas erythroctyes from a small number of sheep rapidly transported inosine (nucleoside-permeable type). Figure 17.8 shows the distribution of inosine permeability in 40 animals of each type. Detailed kinetic analyses of nucleoside transport[50] revealed that nucleoside-permeable cells have a nucleoside transport system with similar properties to that responsible for nucleoside translocation in human cells, although sheep erythrocytes have a substantially lower V_{max}. This system is functionally absent from nucleoside-impermeable erythrocytes. The difference between the two types of erythrocyte is illustrated in Figure 17.9 which shows the concentration dependence of inosine influx in both nucleoside-permeable and impermeable cells. Genetic studies established that nucleoside transport variation was under genetic control with nucleoside-impermeability behaving as if dominant to nucleoside-permeability[54].

What information have we been able to gain from the study of this transport variant?

Physiological significance of nucleoside transport in erythrocytes

The presence of nucleoside transport variation in sheep erythrocytes allows the physiological significance of nucleoside transport in these cells to be assessed. Nucleoside-permeable cells contain 40% more ATP than nucleoside-impermeable erythrocytes, suggesting that the saturable nucleoside transport system participates in the energy metabolism of the cell *in vivo*[50]. This could occur in two ways. First, adenosine may be utilized directly to increase the adenine-nucleotide pool size and second, inosine could be acting as an energy source in addition to glucose. Sheep erythrocytes lack adenosine deaminase and are therefore unable to convert adenosine to inosine[51].

The possibility that adenosine acts as an adenine nucleotide precursor is relevant to mammalian erythrocytes in general. Previous investi-

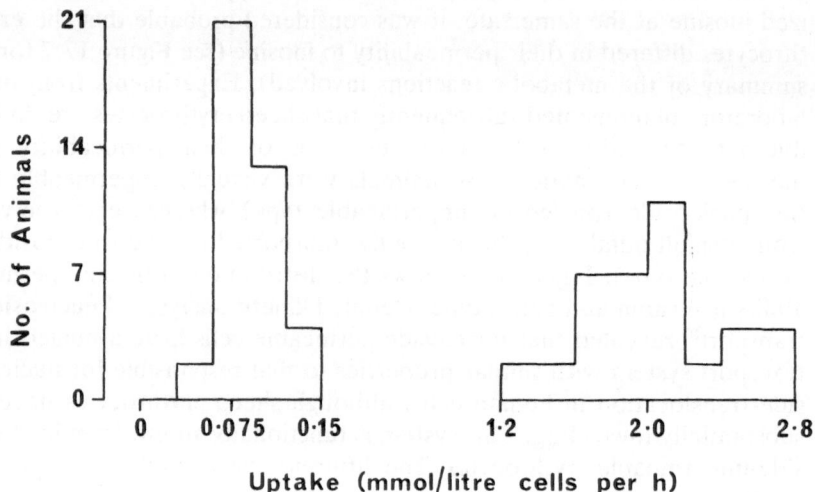

Figure 17.8   Inosine uptake by nucleoside-permeable and nucleoside-impermeable sheep erythrocytes. Initial inosine uptake rates (5 mmol/l, 37°C) were determined in nucleoside-impermeable (left hand histogram) and nucleoside-permeable (right hand histogram) erythrocytes taken from 40 animals of each type of sheep (unpublished data)

gations have demonstrated that the nucleotides of mammalian erythrocytes undergo turnover, as shown by both *in vivo*[55,56] and *in vitro*[57,58] studies. The cells cannot synthesize adenine, and both adenine and adenosine have been considered as possible ATP precursors[59,60]. A key enzyme in the synthesis of adenine nucleotides from adenine is adenine phosphoribosyltransferase. Human erythrocytes with an inherited deficiency of this enzyme have normal ATP levels, indicating that adenine does not significantly contribute to erythrocyte ATP synthesis *in vivo*[61]. Adenosine is therefore the most likely adenine nucleotide precursor.

The possibility that inosine acts as energy substrate is particularly relevant to adult pig erythrocytes which rapidly transport nucleosides, but are unable to utilize glucose due to an inability of the cell membrane to transport sugars[62–66]. Despite considerable study over the last 50 years, the energy substrate of these cells is unknown. Unlike sheep cells, pig erythrocytes usually have adenosine deaminase activity so that adenosine could also be important in this respect. However, pig cells with an inherited deficiency of this enzyme have ATP concentrations similar to those found in normal pig erythrocytes, suggesting that adenosine is not

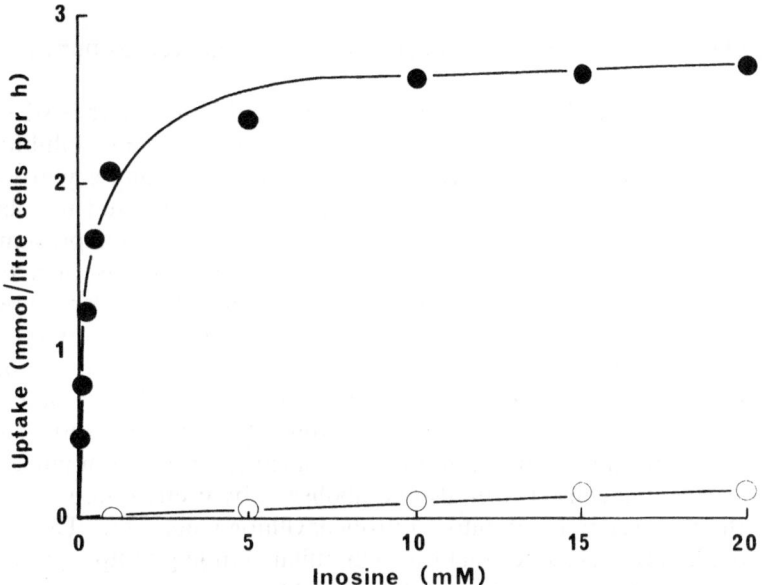

Figure 17.9   Concentration dependence of inosine uptake by nucleoside permeable and nucleoside-impermeable sheep erythrocytes. Initial inosine uptake
rates were determined at 37°C. ●, Nucleoside-permeable cells; ○, nucleoside-
impermeable erythrocytes. The apparent K_m for uptake by the nucleoside-
permeable cells is 0.26 mmol/l (data corrected for the nucleoside-impermeable
linear component). Uptake curves redrawn from Young[50]

an important energy substrate[66]. The inosine concentration of pig plasma
is two orders of magnitude greater than that theoretically required to
maintain the cells' entire energy requirements, strongly supporting the
notion that inosine acts as a major energy source for pig erythrocytes[66].

The removal of vasoactive agents from plasma is an important factor
in the maintenance of circulatory homeostasis. A further possible
physiological role of nucleoside transport in erythrocytes, related to any
involvement in erythrocyte nucleotide turnover, is the removal and subsequent inactivation of adenosine, a potent vasodilator. Various workers
have suggested that pulmonary endothelial cells are the major route for
the removal of circulating adenosine[67,68]. At physiological substrate concentrations, however, adenosine uptake per unit area of cell surface is as
rapid in human and pig erythrocytes as it is in endothelial cells[50,66,68].
Erythrocytes may significantly contribute to the removal of circulating
adenosine in these species.

Mechanism and control of erythrocyte nucleoside transport

Previous studies have shown that nitrobenzylthioinosine (NBMPR), an S-substituted 6-thiopurine ribonucleoside, is a potent inhibitor of nucleoside transport in a variety of cell types including erythrocytes[3]. Binding studies on intact human erythrocytes or isolated membranes using radioactive-NBMPR reveal a high-affinity association presumed to be binding to nucleoside transport sites[69-71]. The results of a typical binding experiment using sheep erythrocyte membranes are shown in Figure 17.10 where the amount of ^{3}H-NBMPR bound is plotted against the equilibrium free concentration of inhibitor in the medium. Nucleoside-permeable cells have two binding components: a high-affinity component with an apparent K_D of approximately 0.7 nmol/l, and a smaller linear association. The saturable component is absent from nucleoside-impermeable cells. It can also be abolished by pretreating membranes with the related inhibitor nitrobenzylthioguanosine[72]. These data provide direct evidence that the high-affinity binding component represents a specific interaction with functional transport sites.

Assuming that each high-affinity NBMPR binding site represents a single nucleoside transport system, it can be calculated that nucleoside-permeable sheep erythrocytes have approximately 20–30 transport sites per cell, giving a turnover number of 600–900 molecules/s per site at 37°C. Nucleoside transport in sheep reticulocytes and fetal erythrocytes is considerably more rapid than in adult nucleoside-permeable cells, with no detectable differences between cells from the two types of animal[73] (unpublished observations). Transport in these cells is mediated by a system with similar properties to that responsible for nucleoside transport in adult nucleoside-permeable erythrocytes. Their increased translocation capacity is associated with increased numbers of NBMPR binding sites. Similarly, human erythrocytes have a 300-fold higher V_{max} for nucleoside transport than mature nucleoside-permeable sheep cells, but proportionately more NBMPR binding sites, so that the translocation capacity for each transport site is similar in the two species[72]. Nucleoside transport acitivity is therefore regulated by variations in the numbers of functional nucleoside transport sites. Radiation inactivation analysis of NBMPR binding to human erythrocyte membranes estimates that the nucleoside transport system has a molecular weight of 128 000[74].

Genetic studies established that nucleoside transport variation in sheep erythrocytes was under genetic control[54]. The results were consistent with the involvement of two allelomorphic genes. In contrast to

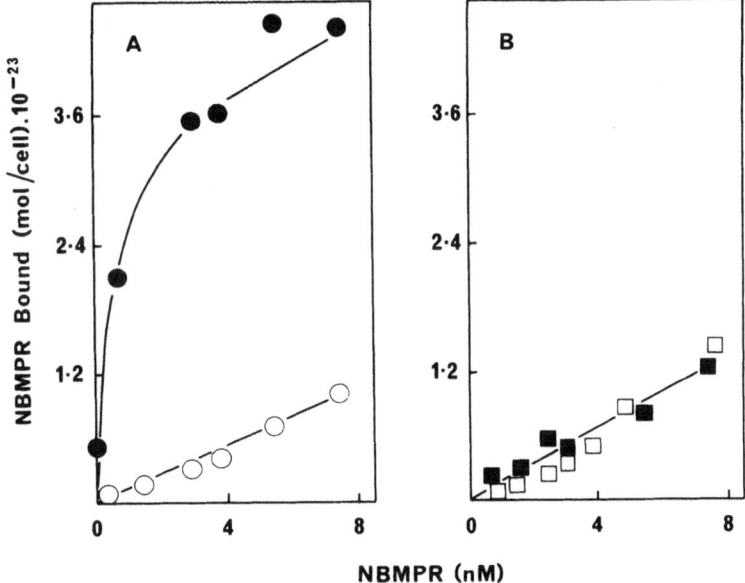

Figure 17.10 Binding of ³H-nitrobenzylthioinosine (NBMPR) to membranes from nucleoside-permeable and nucleoside-impermeable sheep erythrocytes. ³H-Nitrobenzylthioinosine (NBMPR) was incubated at 37°C with nucleoside-permeable (solid symbols) and nucleoside-impermeable (open symbols) erythrocyte membranes in the presence (right hand diagram) and absence (left hand diagram) of 25 μmol/l nitrobenzylthioguanosine. Data from Jarvis and Young[72]. The high-affinity binding component had an apparent K_D of 0.7 nmol/l

amino-acid transport, the gene coding for the functional absence of the nucleoside-transport system is dominant over the gene coding for its presence. Kinetic studies and inhibitor experiments with NBMPR established that the nucleoside-transport system was not present, even in low activity, in heterozygous erythrocytes. This is also unlike the situation for amino-acid transport, where heterozygous cells have an intermediate transport activity. The finding that nucleoside impermeability behaves as if it is dominant to nucleoside permeability suggests that this genetic locus may be some form of regulator locus, perhaps capable of modifying the expression of the structural gene or coding for the presence of a specific inhibitor of nucleoside transport. The genetic control of nucleoside transport could, for example, be similar to that responsible for active K^+ transport variation in this species, where the L-antigen is believed to act as an inhibitor of the Na^+-pump[75]. This form of regulation may be more widespread than is generally believed.

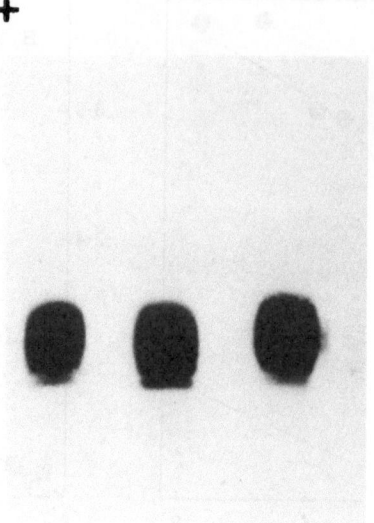

H L H L H

Figure 17.11   Starch gel electrophoresis of lysates from normal and nucleoside-phosphorylase deficient-sheep erythrocytes. After electrophoresis the gel was sliced horizontally and enzyme activity demonstrated by placing the cut surface over a glass plate which had previously been coated with agar containing inosine, phenazine methosulphate, MTT tetrazolium and xanthine oxidase. Zones of enzyme activity stained purple. H, normal cells; L, enzyme-deficient erythrocytes. Reproduced from Tucker and Young[81] with permission

Finally, a number of studies have suggested that nucleoside transport in mammalian systems occurs by group translocation systems involving nucleoside phosphorylase[76-79]. Adenosine deaminase has been implicated in erythrocyte adenosine transport[80]. Fortunately, erythrocytes from some sheep also have an inherited deficiency of purine nucleoside phosphorylase, the enzyme responsible for the cleavage of inosine to ribose-phosphate and hypoxanthine (Figure 17.11)[81]. This lesion is independent of the nucleoside transport variation. Nucleoside-permeable cells which have also inherited the enzyme deficiency show inosine uptake curves indistinguishable from those illustrated in Figure 17.9. Thus nucleoside phosphorylase probably plays no direct role in inosine translocation. Similarly, it has been found that pig erythrocytes with inherited adenosine deaminase-deficiency transport adenosine normally (Jarvis and Young, unpublished observations). These results demonstrate that nucleoside transport is distinct from subsequent metabolism, a view supported by kinetic studies which suggest that purine and pyrimidine nucleosides, including inosine and adenosine, share a common transport pathway[50,66].

CONCLUSIONS

In this chapter we have described studies of inherited amino acid and nucleoside transport variation in sheep erythrocytes. Our investigations have been aided greatly by the parallel discovery of a number of related enzyme deficiencies. The combined study of these transport and enzyme lesions has allowed us to probe a number of important aspects of membrane function. Much of the information gained in these investigations would have been difficult, if not impossible, to obtain by more conventional methods of biochemical analysis. Results obtained to date demonstrate that the sheep has considerable potential for further studies in this area.

The sheep enzyme variants are directly relevant to a large and varied number of human metabolic disorders. For example, GC-S[26], arginase[82] and nucleoside phosphorlyase[83]-deficiency all occur in man. Similarly, pig adenosine deaminase deficiency has a human equivalent[84]. The sheep lesions, however, appear to be restricted to the erythrocyte, whereas the human disorders, with the important exception of some cases of GSH-S deficiency[28], are usually also manifest in other tissues. In one sense this limits the use of sheep as experimental models for the investigation of human metabolic disease. In another, it is a positive advantage and permits the dissection of erythrocyte and tissue effects. Sheep may be particularly useful in the study of human GSH deficiency and related disorders. The increasing numbers of erythrocyte enzyme deficiencies common to the two species make it likely that transport lesions equivalent to those found in sheep may yet be described in man.

References

1. Christensen, H. N. (1979). Exploiting amino acid structure to learn about membrane transport. *Adv. Enzymol.*, **49**, 41
2. Guidotti, G. G., Borgetti, A. F. and Gazzola, G. C. (1978). The regulation of amino acid transport in animal cells. *Biochim. Biophys. Acta*, **515**, 329
3. Berlin, R. D. and Oliver, J. M. (1975). Membrane transport of purine and pyrimidine bases and nucleosides in animal cells. In G. H. Bourne and

J. F. Daniella (eds.). *International Review of Cytology*, Vol. 42, p. 287. (New York; Academic Press)

4. Nyhan, W. L. (1974). *Heritable Disorders of Amino Acid Metabolism*. (New York; Wiley)

5. Stanbury, J. B., Wyngaarden, J. B. and Frederickson, D. S. (eds.). (1978). *Metabolic Basis of Inherited Disease*. (New York; McGraw-Hill)

6. Ellory, J. C., Tucker, E. M. and Deverson, E. V. (1972). The identification of ornithine and lysine at high concentrations in the red cells of sheep with an inherited deficiency of glutathione. *Biochim. Biophys. Acta*, **279**, 481

7. Tucker, E. M. and Kilgour, L. (1970). An inherited glutathione deficiency and a concomitant reduction in potassium concentration in sheep red cells. *Experientia*, **26**, 203

8. Young, J. D., Ellory, J. C. and Tucker, E. M. (1975). Amino acid transport defect in glutathione deficient sheep erythrocytes. *Nature (London)*, **254**, 156

9. Young, J. D. and Ellory, J. C. (1977). Substrate specificity of amino acid transport in sheep erythrocytes. *Biochem. J.*, **162**, 33

10. Young, J. D., Ellory, J. C. and Tucker, E. M. (1976). Amino acid transport in normal and glutathione deficient sheep erythrocytes. *Biochem. J.*, **154**, 43

11. Young, J. D., Jones, S. E. M. and Ellory, J. C. (1979). Amino acid transport in human and sheep erythrocytes. *Proc. R. Soc.*, **B, 209**, 355

12. Tucker, E. M. and Kilgour, L. (1972). A glutathione deficiency in the red cells of certain Merino sheep. *J. Agric. Sci. Cambr.*, **79**, 515

13. Tucker, E. M., Kilgour, L. and Young, J. D. (1976). The genetic control of red cell glutathione deficiency in Finnish Landrace and Tasmanian Merino sheep and in crosses between these breeds. *J. Agric. Sci. Cambr.*, **87**, 315

14. Young, J. D. and Nimmo, I. A. (1975). GSH biosynthesis in glutathione deficient erythrocytes from Finnish Landrace and Tasmanian Merino sheep. *Biochim. Biophys. Acta*, **404**, 132

15. Majerus, P. W., Barumer, M. J., Smith, M. B. and Minnich, V. (1971). Glutathione synthesis in human erythrocytes. II Purification and properties of the enzymes of glutathione biosynthesis. *J. Clin. Invest.*, **50**, 1637

16. Srivastava, S. K. and Beutler, E. (1969). The transport of oxidised glutathione from human erythrocytes. *J. Biol. Chem.*, **244**, 9

17. Wright, P. C., Young, J. D., Mangan, J. L. and Tucker, E. M. (1977). An inherited arginase deficiency in sheep erythrocytes. *J. Agric. Sci., Cambr.*, **88**, 765

18. Young, J. D. and Wright, P. C. (1977). A simple spot test for the detection of erythrocyte arginase deficiency. *Clin. Chim. Acta*, **79**, 611

19. Tucker, E. M., Wright, P. C. and Young, J. D. (1977). Influence of arginase deficiency on amino acid concentrations in sheep erythrocytes with normal and with a defective system for aminoacids. *J. Physiol.*, **271**, 47P

20. Tucker, E. M. (1975). Life span of glutathione-deficient red cells in Tasmanian Merino sheep. *Res. Vet. Sci.*, **19**, 343

21. Tucker, E. M. (1974). A shortened lifespan of sheep red cells with glutathione deficiency. *Res. Vet. Sci.*, **16**, 19

22. Young, J. D., Nimmo, I. A. and Hall, J. G. (1975). The relationship between GSH, GSSG and non GSH thiol in GSH-deficient erythrocytes

from Finnish Landrace and Tasmanian Merino sheep. *Biochim. Biophys. Acta*, **404**, 124

23. Prins, H. K., Oort, M., Loos, J. A., Zürcher, C. and Beckers, T. (1966). Congenital non spherocytic haemolytic anaemia associated with glutathione deficiency of the erythrocytes. Haematological, biochemial and genetic studies. *Blood*, **27**, 145

24. Minnich, V., Smith, M. B. and Brauner, M. J. (1971). Glutathione biosynthesis in the human erythrocytes. I Identification of the enzymes of glutathione synthesis in haemolysates. *J. Clin. Invest.*, **50**, 507

25. Marstein, S., Jellum, E., Halpern, B., Eldjɛrn, L. and Perry, T. L. (1976). Biochemical studies of erythrocytes in a pa'ient with pyroglutamic acidaemia. *N. Engl. J. Med.*, **295**, 406

26. Konrad, P. N., Richards, F., Valentine, 'V. N. and Paglia, D. E. (1972). γ-glutamyl-cysteine synthetase deficiency. *N. Engl. J. Med.*, **286**, 557

27. Hagenfeldt, L., Larsson, A. and Anderson, R. (1978). The γ-glutamyl cycle and amino acid transport. *N. Engl. J. Med.*, **299**, 587

28. Larsson, A. (1981). 5-Oxoprolinuria and other inborn errors related to the γ-glutamyl cycle. This volume, p. 277

29. Tucker, E. M. and Kilgour, L. (1973). The effect of anaemia on sheep with inherited differences in the red cell reduced glutathione (GSH) concentrations. *Res. Vet. Sci.*, **14**, 306

30. Beutler, E. (1972). Disorders due to enzyme defects in the red blood cell. *Adv. Metabol. Disorders*, **6**, 131

31. Luzatto, L. (1974). Annotation: Genetic heterogeneity and pathophysiology of G6PD deficiency. *Br. J. Haematol.*, **28**, 151

32. Stadtman, T. C. (1977). Biological function of selenium. *Nutr. Rev.*, **35**, 161

33. Ellory, J. C. and Young, J. D. (1977). Neutral amino acid transport in erythrocytes from different mammalian species. *J. Physiol.*, **272**, 43P

34. Ellory, J. C. and Young, J. D. (1978). Sodium dependent amino acid transport in human erythrocytes. *J. Physiol.*, **285**, 51P

35. Rosenberg, R. (1979). Zero-trans uptake of L-tryptophan in the human erythrocyte. *J. Neural Transm.*, **15** (Supplement), 153

36. Rosenberg, R., Young, J. D. and Ellory, J. C. (1979). L-Tryptophan transport in human red blood cells. *Biochim. Biophys. Acta*, **598**, 375

37. Young, J. D. and Ellory, J. C. (1979). Transport of tryptophan and other amino acids by mammalian erythrocytes. *J. Neural Transm.*, **15** (Supplement), 139

38. Young, J. D., Wolowyk, M. W., Jones, S. E. M. and Ellory, T. C. (1979). Sodium dependent cysteine transport in human red blood cells. *Nature (London)*, **279**, 800

39. Thomas, E. L. and Christensen, N. H. (1970). Indication of spacial relations among structures recognising amino acids and Na$^+$ at a transport receptor site. *Biochem. Biophys. Res. Commun.*, **40**, 277

40. Tucker, E. M., Dain, A.R. and Young, J. D. (1979). A simple culture technique for studying biochemical changes during reticulocyte maturation *in vitro. Biochem. Soc. Trans.*, **7**, 159

41. Young, J. D. and Ellory, J. C. (1977). In J. C. Ellory and V. L. Lew, (eds). *Membrane Transport in Red Cells*, p. 301. (London, Academic Press)

42. Christensen, H. N. and Handlogten M. E. (1979). Cellular uptake of lithium via amino acid transport system. *J. Neural Transm.*, **15**, (Supplement), 1

43. Agar, N. S., Gruca, M. and Harley, J. D. (1974). Glutathione polymorphism in goat erythrocytes. *Anim. Blood Groups Biochem. Genet.*, **5**, 63

44. Meister, A. (1973). On the enzymology of amino acid transport. *Science*, **180**, 33

45. Palekar, A. G , Tate, S. S. and Meister, A. (1974). Formation of 5 oxoproline from glutathione in erythrocytes by the γ glutamyl transpeptidase–cyclo transferase pathway. *Proc. Natl. Acad. Sci., USA*, **71**, 293

46. Srivastava, S. K., Awasthi, V. C., Miller, S. P., Yoshida, A. and Beutler, E. (1976). Studies on γ glutamyl transpeptidase in human and rabbit erythrocytes. *Blood*, **47**, 645

47. Jackson, R. C. (1969). Studies in the enzymology of glutathione metabolism in human erythrocytes. *Biochem. J.*, **111**, 309

48. Young, J. D., Ellory, J. C. and Wright, P. C. (1975). Evidence against the participation of the γ-glutamyl transferase–γ glutamyl cyclotransferase pathway in amino acid transport by rabbit erythrocytes. *Biochem. J.*, **152**, 713.

49. Young, J. D. (1979). The role of thiol groups in erythrocyte amino acid transport. *Biochem. Soc. Trans.*, **7**, 683

50. Young, J. D. (1978). Nucleoside transport in sheep erythrocytes: genetically controlled transport variation and its influence on erythrocyte ATP concentration. *J. Physiol.*, **277**, 325

51. McManus, T. J. and Lamb, C. (1972). In E. Gerlach, K. Moser, E. Deutch and W. Wilmanns (eds). *International Symposium on Erythrocytes, Thrombocytes and Leucocytes*, p. 135. (Stuttgart: Thieme)

52. Young, J. D. (1976). Nucleoside transport variation in sheep erythrocytes. *J. Physiol.*, **259**, 57P

53. Young, J. D. (1977). Nucleoside transport in inosine permeable and impermeable sheep membrane. *J. Physiol.*, **269**, 46P

54. Jarvis, S. M. and Young, J. D. (1978). Genetic control of nucleoside transport in sheep erythrocytes. *Biochem. Genet.*, **16**, 1035

55. Bishop, C. (1961). Purine metabolism in human blood studied *in vivo* by injection of C^{14} adenine. *J. Biol. Chem.*, **236**, 1778

56. Lowy, B., Ramot, B. and London, I. (1958). Adenosine triphosphate metabolism in the rabbit erythrocyte *in vivo*. *Nature (London)*, **181**, 324

57. Bishop, C. (1960). Purine metabolism in human and chicken blood, *in vitro*. *J. Biol. Chem.*, **235**, 3228

58. Lowy, B., Ramot, B. and London, I. (1960). The biosynthesis of adenosine triphosphate and guanosine triphosphate in the rabbit erythrocyte *in vivo* and *in vitro*. *J. Biol. Chem.*, **235**, 2920

59. Brewer, G. J. (1974). In D. Surgenor (ed). *The Red Blood Cell*, Vol. 1, p. 387. (New York: Academic Press)

60. Meyskens, F. L. and Williams, H.. (1971). Adenosine metabolism in human erythrocytes. *Biochim. Biophys. Acta*, **240**, 170

61. Dean, B. M., Perrett, D., Simmonds, H. A., Saliota, A. and Van Acker, K. J. (1978). Adenine and adenosine metabolism in intact erythroctyes deficient in adenosine monophosphate pyrophosphate phospho-

ribosyl transferase: a study in two families. *Clin. Sci. Mol. Med.*, **55**, 407
62. Engelhardt, W. A. and Ljubinova, M. (1930). Glucolysis and phosphoric acid production in the red blood cells of different species. *Biochem. Z.*, **227**, 6
63. Kolotilova, A. I. and Engelhardt, W. R. (1937). Glycolytic activity of red blood cells of mammals. *Biokhimja*, **2**, 387
64. Laris, P. C. (1958). Permeability and utilisation of glucose in mammalian erythrocytes. *J. Cell. Comp. Physiol.*, **51**, 273
65. Kim, H. D. and McManus, T. J. (1971). Studies on the energy metabolism of red cells. 1. The limiting roles of membrane permeability in glycolysis. *Biochim. Biophys. Acta*, **230**, 1
66. Jarvis, S. M., Young, J. D., Ansay, M., Archibald, A. L., Harkness, R. A. and Simmonds, R. J. (1979). Is inosine the physiological energy source of pig erythrocytes. *Biochim. Biophys. Acta*, **597**, 183
67. Kolassa, N., Pfleger, K. and Tram, M. (1971). Species differences in action and elimination of adenosine after dipyridamole and hexobendine. *Eur. J. Pharmacol.*, **13**, 320
68. Pearson, J. D., Carleton, J. S., Hutchings, A. and Gordon, J. L. (1978). Uptake and metabolism of adenosine by pig aortic endothelial and smooth muscle cells in culture. *Biochem. J.*, **170**, 265
69. Cass, E., Gaudette, L. A. and Paterson, A. R. P. (1974). Mediated transport of nucleosides in human erythrocytes. Specific binding of the inhibitor nitrobenzyl thioinosine to nucleoside transport sites in the erythrocyte membrane. *Biochim. Biophys. Acta*, **345**, 1
70. Pickard, M. A., Brown, R. P., Paul, B. and Paterson, A. R. P. (1973). Binding of nucleoside inhibitor 4 nitrobenzyl thioinosine to erythrocyte membranes. *Can. J. Biochem.*, **51**, 666
71. Pickard, M. A. and Paterson, A. R. P. (1976). Fractionation of human erythrocyte membranes. Presence of the nucleoside transport complex in an insoluble residue. *Biochim. Biophys. Acta*, **455**, 817
72. Jarvis, S. M. and Young, J. D. (1978). Direct evidence for the specific interaction of nitrobenzyl thioinosine with functional nucleoside transport sites in sheep erythrocyte membranes. *J. Physiol.*, **284**, 96P
73. Mooney, N. A. and Young, J. D. (1978). Nucleoside and glucose transport in erythrocytes from new-born lambs. *J. Physiol.*, **284**, 229
74. Ellory, J. C., Green, J. R., Jarvis, S. M. and Young, J. D. (1979). Measurement of the apparent molecular volume of membrane-bound transport systems by radiation inactivation. *J. Physiol.*, **295**, 10P
75. Ellory, J. C. (1977). In J. C. Ellory and V. L. Lew (eds). *Membrane Transport in Red Cells*, p. 363 (London: Academic Press)
76. Li, C. C. and Hochstadt, J. (1976). Membrane associated enzymes involved in nucleoside processing by plasma membrane vesicles isolated from L_{929} cells grown in defined medium. *J. Biol. Chem.*, **251**, 1181
77. Quinlan, D. C. and Hochstadt, J. (1976). Group translocation of the ribose moiety of inosine by vesicles of plasma membrane from 3T3 cells transformed by Simian virus 40. *J. Biol. Chem.*, **251**, 344
78. Cohen, A. and Martin, D. W. (1977). Inosine uptake by cultured fibroblasts from normal and purine nucleoside phosphorylase deficient humans. *J. Biol. Chem.*, **252**, 4428

79. Dowd, D. J., Quinlan, D. C. and Hochstadt, J. (1977). Mechanism of purine nucleoside handling and transport in isolated membrane vesicles from polyoma transformed BHK/21 cells. *Biochemistry*, **16,** 4526
80. Aqarwal, R. P. and Parks, R. E. (1975). A possible association between the nucleoside transport system of human erythrocytes and adenosine deaminase. *Biochem. Pharmacol.*, **24,** 547
81. Tucker, E. M. and Young, J. D. (1976). Genetic variations in the purine nucleoside phosphorylase of sheep red cells. *Anim. Blood Groups Biochem. Genet.*, **7,** 109
82. Terhaggen, H. G., Lavinha, F. and Colombo, J. P. (1972). Familiar argininaemia. *J. Genet. Hum.*, **20,** 69
83. Stoop, J. N., Zegers, B. J. M., Hendrick, G. F. M., Seegenbeck, L. H., Staal, G. E. J., de Bree, P. K., Wadman, S. K. and Ballieux, R. E. (1977). Purine nucleoside phosphorylase deficiency associated with selective cellular immunodeficiency. *N. Engl. J. Med.*, **296,** 651
84. Giblett, E. R., Anderson, J. E., Cohen, F., Pollara, B. L. and Meuwissen, H. J. (1972). Adenosine deaminase deficiency in two patients with severely impaired cellular immunity. *Lancet,* **ii,** 1067
85. Lowy, B. A. and Dorfman, B. Z. (1970). Adenylosuccinase activity in human and rabbit erythrocyte lysates. *J. Biol. Chem.*, **245,** 3043

Index